Other Best-selling Books

FINE NEEDLE ASPIRATION CYTOLOGY

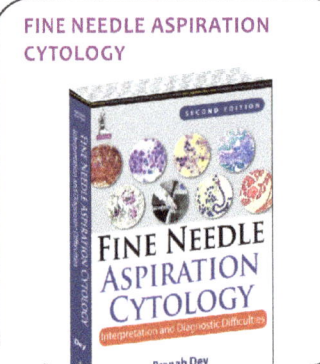

Pranab Dey

Two Colour | Soft Cover | 2/e, 2015 | 8.5" x 11" | 590 Pages | 9789351526087

- In this book the author has described the characteristic diagnostic features and differential diagnosis of various lesions on fine needle aspiration cytology.
- This book contains all the recent information in the field of cytology.
- A simple, concise and illustrative book.
- There are a large number of tables, boxes, and microphotographs in every chapter.
- The review section of the book (case studies) is helpful for self-assessment.
- This is a complete book on fine needle aspiration cytology and will be very helpful to all the students, practicing cytologists and pathology residents.

DIAGNOSTIC CYTOLOGY

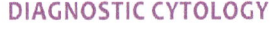
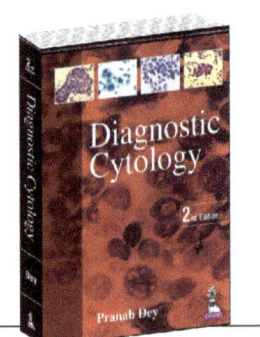

Pranab Dey

Four Colour | Hard Cover | 2/e, 2017 | 8.5" x 11" | 668 Pages | 9789352701209

- In this book, the author has described general cytology, clinical cytology (exfoliative cytology and fine needle aspiration cytology), and laboratory techniques in cytology.
- Contains all the recent information in the field of cytology
- This is a simple, concise and illustrative book.
- Includes large number of tables, boxes, line arts and microphotographs in every chapter.
- All the important information is specially highlighted in small boxes.
- This book is both a theoretical and practical resource for the trainees and the practicing cytopathologists.

CASE-BASED APPROACH IN EXFOLIATIVE CYTOLOGY

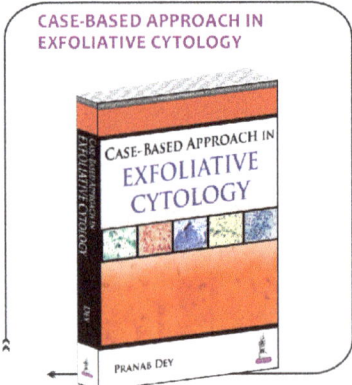

Pranab Dey

Full Colour | Soft Cover | 1/e, 2017 | 6.75" x 9.5" | 382 Pages | 9789386261892

- Case-by-case learning of exfoliative cytology
- Provides 215 real cases of exfoliative cytology supplemented with clinical details and multiple microphotographs
- Discussed diagnostic features as well as differential diagnosis
- Special emphasis on cervical cytology and abundant microphotographs of liquid-based cytology (LBC)
- Includes recent classification of lung tumors and urinary cytolog.

AUTOPSY PRACTICES

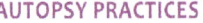
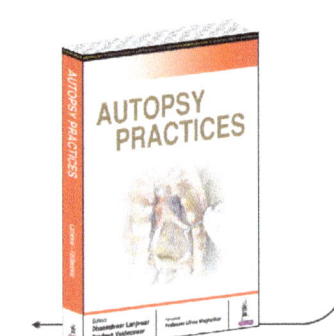

Dhaneshwar Lanjewar, et al.

Full Colour | Soft Cover | 1/e, 2017 | 6.5" x 9.75" | 196 Pages | 9789386056160

- This book emphasizes the practical procedures of dissecting and describing various organ systems.
- All the topics are written in conventional pattern, designed to offer practical guidelines that will lead pathologists to identify, interpret and correlate the autopsy findings.
- A topic on "Autopsy and Law" will be useful for the postgraduates in Forensic Medicine and Toxicology.
- It has been contributed by stalwarts carefully selected from different prominent centers of the country.
- Users of the book will realize the truth behind the quote: Pathology can be taught but cannot be learnt without autopsies.

JAYPEE
The Health Sciences Publisher

Please visit our website
www.jaypeebrothers.com or Scan the QR Code

RENAL BIOPSY INTERPRETATION

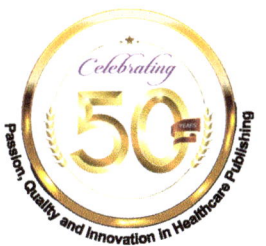

RENAL BIOPSY INTERPRETATION

Anila Korula
MBBS MD (Pathology)
Professor
Department of Pathology
Pushpagiri Institute of Medical Sciences
Thiruvalla, Kerala, India

Formerly, Professor and Head
Department of Pathology
Christian Medical College and Hospital
Vellore, Tamil Nadu, India

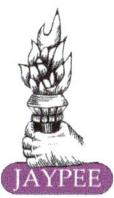

JAYPEE BROTHERS MEDICAL PUBLISHERS
The Health Sciences Publisher
New Delhi | London | Panama

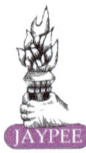 Jaypee Brothers Medical Publishers (P) Ltd

Headquarters
Jaypee Brothers Medical Publishers (P) Ltd
4838/24, Ansari Road, Daryaganj
New Delhi 110 002, India
Phone: +91-11-43574357
Fax: +91-11-43574314
Email: jaypee@jaypeebrothers.com

Overseas Offices

J.P. Medical Ltd
83 Victoria Street, London
SW1H 0HW (UK)
Phone: +44 20 3170 8910
Fax: +44 (0)20 3008 6180
Email: info@jpmedpub.com

Jaypee-Highlights Medical Publishers Inc
City of Knowledge, Bld. 235, 2nd Floor
Clayton, Panama City, Panama
Phone: +1 507-301-0496
Fax: +1 507-301-0499
Email: cservice@jphmedical.com

Jaypee Brothers Medical Publishers (P) Ltd
Bhotahity, Kathmandu, Nepal
Phone: +977-9741283608
Email: kathmandu@jaypeebrothers.com

Website: www.jaypeebrothers.com
Website: www.jaypeedigital.com

© 2019, Jaypee Brothers Medical Publishers

The views and opinions expressed in this book are solely those of the original contributor(s)/author(s) and do not necessarily represent those of editor(s) of the book.

All rights reserved. No part of this publication may be reproduced, stored or transmitted in any form or by any means, electronic, mechanical, photocopying, recording or otherwise, without the prior permission in writing of the publishers.

All brand names and product names used in this book are trade names, service marks, trademarks or registered trademarks of their respective owners. The publisher is not associated with any product or vendor mentioned in this book.

Medical knowledge and practice change constantly. This book is designed to provide accurate, authoritative information about the subject matter in question. However, readers are advised to check the most current information available on procedures included and check information from the manufacturer of each product to be administered, to verify the recommended dose, formula, method and duration of administration, adverse effects and contraindications. It is the responsibility of the practitioner to take all appropriate safety precautions. Neither the publisher nor the author(s)/editor(s) assume any liability for any injury and/or damage to persons or property arising from or related to use of material in this book.

This book is sold on the understanding that the publisher is not engaged in providing professional medical services. If such advice or services are required, the services of a competent medical professional should be sought.

Every effort has been made where necessary to contact holders of copyright to obtain permission to reproduce copyright material. If any have been inadvertently overlooked, the publisher will be pleased to make the necessary arrangements at the first opportunity. The **CD/DVD-ROM** (if any) provided in the sealed envelope with this book is complimentary and free of cost. **Not meant for sale.**

Inquiries for bulk sales may be solicited at: jaypee@jaypeebrothers.com

Renal Biopsy Interpretation

First Edition: **2019**

ISBN 978-93-5270-600-6

Preface

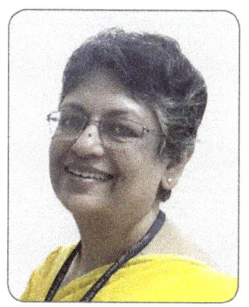

The book has been written to target and facilitate the routine diagnostic reporting of renal biopsies by postgraduate residents, fellows and consultants in the Departments of Pathology, Nephrology and Pediatric Nephrology.

The respective chapters begin with the normal histology of glomerular, tubulointerstitial and vascular compartments of the renal parenchyma and succinctly details the pathognomonic light microscopic, immunofluorescent and electron microscopic features of the various renal diseases. The text is comprehensively elucidated with excellent photomicrographs. Diagnostic features of renal allograft biopsies and rarer entities are highlighted to provide immediate and vital details that lead to the final diagnosis at the work bench beside the microscope.

The book also includes the recent classifications and scoring systems of some of the primary and secondary systemic renal diseases that have been currently validated at the Christian Medical College and Hospital, Vellore, Tamil Nadu, India.

I am really grateful for the vast experience and skilled expertise that I have gained at the Christian Medical College and Hospital, Vellore in the 26 years that I have been reporting renal biopsies. The sabbatical leave granted to me by the administration has enabled me to fulfil the commitment to complete this manuscript.

I sincerely hope that this will become a valuable resource for pathology and nephrology trainees and faculty involved in the discipline.

Anila Korula

Acknowledgments

I wish to first express my heartfelt gratitude to God Almighty and our Savior for the teaching, instruction and invaluable experience I have gained in all aspects of renal pathology.

I am very thankful to my beloved husband, Dr Roy John Korula; loving children, Pritish and Ashika, and my mother Dr Rachel Chacko, for their constant, prayerful support and great encouragement from the start to completion of this book.

I am grateful for the excellent postgraduate training I received at the Christian Medical College, Vellore, one of the premier institutes in India. I am also truly indebted to all my Professors, now retired from service, and all my colleagues in the Department of Pathology, CMC Vellore, whom I had the privilege to work with during my time there. I am also truly grateful to all my students who encouraged and motivated me to share my experience, and write this book.

I acknowledge with gratitude, the electron micrographs provided previously from Dr Larson, a Visiting Nephropathologist from USA, the central electron microscopic facility, including the present pathologists, Dr Anna Pulimood and Dr Smitha Mary Matthai and the currently available open access Internet resources.

Contents

1. **Introduction**   1
2. **Indications for Biopsy Proven Categories of Renal Diseases**   3
3. **Histopathologic Evaluation**   5
   - ❏ Normal Structure of Glomerulus   5
   - ❏ Ultrastructure of Glomerular Capillary Lobule   6
   - ❏ Reporting of the Renal Biopsy   8
4. **Glomerular Diseases**   10
   - ❏ Primary Glomerulonephritis   10
   - **Non-proliferative Glomerulonephritis**   10
   - ❏ Minimal Change Disease   10
   - ❏ Variants of Minimal Change Disease   12
   - ❏ Focal Segmental Glomerulosclerosis   16
   - ❏ Membranous Nephropathy   25
   - **Proliferative Glomerulonephritis**   32
   - ❏ Diffuse Predominantly Endocapillary Proliferative Glomerulonephritis   32
   - ❏ IgA Nephropathy   36
   - ❏ Non-IgA Mesangial Proliferative Glomerulonephritis   42
   - ❏ Crescentic Glomerulonephritis   44
   - ❏ Membranoproliferative Glomerulonephritis   46
   - ❏ C3 Glomerulopathy   54
   - ❏ C1Q Glomerulopathy   59
   - ❏ Focal (Segmental) Proliferative Glomerulonephritis   60
5. **Systemic Glomerular Diseases**   61
   - **Collagen Vascular Diseases**   61
   - ❏ Systemic Lupus Erythematosus   61
   - ❏ ISN/RPS Classification of Lupus Nephritis (LN) (2003)   62
   - ❏ Mixed Connective tissue Disease   77
   - ❏ Systemic Sclerosis   78
   - ❏ Sjogren's Syndrome   80
   - ❏ Rheumatoid Arthritis   81
6. **Diabetic Nephropathy**   83
   - ❏ Glomerular Classification of Diabetic nephropathy   85
7. **Systemic and Renal Limited Vasculitides**   89
   - **Major Categories of Non-infectious Vasculitis**   90
   - ❏ ANCA-associated Small Vessel Vasculitis   90
   - ❏ Large Vessel Vasculitis   96

- Medium-sized Vessel Vasculitis   96
- Henoch-Schonlein Purpura Nephritis   98

8. **Anti-glomerular Basement Membrane Disease** — 100
9. **Paraproteinemias/Dysproteinemias-associated Renal Disease** — 103
   - Amyloidosis   103
   - Monoclonal Immunoglobulin Deposition Disease   108
   - Light Chain Cast Nephropathy   111
   - Proliferative Glomerulonephritis with Monoclonal Immunoglobulin Deposits   112
10. **Glomerulonephritis with Organized Immune Deposits** — 114
    - Fibrillary Glomerulopathy   114
    - Immunotactoid Glomerulopathy   117
    - Cryoglobulinemic Glomerulonephritis   120
11. **HIV-associated Nephropathy** — 124
12. **Heredofamilial Glomerulopathies** — 128

    Collagen Nephropathies   128

    Type IV Collagen Nephropathies   128
    - Alport's Syndrome   129
    - Thin Basement Membrane Disease/Benign Familial Hematuria   132

    Type III Collagen Nephropathy   134
    - Collagenofibrotic Glomerulopathy   134
    - Nail-Patella Syndrome (Hereditary Osteo-onychodysplasia)   136

    Fibronectin Glomerulopathy   139

    Lipid Storage Diseases   142
    - Fabry's Disease   142
    - Familial Lecithin Cholesterol Acyltransferase Deficiency   145
    - Lipoprotein Glomerulopathy   146

    Congenital Nephrotic Syndrome and Podocytopathies   148
    - Finnish Type Congenital Nephrotic Syndrome   148
    - Diffuse Mesangial Sclerosis   149
    - Minimal Change Nephrotic Syndrome   150
    - Focal Segmental Glomerulosclerosis   150
    - Collapsing Glomerulopathy   151
    - Podocytopathies   151
13. **Tubulointerstitial Diseases** — 154
    - Normal Structure   154
    - Acute Tubular Injury/Necrosis   156
    - Nephrotoxic Acute Tubular Necrosis   157
    - Tubulointerstitial Nephritis   157
    - Acute Tubulointerstitial Nephritis   158
    - Chronic Tubulointerstitial Nephritis   159
    - Granulomatous Interstitial Nephritis   160

- ❏ IgG4-related Tubulointerstitial Nephropathy   161
- ❏ Metabolic Disorders (Crystallopathies)   163
- ❏ Cystinosis   165
- ❏ Mitochondriopathies   166
- ❏ Hyperuricemia and Urate Nephropathy   166
- ❏ Hypercalcemic Nephropathy   167

14. Vascular Renal Diseases — 171
- ❏ Normal Structure of Renal Vasculature   171
- ❏ Juxtaglomerular Apparatus   172
- ❏ Malignant Hypertensive Nephrosclerosis   174
- ❏ Thrombotic Microangiopathy   176
- ❏ Antiphospholipid Antibody Syndrome   182
- ❏ Pre-eclamptic Toxemia and Eclampsia   183

15. Renal Transplant Diseases — 186
- ❏ Revised Banff 2017 Classification   186
- ❏ Acute/Active Antibody-mediated Rejection   187
- ❏ Chronic Active Antibody-mediated Rejection   194
- ❏ Acute/Active T cell-mediated Rejection   197
- ❏ Chronic active T cell-mediated Rejection (GRADE II)   200
- ❏ Calcineurin Inhibitor Toxicity   202
- ❏ Infections in Renal Allograft   204
- ❏ Polyomavirus Nephropathy   204
- ❏ Cytomegalovirus Nephropathy   208
- ❏ Adenovirus Nephropathy   209
- ❏ Recurrent Glomerulonephritis   210
- ❏ De novo Glomerular Diseases   212
- ❏ Post-transplant Lymphoproliferative Disorder   213

Index — *219*

CHAPTER 1

Introduction

> **ABSTRACT**
>
> Renal biopsies are invaluable in the diagnosis and management of both adult and pediatric renal diseases and have become the gold standard in the detection and categorization of primary and secondary glomerular diseases. Renal biopsy interpretation is vitally important for the final diagnosis, to categorize and classify types of renal diseases, to assess the extent of their activity, severity and chronicity, and determine prognosis and response to treatment.
>
> This book comprehensively documents the diagnostic features and current perspectives of rarer entities such as Renal-limited and systemic ANCA-mediated vasculitis, thrombotic microangiopathies, C3 glomerulopathy, paraproteinemias with organized glomerular immune deposits and HIV-associated nephropathy, IgG4 related nephritis and lupus nephritis. Biopsy interpretation of heredofamilial nephropathies and newer classifications in IgA nephropathy, diabetic nephropathy and transplant renal diseases have been elucidated.
>
> The light microscopic, immunofluorescent and electron microscopic details in this book are intended to facilitate routine diagnostic reporting of renal biopsies by postgraduate residents, fellows and consultants, in the Departments of Pathology, Nephrology and Pediatric Nephrology.

Renal biopsies are invaluable in the diagnosis and management of both adult and pediatric renal diseases and have become the gold standard in the detection and categorization of primary and secondary glomerular diseases. The vast experience I have gained with God's guidance, from reporting renal biopsies for the Department of Pathology at the Christian Medical College (CMC) and Hospital, Vellore, from 1990 to the current date has yielded the skilled expertise required for their interpretation. The renal biopsy is vitally important for the final diagnosis, to categorize and classify types of renal diseases, to assess the extent of their activity, severity and chronicity, and determine prognosis and response to treatment.

The Christian Medical College at Vellore is a Tertiary Referral Medical Centre in South India. Therefore, renal biopsies from this institution, represent the types of renal disease prevalent in the Eastern, North Eastern and Southern states of India as well as neighboring countries and not exclusively from Vellore. Dr Anand Date pioneered renal biopsy reporting in India, and the Department of Pathology started its renal biopsy service over 4 decades ago. We currently report 2600 renal biopsies, each year, including renal transplant biopsies and referral biopsies.

A comparison of retrospective analysis of adult renal biopsies performed at CMC from 1986 to 2002 and an earlier cohort from 1971 to 1985, over 31 years, in the largest published Indian data[1,2] has shown a statistically significant increase in the prevalence of focal segmental sclerosis, membranous and post infectious glomerulonephritis among the primary glomerular diseases. Minimal change disease predominated in biopsy proven pediatric renal disease, in another case series from CMC including children and adults,[3] with an increase in IgA nephropathy, and a decreasing trend in the frequency of crescentic glomerulonephritis, membranoproliferative glomerulonephritis and focal proliferative glomerulonephritis. A decreasing trend was also reported in the occurrence of lupus nephritis, diabetic nephropathy, benign arteriolonephrosclerosis and amyloidosis among the systemic renal diseases in this series. The current prevalence and changing pattern of biopsy proven pediatric renal diseases in South Asia has been documented in a recent article from CMC.[4]

The present book aims to highlight the diagnostic features of renal diseases, including rarer entities such as Renal-limited and systemic ANCA-mediated vasculitis, thrombotic microangiopathies, C3 glomerulopathy, paraproteinemias with organized glomerular immune deposits and HIV-associated nephropathy. Biopsy interpretation of heredofamilial nephropathies with features of Alport's syndrome and lipid storage diseases, congenital nephrotic syndrome, podocytopathies and primary oxalosis have been elucidated. Diagnostic criteria for autoimmune diseases, such as subclasses of lupus nephritis and IgG4 sclerosing tubulointerstitial nephritis are detailed. Newer international classifications have been applied here that are useful to determine the predictive prognostic value of semi-quantitative scoring systems currently available for validation, of renal pauci-immune vasculitis, IgA nephropathy and diabetic nephropathy. The Banff diagnostic categories with current updates on acute and chronic antibody mediated rejection, scoring of T cell-mediated rejection and polyoma virus nephropathy in the allograft have also been comprehensively described in the interests of postgraduates.

The light microscopic, immunofluorescent and electron microscopic details in this book are intended to facilitate routine diagnostic reporting of renal biopsies by postgraduate residents, fellows and consultants in the Departments of Pathology, Nephrology and Pediatric Nephrology.

REFERENCES

1. Narasimhan B, Chacko B, John GT, Korula A, Kirubakaran MG, Jacob CK. Characterization of kidney lesions in Indian adults: towards a renal biopsy registry. J Nephrol. 2006;19:205-10.
2. Date A, Raghavan R, John TJ, Richard, Kirubakaran MG, Shastry JCM. Renal disease in adult Indians: a clinicopathological study of 2827 patients. Q J Med. 1987;64:729-37.
3. Balakrisnan N, John GT, Korula A, Visalakshi J, Talauikar GS, Thomas PP, et al. Spectrum of biopsy proven renal disease and changing trends at a Tropical Tertiary Care Centre,1990-2001. Indian J Nephrol. 2003;13;29-35.
4. Mohapatra AM, Kakde S, Annapandian VM, Valson AT, Duhli N, Korula A, et al. Spectrum of biopsy proven renal disease in South Asian children: two decades at a tropical tertiary care centre. Nephrology(Carlton).2017 August. Accepted for publication doi:10.1111/nep.13160 (epub ahead of print).

CHAPTER 2

Indications for Biopsy Proven Categories of Renal Diseases

ABSTRACT

The categories of renal diseases, commonly associated with clinical syndromes, are enlisted in this chapter for both pathologists and nephrologists. This includes the various forms of primary glomerulonephritis presenting with nephrotic syndrome or nephritic syndrome and tubulo-interstitial and parenchymal lesions associated with acute and chronic renal failure. The systemic renal diseases typically present with hematuria and/or persistent proteinuria and renal dysfunction, and include autoimmune diseases, diabetic nephropathy, vasculitides, antiglomerular basement membrane disease and paraproteinemias/glomerulonephritis with organized immune deposits and HIV-associated nephropathy. Heredofamilial nephropathies include the collagenopathies, thin basement membrane disease, lipid storage diseases and podocytopathies. The vascular diseases of benign and malignant hypertension and thrombotic microangiopathies constitute a distinct subset as well as transplant renal diseases. The latter mainly comprise the categories of T cell mediated and antibody mediated rejection, recurrent forms of glomerulonephritis, polyoma virus nephropathy calcineurin inhibitor toxicity and post-transplant lymphoproliferative disorders.

The common indications for a renal biopsy are categorized as follows:[1-4]

Nephrotic syndrome:
- Minimal change disease
- Focal and segmental glomerulosclerosis
- Membranous nephropathy
- Mesangial proliferative glomerulonephritis
- Membranoproliferative glomerulonephritis
- C3 glomerulopathy
- C1q nephropathy.

Nephritic syndrome:
- Diffuse endocapillary proliferative glomerulonephritis
- IgA nephropathy
- Crescentic glomerulonephritis (Rapidly progressive glomerulonephritis)
- Focal proliferative glomerulonephritis.

Acute renal failure:
- Acute tubular necrosis
- Cortical necrosis
- Acute interstitial nephritis
- Acute thrombotic microangiopathy (hemolytic uremic syndrome).

Chronic renal failure:
- Chronic glomerulonephritis (or end-stage diffuse sclerosing primary/secondary glomerulonephritis)
- Chronic interstitial nephritis
- Granulomatous interstitial nephritis.

Hematuria and/or persistent proteinuria*/renal dysfunction:
Systemic renal diseases:
- Systemic lupus erythematosus and other collagen vascular diseases: Mixed connective tissue disease, scleroderma, rheumatoid arthritis and Sjögren syndrome (***subnephrotic to nephrotic range**)
- Diabetic nephropathy
- Vasculitis: ANCA-mediated vasculitides (Wegener's granulomatosis or granulomatous polyangiitis, microscopic polyangiitis and Churg-Strauss disease) and Henoch-Schonlein purpura
- Good Pasture's syndrome (Antiglomerular basement membrane disease)
- Paraproteinemias and/or organized glomerular immune deposits including:
  - Amyloidosis, monoclonal immunoglobulin deposition disease (light and heavy chain deposition disease), fibrillary/immunotactoid glomerulopathy and cryoglobulinemic glomerulonephritis
- HIV-associated nephropathy.

Heredofamilial nephropathies:
- Collagenopathies including Alport's syndrome
- Thin basement membrane disease
- Lipid storage diseases:
  - Fabry's disease, LCAT deficiency and lipoprotein glomerulopathy
- Congenital nephrotic syndrome and podocytopathies.

Vascular diseases:
- Benign and malignant nephrosclerosis
- Thrombotic microangiopathies.

Transplant renal diseases.

REFERENCES

1. Narasimhan B, Chacko B, John GT, Korula A, Kirubakaran MG, Jacob CK. Characterization of kidney lesions in Indian adults: towards a renal biopsy registry. J Nephrol. 2006;19:205-10.
2. Balakrisnan N, John GT, Korula A, Visalakshi J, Talauikar GS, Thomas PP, et al. Spectrum of biopsy proven renal disease and changing trends at a Tropical Tertiary Care Centre, 1990-2001. Indian J Nephrol. 2003;13;29-35.
3. Das U, Prayaga A, Dakshinamurthy KV. Pattern of renal disease in a single centre of South India: 19 years experience. Indian J Nephrol. 2011;21:250-7.
4. Jennette JC, Falk RJ. Glomerular clinicopathologic syndromes. In: Greenberg A, Cheung AK, Coffman TM, Falk RJ, Jennette JC, (Eds). Primer on Kidney Diseases, 5th Edition National Kidney Foundation; 2009.

CHAPTER 3

Histopathologic Evaluation

> **ABSTRACT**
> This chapter deals with the normal structure of glomeruli by light microscopy and electron microscopy required for evaluation of glomerular lesions. The standard histopathologic technique, fixatives used and optimal thickness of renal biopsy serial sections including routine and special stains and immunofluorescence is emphasized.
>
> The reporting protocol with detailed, systematic and semiquantitative assessment of the glomerular, tubulointerstitial and vascular compartments is included for the benefit of postgraduate trainees and consultants in order to accurately interpret microscopic features for a diagnosis. This would serve as a guide to further detailed and comprehensive analysis of primary and systemic renal diseases in the subsequent chapters of the book.
>
> The relevant laboratory investigations required, that are supportive of the renal biopsy diagnosis are also considered. The careful evaluation and integration of these pathologic details with clinical syndromes and laboratory data leads to the identification of the primary site of the disease and the secondary or concomitant tubulointerstitial and vascular lesions.

Recapitulation of the normal structure of the major glomerular component is primarily required for comprehensive evaluation of glomerular lesions.[1-5] The normal histology of tubulo-interstitial and vascular components and their diseases will be individually detailed in the respective later chapters.

NORMAL STRUCTURE OF GLOMERULUS (FIG. 3.1)

A glomerulus is composed of a tuft of anastomosing capillaries, projecting into the Bowman's space (BS) and supported by the mesangium in the intercapillary region. Each glomerulus has an endocapillary compartment and an extracapillary compartment separated by the glomerular basement membrane (GBM). The endocapillary compartment comprises the endothelial cells, mesangial cells, and any leukocytes in the capillary lumens or mesangium. Normally, in a 3–4 µm histologic section, one or rarely two endothelial nuclei per capillary lumen are present with one to two mesangial cell nuclei in a peripheral segment of contiguous mesangial matrix. The mesangium merges with the vascular pole of the glomerulus, and there may be more than four nuclei in the contiguous matrix at this location. The extracapillary compartment normally includes a single layer of visceral epithelium (the podocyte) that covers the external surface of the capillaries and the para mesangial region of the GBM. The podocyte is continuous at the glomerular hilum with the parietal epithelium that lines the Bowman's capsule (BC). The parietal epithelium is continuous at the tubular pole with the columnar proximal tubular epithelial cells. The normal glomerulus contains minimal extracellular matrix that comprises the GBM, the

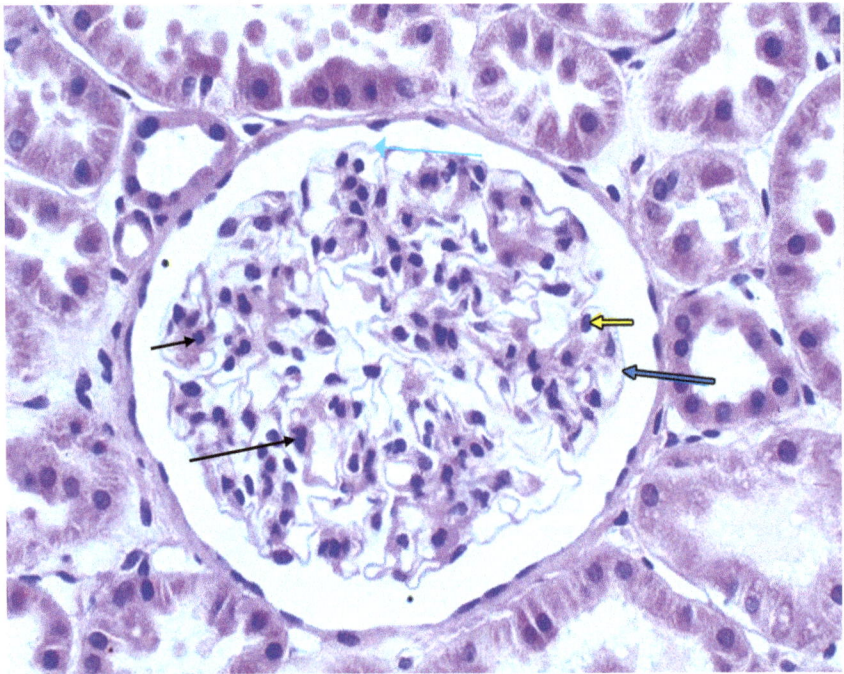

Figure 3.1: Light micrograph of a normal glomerulus with 1 or 2 mesangial cell nuclei (black arrows), in mesangial matrix, one endothelial cell nucleus (yellow arrow) and normal thickness of capillary wall (blue arrows)

mesangial matrix, and the basement membrane of Bowman's capsule. The afferent arteriole enters the glomerulus and branches to form the capillary lobules, while the efferent capillaries converge at the hilum to become the efferent arteriole. The afferent arteriole has a larger diameter than the efferent arteriole with a thicker media and wider lumen.

ULTRASTRUCTURE OF GLOMERULAR CAPILLARY LOBULE (FIG. 3.2)

The mesangium forms the central core of the capillary lobule consisting of the mesangial cells (M) and matrix (MM). The mesangial cell has cytoplasmic processes that can extend into the capillary loops subjacent to the endothelium. The endothelium (E) consists of a thin layer with fenestrated (F) cytoplasm and an oval nucleus located adjacent to the mesangium. The glomerular basement membrane (Fig. 3.3) is trilaminar, measuring 300–350 nm in thickness and composed of an inner lamina rara interna, central lamina densa and outer lamina rara externa. The podocyte (P_1) has a cell body with primary cytoplasmic processes and terminal interdigitating foot processes (P_2) known as pedicles arranged perpendicular to the GBM. The intervening slits of uniform width between the pedicles are bridged by slit diaphragms that form the filtration barrier.

Histopathologic Technique

Renal biopsies are fixed in 10% neutral buffered formalin and serial paraffin sections, of 2–3 micrometers thickness, are routinely stained with hematoxylin and eosin (H & E), periodic acid-Schiff reagent, Jones methenamine silver (JMS), on consecutive slides. Special stains include

Histopathologic Evaluation

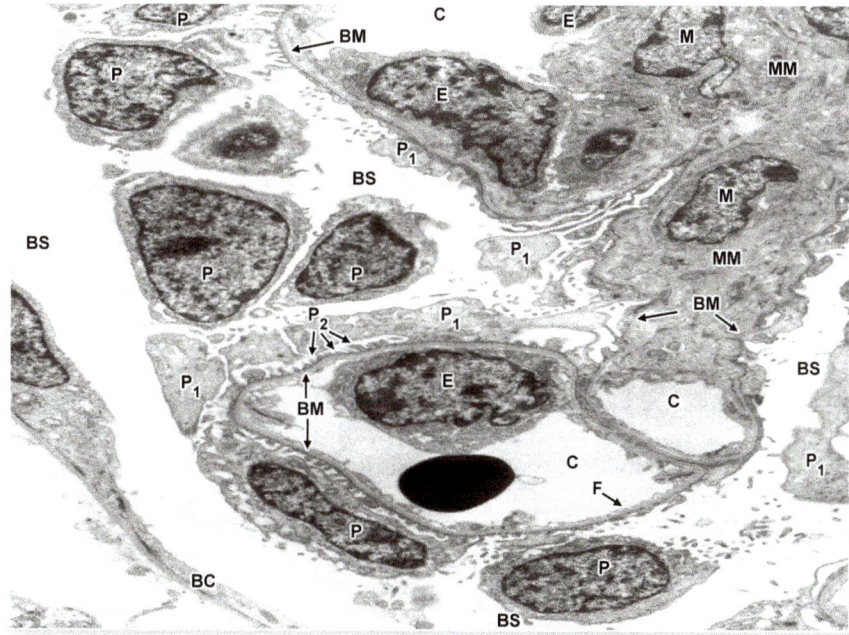

Figure 3.2: Electron micrograph of normal glomerulus. For labeling see text (Internet Resource)

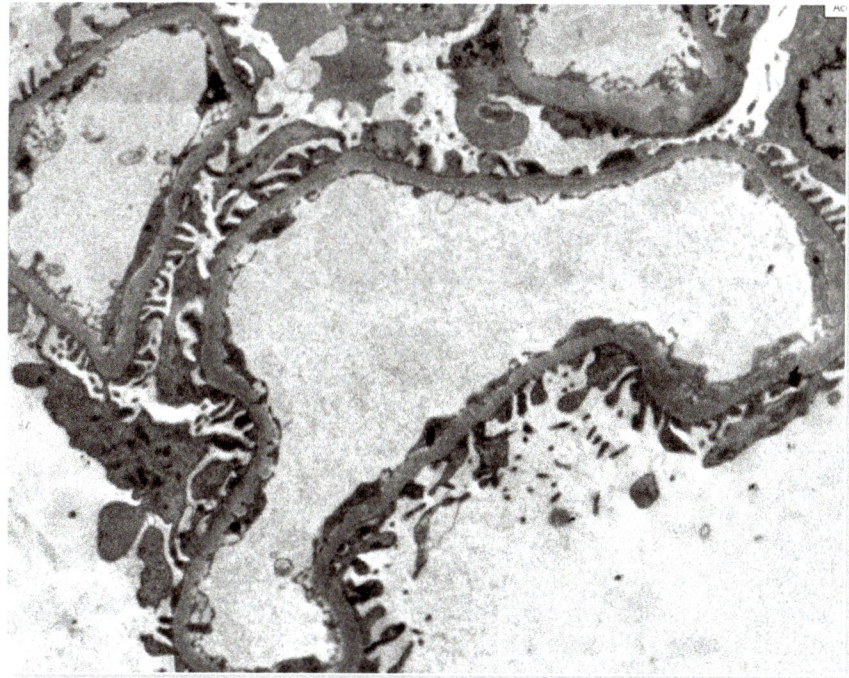

Figure 3.3: Glomerular basement membrane (EM × 4200)

Masson trichrome stain (for type III collagen), Martius Scarlet blue (for fibrin) and Congored/thioflavine-T (for amyloid), when required. Standard immunofluorescent stains are done on cryostat sections with FITC-labelled IgG, IgA, IgM, C3, C1q, or kappa and lambda conjugated antisera (DAKO reagents) of all biopsies. Immunohistochemical staining for C4d is routinely done on transplant renal biopsies. Electron microscopy is performed in selected cases with 2–3% glutaraldehyde as the fixative. After a preview of 1 micron sections with toluidine blue, representative ultrathin sections of identified glomeruli and other components are stained with lead citrate and uranyl acetate, for this purpose.

REPORTING OF THE RENAL BIOPSY

Microscopic details of the four major components: glomerular, tubulointerstitial and vascular compartments are methodically described and the diagnostic report, including the immunofluorescence report is released electronically to the clinicians. Semiquantitative assessment is done of these details for prognostication and clinicopathologic correlations with the biopsy request form and relevant laboratory investigations. A definitive final diagnosis and classification of disease category can be made with careful integration of the light microscopic features with immunofluorescence and electron microscopic findings. Interdepartmental clinicopathologic weekly meetings or conferences across a multiheaded microscope are very useful for case discussions of selected problematic cases with appropriate clinical information, comparison of previous biopsies, differential diagnosis and therapeutic aspects.

Light microscopic features noted are as displayed in a renal biopsy and described in order as follows:

- Glomeruli:
  - Number in a biopsy including globally sclerosed tufts
  - Adequacy (6–10 glomeruli)
  - Enlargement of the glomerular tufts and lobular expansion
  - Cellularity (in <25%, 26–50% and >50% glomeruli) of the intrinsic cells
  - Mesangial, capillary endothelial cells and hyperplasia of extracapillary cells (visceral and parietal epithelial cells), crescents
  - Leukocytic infiltration
  - Matrix expansion or condensation with sclerosis and capsular synechiae (on PAS and JMS special stains for type IV collagen)
  - Capillary luminal patency, narrowing, occlusion and/or obliteration, thrombi
  - Capillary wall thickening with duplication and double contours (on PAS and JMS special stains)
  - Capillary tuft: wrinkling, collapse, retraction, sclerosis, (JMS stain), hyalinosis, fibrinoid necrosis (MSB stain) and karyorrhectic nuclei.
- Tubules:
  - Dilatation, atrophy, necrosis and casts (hyaline, erythrocyte, leukocyte and light chain casts) or crystals
  - Epithelial flattening with attenuation of brush border and regeneration (PAS stain)
  - Viral inclusions
  - Hyaline droplet degeneration and pigment deposits
  - Thickening of basement membranes (PAS stain)
  - Hydropic or fatty change/isometric or coarse vacuolization.

- Interstitium:
  - Edema
  - Inflammatory cell infiltrates with neutrophils, lymphocytes, eosinophils, plasma cell, histiocytes and foam cells or granulomas
  - Fibrosis.
- Vascular:
  - Arteriolar hyalinosis or sclerosis (PAS stain)
  - Interlobular and arcuate arteries: Intimal fibrosis (< or > than media)
  - Reduplication of internal elastic lamina (JMS stain)
  - Medial hyperplasia
  - Mural fibrinoid necrosis (Masson trichrome/MSB stains)
  - Luminal thrombosis and atheroemboli with cholesterol clefts.

Immunofluorescence report contains the following details:

Intensity (1 to 3+), patterns exhibited (fine/coarsely granular, confluent, granular and clumped, linear or interrupted linear) and localization of immune deposits whether mesangial, mesangial and capillary wall or capillary wall with segmental or lobular accentuation. Nonspecific trapping of IgM and/ or C3 in segments of sclerosis are noted.

Electron microscope report includes structural details of the major components as follows:
Glomerular endothelium, basement membrane thickening, thinning with attenuation or lamellation and the exact measurement, mesangial expansion with interposition, localization and extent of immune deposits (mesangial, paramesangial, subepithelial, subendothelial or intramembranous) with organized substructure (fibrillar or microtubular and size in nanometers), podocyte foot process effacement, hypertrophy or microvillous transformation are noted. Diagnostic intracellular, laminated lysosomal myelin inclusions, tubuloreticular inclusions and extracellular structures (amyloid fibrils) with their localization provide important confirmatory evidence in a renal biopsy. Tubulo-interstitial and vascular components are also examined, as and when appropriate for the diagnosis. Electron micrographs are taken and attached to the report with a conclusive diagnosis, integrated with the light and immunofluorescent microscopic features and clinical correlations.

The **various terminologies and the nomenclature utilized** in the reporting of renal biopsies are defined clearly and precisely in the respective chapters of this book.

Relevant laboratory investigations required include serum creatinine, blood urea, 24-hour urinary protein, urine sediment, UP/UC ratio, serum complement (C3 and C4) antinuclear antibody and dsDNA ANCA levels, hepatitis B and C and HIV viral screening, that are supportive of the diagnosis on a renal biopsy.

REFERENCES

1. Bonsib SM. Renal anatomy and renal histology in Heptinstall's pathology of the kidney, 6th edition. Lippincott Williams and Wilkins; 2007.
2. Young B, Woodford P, O'Dowd G. Wheater's functional histology: a text and color atlas, 6th edition. Elsevier-Health Science Division; 2013.
3. Mills SE. Histology for pathologists, 3rd Edition. Lippincott, Williams and Wilkins: Philadelphia; 2007
4. Mills SE, Carter D, Greenson JK, Reuter VE, Stoler MH. Sternberg's Diagnostic Surgical Pathology, 5th Edition, Lippincott Williams and Wilkins. 2009.
5. Rosai J. Rosai and Ackerman's surgical pathology, 10th edition. Mosby; 2011.

CHAPTER 4

Glomerular Diseases

ABSTRACT

This chapter categorizes this entity into non-proliferative and proliferative glomerulonephritis, and includes the incidence in CMCH, Vellore, relevant pathogenesis, light microscopic, immunofluorescence and electron microscopic features of each subtype, with the differential diagnosis, course and prognosis. The non-proliferative forms comprise minimal change disease, focal and segmental glomerulosclerosis (FSGS) and membranous nephropathy. Minimal change disease with its variants and inherited forms are dealt with concisely in perspective as "podocytopathies". The classification of FSGS and differentiation from secondary FSGS is delineated with pertinent details. The important stages of membranous nephropathy by light and electron microscopy are clearly highlighted along with the detection of glomerular expression of PLA2R as the major target antigen by immunohistochemistry.

The proliferative glomerulonephritis (GN) classified as focal or diffuse is further elucidated comprising details of the endocapillary, mesangial IgA (with the Oxford classification and MEST score) crescentic, membranoproliferative, (MPGN), C3GN and C1q glomerulopathy. The rarer forms of MPGN with electron microscopic features as reported in our center are clearly depicted.

PRIMARY GLOMERULONEPHRITIS

Primary glomerulonephritis comprises two major categories:
1. Non-proliferative
2. Proliferative.

Non-proliferative Glomerulonephritis

Non-proliferative glomerulonephritis comprises three major entities, that are associated with podocyte injury but do not exhibit significant proliferation of intrinsic glomerular cells, as follows:
1. Minimal change disease
2. Focal and segmental sclerosis
3. Membranous nephropathy.

MINIMAL CHANGE DISEASE

Minimal change disease accounts for 90% of primary nephrotic syndrome in children presenting with highly selective proteinuria of >3.5 g/day. The peak incidence is 2 to 3 years of age and median age is 2.5 years. Our biopsy series in the pediatric age showed a prevalence of 47.2%,[1] and

Glomerular Diseases

this is the most common category in children.[2, 3] This entity has a normal morphology by light microscopy and has ultrastructural features of a "podocytopathy" defined by effacement of foot processes and normal podocyte numbers. There are idiopathic, reactive and genetic forms of minimal change nephropathy (MCN). It is postulated that an associated T cell dysfunction, with release of cytokines initiates podocyte transformation. The latter process is mediated by signal transduction through the slit diaphragm, increased lysosomal proteinases, loss of cell polarity and loss of anionic podocyte proteins, resulting in proteinuria. As there are alterations in podocyte structure and no podocyte loss, these changes are potentially reversible with corticosteroids.[4]

Light Microscopic Features

- Normocellular glomeruli of standard normal size with patent capillary lumina in the majority (Fig. 4.1)
- Focal mild increase in mesangial cellularity with 3 mesangial cells in mesangial zone, in a minority
- No significant expansion of mesangial matrix
- Capillary walls of normal thickness
- Tubulointerstitial and vascular compartments are normal.

Immunofluorescent Features

- Negative for immunoglobulins and complement
- Mesangial IgM 1+ in occasional biopsies.

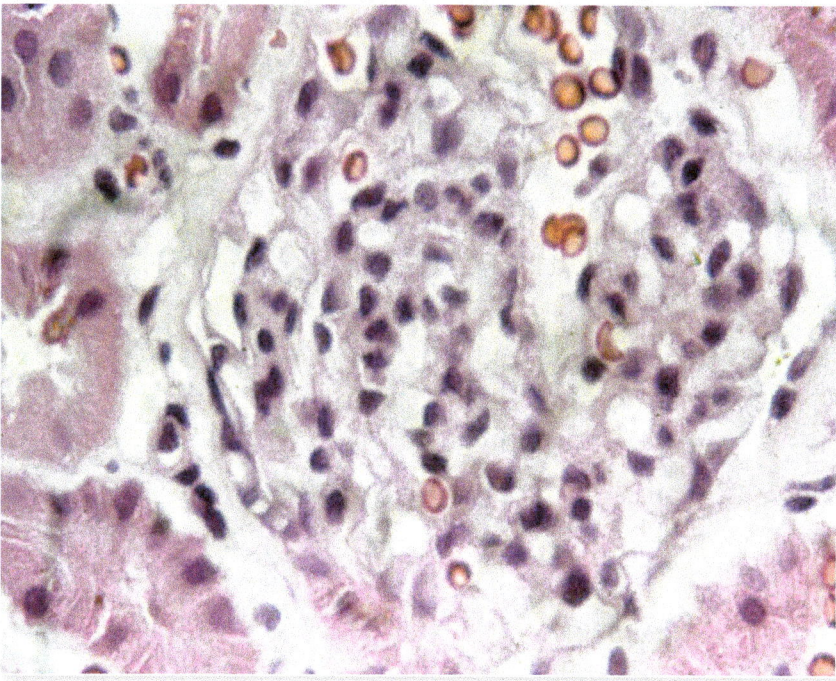

Figure 4.1: Minimal change disease (H&E x 400)

12 Renal Biopsy Interpretation

Electron Microscopic Features

Diffuse effacement of foot processes of podocytes with retraction, widening and shortening of foot processes and normal numbers of podocytes (Figs 4.2A and B).

Prognosis

Remission of proteinuria is usually seen in 8 weeks of treatment with steroids in 90–95% of cases. Frequent relapses with steroid dependence occur in the remaining cases.

Glomerular hypertrophy with glomerular tuft area up to 1.75 times and greater than that of glomeruli from age matched normal controls or minimal change disease is associated with the risk of developing focal and segmental sclerosis, which can be detected on repeat biopsies.[5] Serial deeper sections of the entire paraffin block are required for the detection of an incipient focus of early tuft sclerosis and differentiation from minimal change disease in our experience.

VARIANTS OF MINIMAL CHANGE DISEASE

Diffuse Mesangial Hypercellularity

Diffuse mesangial hypercellularity accounts for 3% of pediatric nephrotic syndrome.

Light Microscopic Features (Fig. 4.3)

- Diffuse mesangial cellularity, with >4 mesangial cells per mesangial region, involving 80% of glomeruli, by International Study of Kidney Disease in Childhood (ISKDC) criteria[6,7]
- No evidence of mesangial matrix expansion or occlusion of capillary lumina.

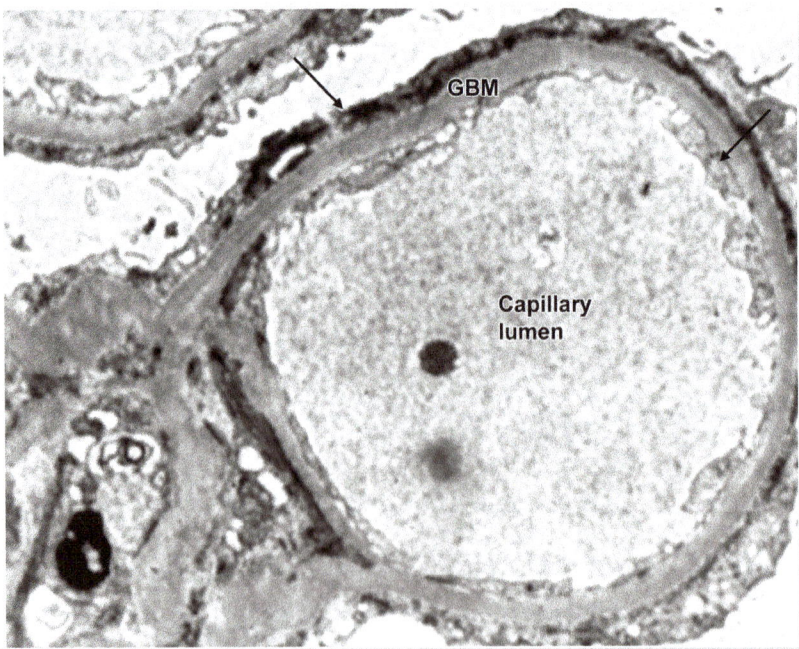

Figure 4.2A: Foot process effacement in minimal change disease (arrows)

Glomerular Diseases

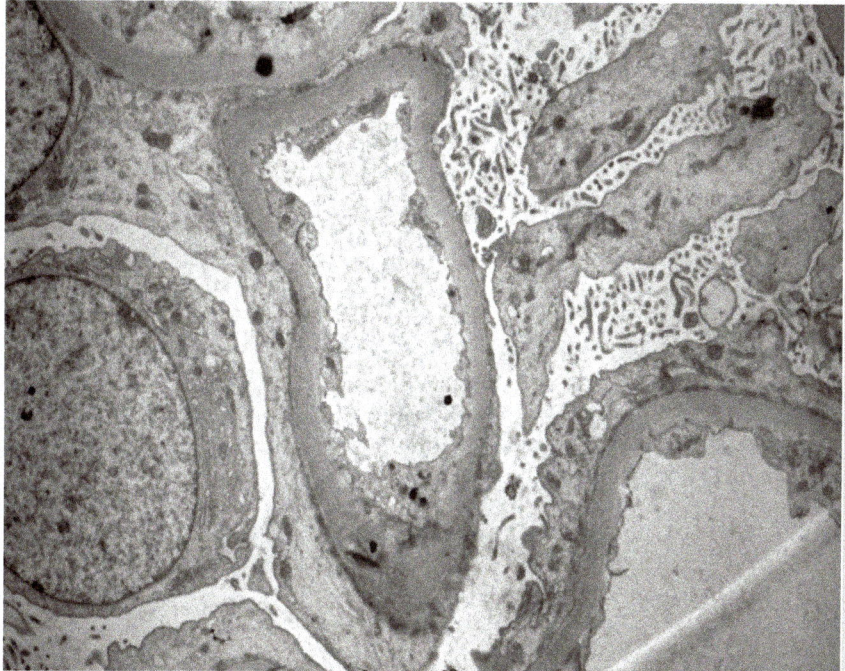

Figure 4.2B: Foot process effacement with microvillous hypertrophy in MCD (EM x 4200)

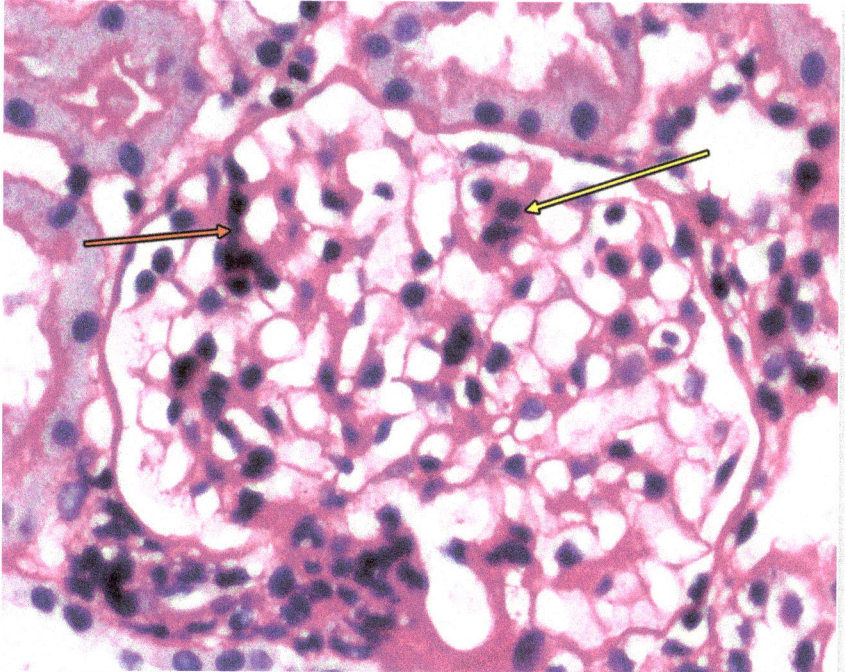

Figure 4.3: Mild (yellow arrow) to moderate (red arrow) mesangial hypercellularity (PAS x 400)

Grades of Mesangial Hypercellularity: South West Pediatric Nephrology Study[8]

Mesangial hypercellularity is graded according to the number of mesangial cells/mesangial area as follows:
- Mild mesangial hypercellularity: 3 mesangial cell nuclei, per mesangial area
- Moderate mesangial hypercellularity: 4 mesangial cell nuclei, per mesangial area
- Severe mesangial hypercellularity: ≥5 mesangial cell nuclei, per mesangial area.

Prognosis

Diffuse mesangial hypercellularity and grades of mesangial hypercellularity, from mild to severe, are associated with poor response to 8 weeks course of intensive corticosteroid therapy.[9] There are reportedly no significant differences in long term outcome of diffuse mesangial hypercellularity, after 52 weeks of steroid therapy, from minimal change disease. Late steroid non-responsiveness is not related to the initial severity of mesangial hypercellularity and does well with alternative forms of immunosuppression.[9]

IgM Variant (IgM Nephropathy)

Light Microscopic Features

It can be similar to minimal change disease:
- Variable increase in mesangial cellularity is seen
- Progression to diffuse mesangial cell and matrix proliferation and focal and segmental sclerosis.[10-15]

Immunofluorescent Features

Diffuse mesangial deposition of IgM 2+ or 3+ with C3 deposits (in 30–100% cases).

Electron Microscopic Features

Extensive foot process effacement with small mesangial electron dense deposits in paramesangial areas in 50% cases.

Differential Diagnosis

Diffuse mesangial proliferative glomerulonephritis that is associated with diffuse mesangial matrix and cell proliferation and is often immunofluorescence negative.

Prognosis

Steroid dependence or resistance has been noted in 25–50% cases and progression to focal and segmental sclerosis on repeat serial biopsies. As the prognosis differs from minimal change disease this is considered as a different and distinct entity by some nephropathologists.

Inherited forms of MCNS that are steroid resistant have been reported with genetic mutations and include:

- Non-syndromic type associated with the *podocin (NPHS2) gene*
- Syndromic type with *dysferlin (DYSF) gene* of limb-girdle muscular dystrophy, 2B mutation.[4,16]

Reactive forms of MCN are associated with malignancy (Hodgkin's lymphoma), immune dysregulation and are induced by medication (non-steroidal anti-inflammatory drugs penicillamine, interferon).

Minimal change disease in adults occurs in 10–15% cases[17] with 11.6% in our case series from CMC, Vellore.[18] A higher incidence of 21.8% has been recently reported, inclusive of children and adults from South India.[19] This is usually secondary or reactive associated with drugs, neoplasms, infections, allergies and other concurrent glomerular and extraglomerular diseases.

REFERENCES

1. Balakrisnan N, John GT, Korula A, Visalakshi J, Talauikar GS, Thomas PP, et al. Spectrum of biopsy proven renal disease and changing trends at a Tropical Tertiary Care Centre, 1990-2001. Indian J Nephrol. 2003;13; 29-35.
2. Habib R, Kleinknecht C. The primary nephrotic syndrome of childhood: Classification and clinicopathologic study of 406 cases. Pathol Ann.1971;6:417-74.
3. Churg J, Habib R, White RHR. Pathology of the nephrotic syndrome in children: a report of the International Study of Kidney Disease in Children. Lancet. 1970;1:1299-302.
4. Lane JC, Kaskel FJ. Pediatric nephrotic syndrome. From the simple to the complex. Seminars In Nephrology. 2009;29:389-98.
5. Fogo A, Hawkins EP, Berry PL, et al. Glomerular hypertrophy in minimal change disease predicts subsequent progression to focal glomerular sclerosis. Kidney Int. 1990;38:115-23.
6. Primary nephrotic syndrome in children: clinical significance of histopathologic variants of minimal change and of diffuse mesangial hypercellularity. A Report of the International Study of Kidney Disease in Children. Kidney Int. 1981;20(6):765-71.
7. Report of the International Study of Kidney Disease in Children. The primary nephrotic syndrome in children. Identification of patients with minimal change nephrotic syndrome from initial response to prednisone. J Pediatr. 1981;98:561-4.
8. Childhood nephrotic syndrome associated with diffuse mesangial hypercellularity. A report of the Southwest Pediatric Nephrology Study Group. Kidney Int. 1983;24(1):87-94.
9. Bernstein J, Edelmann CM. Minimal change nephrotic syndrome. Histopathology and steroid- responsiveness. Archives of Disease in Childhood. 1982;57:816-7.
10. Cohen AH, Border WA, Glassock RJ. Nephrotic syndrome with glomerular mesangial IgM deposits. Lab Invest. 1978;38:610-9.
11. Swartz SJ, Eldin KW, Hicks MJ, Feig DI. Minimal change disease with IgM+ immunofluorescence: a subtype of nephrotic syndrome. Pediatr Nephrol. 2009;24(6):1187-92. doi: 10.1007/s00467-009-1130-0. Epub 2009.
12. Zeis PM, Kavazarakis E, Nakopoulou L, Moustaki M, Messaritaki A, Zeis MP, et al. Glomerulopathy with mesangial IgM deposits: long-term follow-up of 64 children. Pediatr Int. 2001;43:287-92.
13. Al Eisa, et al. Childhood IgM nephropathy: comparison with minimal change disease. Nephron. 1996;72:37-43.
14. Hirszel P, et al. Mesangial proliferative glomerulonephritis with IgM deposits. Nephron.1984;32(2):100-8.
15. Little MA, Dorman A, et al. Glomerulonephritis with IgM deposits: Clinical characteristics and outcome. Renal Failure. 2000;22(4):445-57.
16. Caridi G, et al. Familial forms of nephrotic syndrome. Pediatr Nephrol. 2010;25:241-52L.
17. Rathi M, Bhaghat RL, Mukhopadhyay P, Kohli HS, Jha V, Gupta KL. Changing histologic spectrum of adult nephrotic syndrome over five decades in north India: A single center experience. Indian J Nephrol. 2014;24(2):86-91.
18. Narasimhan B, Chacko B, John GT, Korula A, Kirubakaran MG, Jacob CK. Characterization of kidney lesions in Indian adults: towards a renal biopsy registry. J Nephrol. 2006;19: 205-10.
19. Das U, Prayaga A, Dakshinamurthy KV. Pattern of renal disease in a single centre of South India:19 years experience. Indian J Nephrol. 2011;21:250-7.

FOCAL SEGMENTAL GLOMERULOSCLEROSIS

Focal segmental glomerulosclerosis (FSGS) is a leading cause of nephrotic syndrome in adults and the most common biopsy proven category in the age groups >15 years in our experience, comprising 16.8-17% in a series of cases. By definition, this lesion is "focal", involving <50% of glomeruli in a biopsy and "segmental", affecting part of the circumference of a glomerular tuft. Diffuse effacement of podocyte architecture is a defining ultrastructural feature, with reduction in numbers of podocytes. Loss of podocytes through detachment or apoptosis, leads to denudation of the GBM, adhesions to Bowman's capsule with segmental sclerosis. Phenotypic changes in podocyte structure with epithelial mesenchymal transition and foot process effacement with loss of function of slit diaphragms and glomerular filtration barrier lead to proteinuria. These changes become progressive and irreversible in FSGS.[1-3] Circulating permeability factors including elevated serum levels of soluble urokinase receptor have been postulated to induce foot process effacement through the activation of podocyte B3 integrin, but the exact source and stimulants of this receptor is unknown.[4]

There are primary and secondary forms of FSGS with 5 morphologic variants in order of frequency in the Columbia classification,[2] as follows:
1. FSGS, not otherwise specified [FSGS (NOS)]
2. Perihilar variant
3. Cellular variant
4. Tip variant
5. Collapsing variant.

FSGS, Not Otherwise Specified

It is the classic or usual type, involves at least one glomerulus and requires the exclusion of other morphologic categories:[5-8]

Light Microscopic Features (Fig. 4.4)

- Discrete segmental increase and condensation of extracellular matrix
- Obliteration of glomerular capillary lumina
- Early involvement of peripheral segments of juxtamedullary glomeruli
- Associated hyalinosis, known as "plasmatic insudation" comprising: amorphous, eosinophilic, PAS positive nonargyrophilic and trichrome red material
- Diffuse mesangial hypercellularity (in pediatric cases)
- Capsular adhesions or synechiae to Bowman's capsule
- Cellular cap formed by podocytes over the segment
- Detachment of podocytes with intervening weakly positive PAS positive matrix.

Immunofluorescent Features (Fig. 4.5)

Focal and segmental trapping of IgM and C3 in sclerotic tufts.

Electron Microscopic Features (Figs 4.6A and B)

- Retraction of glomerular basement membrane in sclerotic segments
- Obliteration of lumen by matrix material

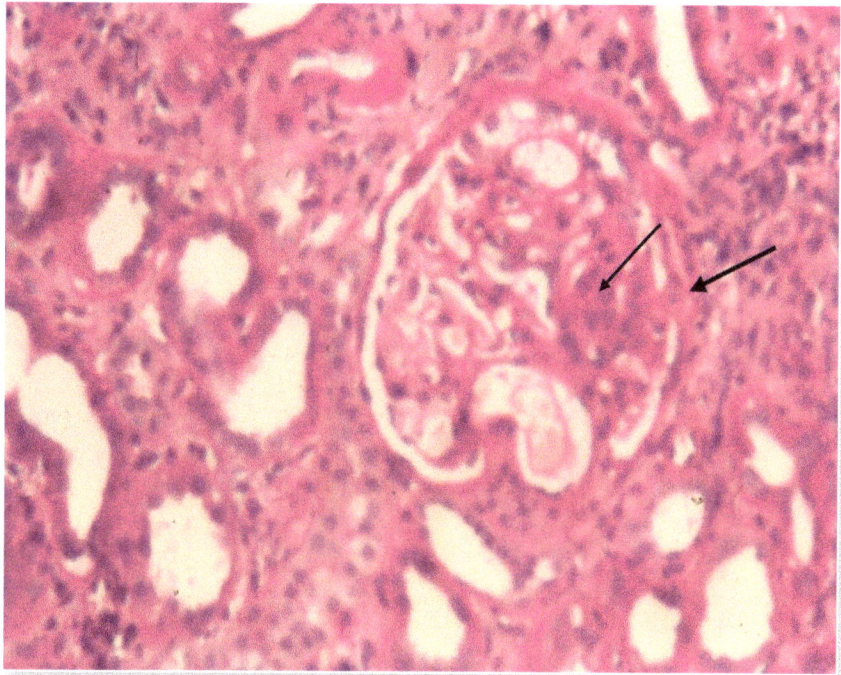

Figure 4.4: Focal segmental sclerosis-NOS (PAS x 400) with condensation of matrix (thin arrow) and capsular synechiae (thick arrow) (PAS x 400)

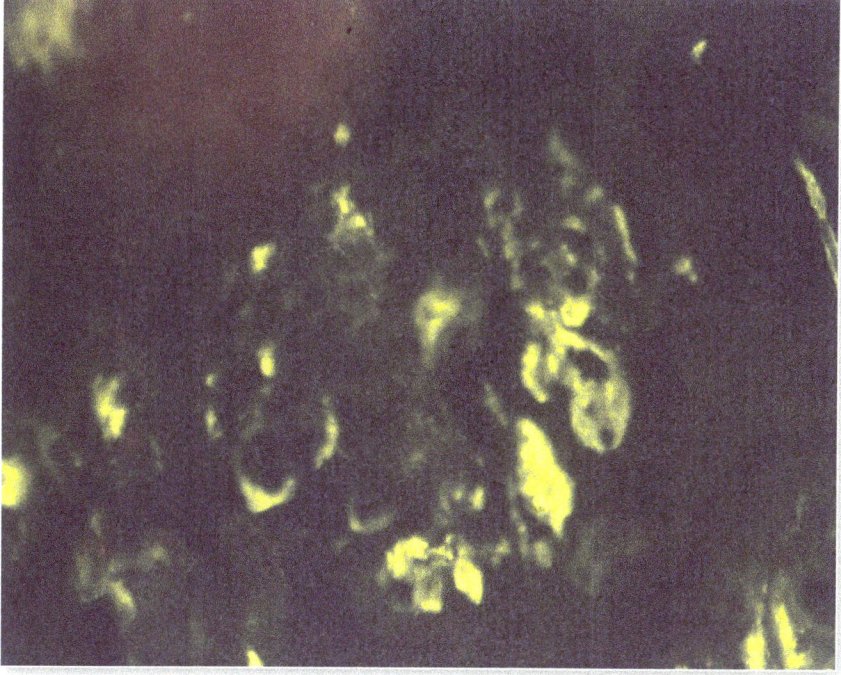

Figure 4.5: Focal segmental trapping of IgM in sclerotic tufts (IF x 400)

18 Renal Biopsy Interpretation

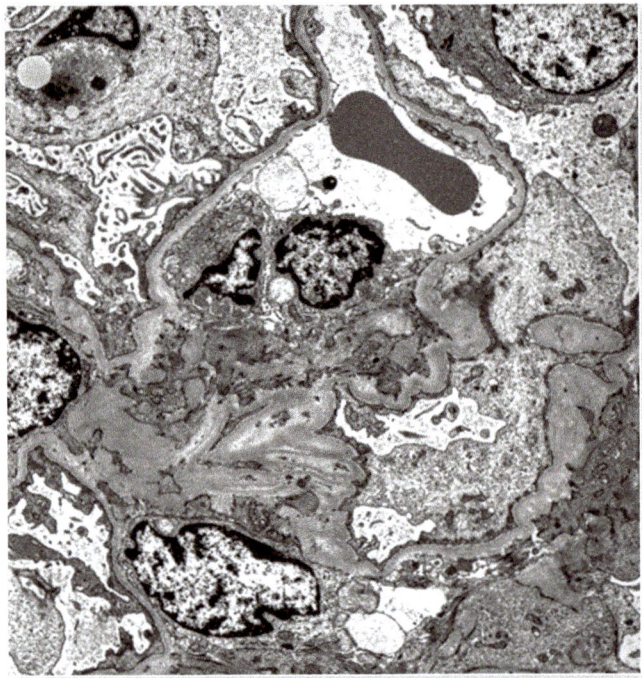

Figure 4.6A: FSGS (NOS) with diffuse effacement of foot processes of podocytes and microvillous processes (EM)

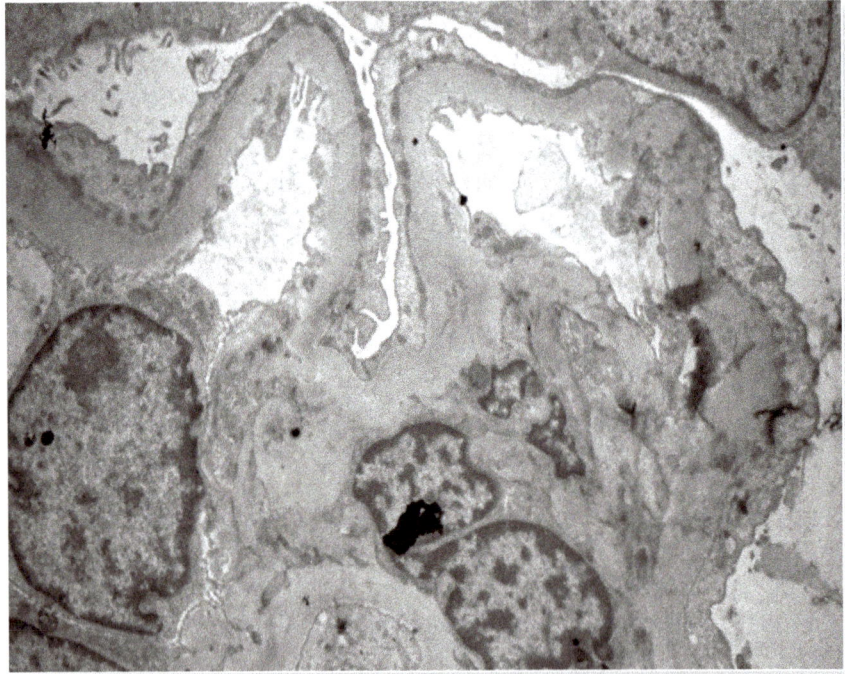

Figure 4.6B: FSGS (NOS) with diffuse effacement of foot processes (EM x 6000)

Glomerular Diseases

- Electron dense hyaline material in lumen between endothelial cell and GBM
- Diffuse effacement of foot processes of podocytes (>50% of glomerular capillary surface area)
- Loss of primary cytoplasmic processes and slit diaphragms noted
- Detachment and hypertrophy of podocytes with microvillous processes, on luminal aspect
- Lamellated neomembrane between denuded GBM and detached podocyte.

Perihilar Variant

It is more common with secondary forms of FSGS, mediated by an adaptive response to increased capillary pressures with reduced number of functioning nephrons.[1]

Microscopic Features

- Sclerosis at and adjacent to vascular pole as the predominant lesion (Fig. 4.7)
- Involving >50% of segmentally sclerotic glomeruli
- Glomerulomegaly with capsular synechiae and arteriolar hyalinosis
- Podocyte hypertrophy and hyperplasia less frequent
- Other glomeruli can display segmental and/or global sclerosis of classical (NOS) type.

Cellular Variant[5,9-11]

Microscopic Features

- Segmental endocapillary hypercellularity of at least 25% of the tuft (Fig. 4.8)
- Peripheral or hilar segment involved with condensation of matrix

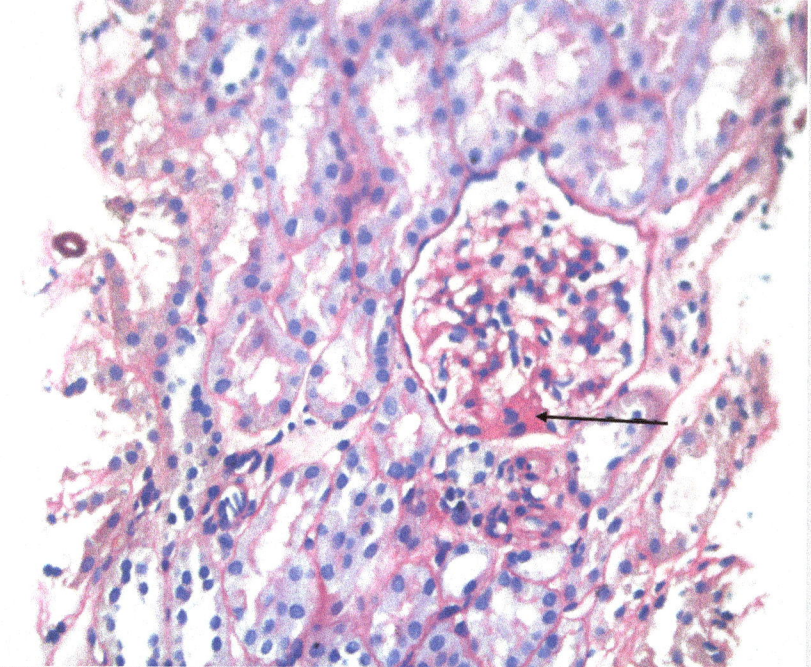

Figure 4.7: Focal segmental sclerosis—perihilar variant (PAS × 200, arrow)

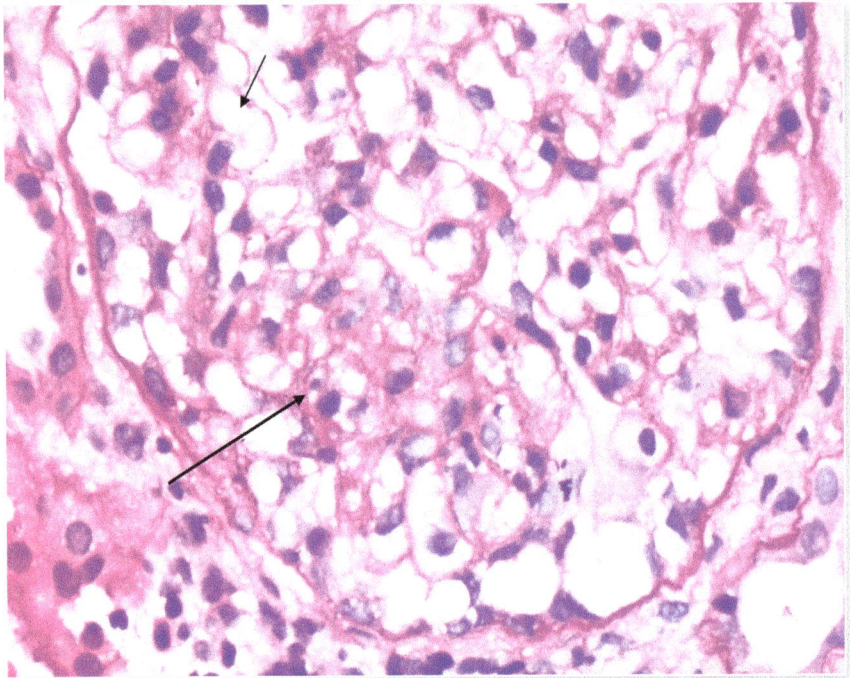

Figure 4.8: Focal segmental glomerulosclerosis—cellular variant (PAS × 400, arrow)

- Endocapillary cells include leukocytes (monocytes, **foamy macrophages, lymphocytes or neutrophils**)
- **Karyorrhexis** without rupture of glomerular basement membrane
- Often associated with lesions of classical, focal segmental (NOS) and global glomerulosclerosis
- Can be differentiated from focal segmental proliferative glomerulonephritis
- By immunofluorescence, glomeruli are negative for immune complex deposits.

Tip Variant[5,12,13]

Microscopic Features

- Focal condensation of matrix in tip domain, adjacent to origin of proximal tubule (Figs 4.9 and 4.10)
- Involves 25% of at least one glomerulus opposite the vascular pole
- Confluence of enlarged podocytes with parietal cells or tubular epithelial cells
- Intracapillary foam cells and capsular synechiae of the tuft at tubular pole
- Collapsing variant and perihilar sclerosis have to be excluded
- Peripheral segments of sclerosis or endocapillary hypercellularity in other glomeruli can be present.

Collapsing Variant (Collapsing Glomerulopathy)

The podocyte expresses a dysregulated phenotype with increased rate of proliferation and loss of mature podocyte markers including synaptopodin, WT-1, podocalyxin, GLEPP-1 (glomerular

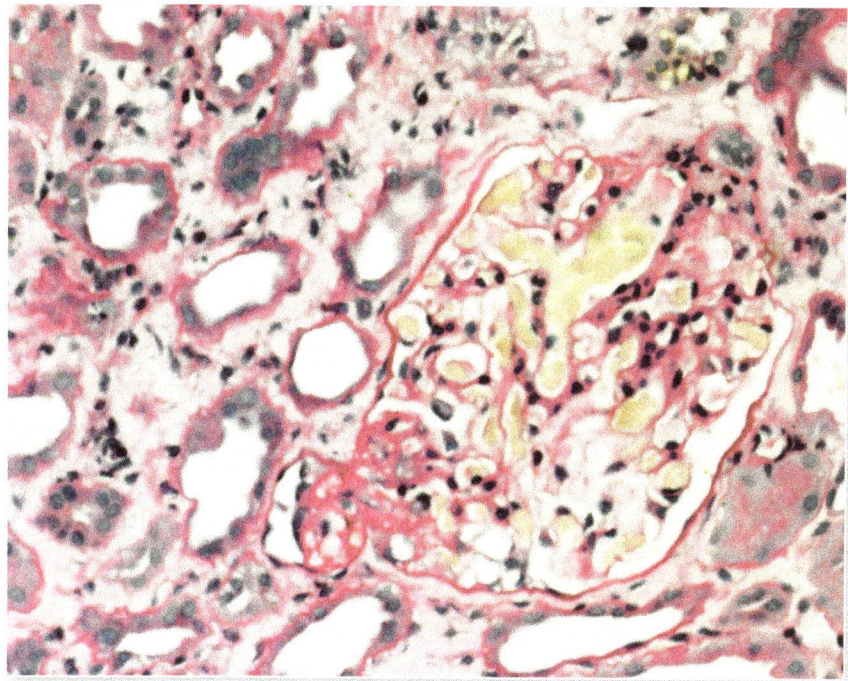

Figure 4.9: FSGS—tip variant (H&E x 200)

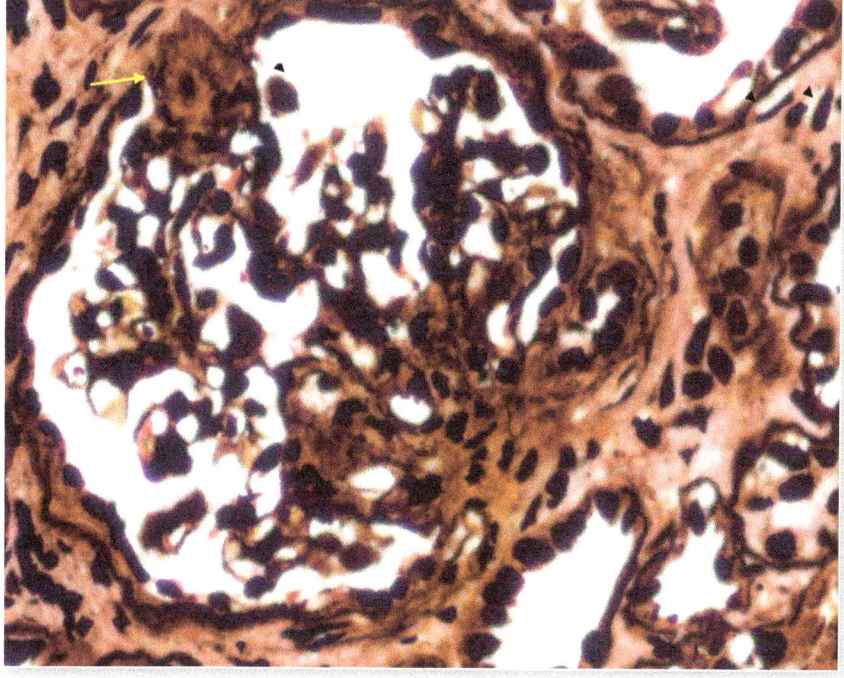

Figure 4.10: FSGS—tip variant (JMS x 400, arrow)

epithelial protein), C3b receptor and CALLA (CD10), and re-expression of proliferative markers and cytokeratins. As the podocytes re-enter the cell cycle, there is associated reduced expression of cell cycle inhibitors.[14-17]

Microscopic Features

- Implosive wrinkling and collapse of glomerular basement membrane (on the PAS and Jones methenamine stains) of at least one glomerulus (Fig. 4.11)
- Segmental or global obliteration of capillary lumina
- No appreciable increase in intracapillary or mesangial matrix
- Marked podocyte hypertrophy and hyperplasia, forming "pseudocrescents"
- Comprised of discohesive rounded cells (not spindled) devoid of pericellular matrix
- Detached from intact Bowman's capsule
- Enlarged podocytes have vesicular nuclei and prominent nucleoli
- Occasional binucleate forms and mitoses are found
- Pseudocrescents contain prominent intracytoplasmic protein resorption droplets.

Immunohistochemistry: Negative for WT-1, positive for Ki67, PAX2 and cytokeratins (CK8, 18, CK19 and CAM 5.2).

Collapsing glomerulopathy can be idiopathic, reactive, secondary to HIV nephropathy or other viral infections, including parvovirus B19, CMV, bacterial and parasitic infections, autoimmune diseases (SLE, mixed connective tissue disease), thrombotic microangiopathy, hematologic malignancy, drugs (interferon, biphosphonates, valproic acid, calcineurin inhibitors) or associated with genetic mutations with dysregulation of mitochondrial activity.

Electron Microscopy

- Folded, corrugated, collapsed GBM with occlusion of capillary lumen
- Focal detachment of podocytes with interposed matrix
- Extensive foot process effacement
- Loss of primary processes
- Cuboidal podocytes with pale cytoplasm and protein reabsorption droplets
- Loss of fenestration of endothelial cells.

Prognosis

The collapsing variant has a rapid rate of progression to end stage renal disease when compared to the tip variant, which is an early lesion and the cellular variant that has an intermediate prognosis. The outcome of the perihilar and NOS variants depends on the degree of interstitial fibrosis rather than the percentage of glomerular involvement by segmental/global scars, which does not have an independent predictive value.

Differential Diagnosis[1,18,19]

Secondary Focal Segmental Glomerulosclerosis

It is caused by numerous factors such as:

Glomerular Diseases 23

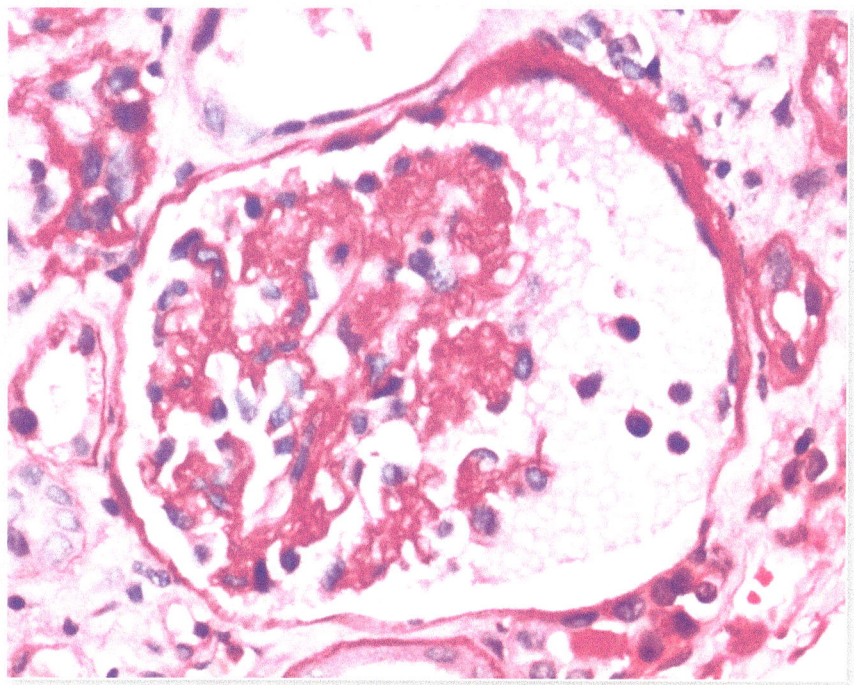

Figure 4.11: FSGS—collapsing variant (PAS x 200)

Infections: HIV

Drugs and toxins: Heroin and pamidronate.

Genetic autosomal mutations: Alpha-actinin 4 and podocin mutations and mitochondrial cytopathies.

Adaptive structural-functional response to hyperfiltration and nephron loss: Reflux nephropathy, unilateral renal agenesis, diabetes mellitus, hypertension and morbid obesity.

Nonspecific scarring: As in focal proliferative/necrotizing glomerulonephritis, membranous nephropathy, hereditary nephritis and thrombotic microangiopathies.

Microscopic Features

- Glomerular hypertrophy with discrete segmental scars
- Involvement of perihilar regions
- Podocyte hypertrophy and hyperplasia, less frequent
- Ischemic atrophy of glomerular tufts with microcystic dilatation in hypertensive segmental sclerosis.

Electron Microscopy

Degree of foot process effacement is usually <50% of total glomerular capillary surface area.

REFERENCES

1. Lane JC, Kaskel FJ. Pediatric nephrotic syndrome: from the simple to the complex. Seminars in nephrology. 2009;29:389-98.
2. Fogo AG. Causes and pathogenesis of focal segmental glomerulosclerosis Nature reviews. Nephrology. 2014 doi:10. 1038/nrneph. 2014. 216.
3. D'Agati VD, Kaskel FJ, Falk RJ. Focal segmental glomerulosclerosis. N Engl J Med. 2011;365:2398-411.
4. McCarthy ET, Sharma M, Savin VJ. Circulating permeability factors in idiopathic nephrotic syndrome and focal segmental glomerulosclerosis. Clin J Am Soc Nephrol. 2010;5:2115-21.
5. Vivette D'Agati. Pathologic classification of focal segmental glomerulosclerosis. Seminars in Nephrology. 2003; 23:117-34.
6. D'Agati VD, Fogo AB, Bruijn JA, Jennette JC. Pathologic classification of FSGS: a working proposal. Am J Kidney Dis. 2004;43:368-82.
7. Thomas DB, Franceschini N, Hogan SL, et al. Clinical and pathologic characteristics of focal segmental glomerulosclerosis, pathologic variants. Kidney Int. 2006; 69(5): 920-6.
8. Thomas DB. Focal segmental glomerulosclerosis, a morphologic diagnosis in evolution. Arch Pathol Lab Med. 2009;133:217-23.
9. D'Agati VD. The spectrum of focal segmental glomerulosclerosis: new insights. Curr Opin Nephrol Hypertens. 2008;17:271-81.
10. Schwartz MM, Lewis EJ. Focal segmental glomerular sclerosis: the cellular lesion. Kidney Int. 1985;28:968-74.
11. Schwartz MM, Evans J, Bain R, et al. Focal segmental glomerulosclerosis: prognostic implication of the cellular lesion. J Am Soc Nephrol. 1999;10:1900-7.
12. Howie AJ, Brewer DB. The glomerular tip lesion: a previously undescribed type of segmental glomerular abnormality. J Pathol. 1984;142:205-20.
13. Huppes W, Hene RJ, Kooiker CJ. The glomerular tip lesion: a distinct entity or not? J Pathol. 1988;154:187-90.
14. Detwiler RK, Falk RJ, Hogan SL, et al. Collapsing glomerulopathy: a clinically and pathologically distinct variant of focal segmental glomerulosclerosis. Kidney Int. 1994;45:1416-24.
15. Valeri A, Barisoni L, Appel GB, et al. Idiopathic collapsing focal segmental glomerulosclerosis: a clinico-pathologic study. Kidney Int. 1996;50:1734-46.
16. Albaqumi M, Barisoni L. Current views on collapsing glomerulopathy. J Am Soc Nephrol. 2008;19:1276-81.
17. Daskalakis N, Winn MP. Focal and segmental glomerulosclerosis: varying biologic mechanisms underlie a final histopathologic end point seminars in nephrology. 2006;26(2):89-94.
18. D'Agati V: The many masks of focal segmental glomerulosclerosis. Kidney Int. 1994;46:1223-41.
19. Rennke H, Klein PS. Pathogenesis and significance of non-primary focal and segmental glomerulosclerosis. Am J Kidney Dis. 1989;13:443-55.

Glomerular Diseases

MEMBRANOUS NEPHROPATHY

Membranous nephropathy is the second common cause of nephrotic syndrome in adults above the age of 40 years with a male predilection and a relative frequency of 9.8% in adults, in our experience.[1] There are primary and secondary forms of this entity; the former (idiopathic–IMN) is an autoimmune disease with glomerular immune deposits directed against endogenous antigens expressed on the podocyte foot processes. **The M-type phospholipase A2 receptor (PLA2R), a transmembrane receptor expressed on the podocyte has recently been identified as the major antigen in human IMN associated with circulating autoantibodies to PLA2R** that were detected in 70% of patients in their sera and correlating with disease activity,[2-4] mainly in adults. **The subepithelial deposits are the defining features leading to varying degrees of glomerular basement membrane thickening.**

Primary Membranous Nephropathy

Microscopic Features[5,6]

- Uniform thickening of glomerular capillary walls accentuated on the PAS stain (Fig. 4.12)
- No increase in mesangial and endocapillary cellularity or matrix
- Subepithelial deposits with spikes of glomerular capillary basement membranes (on PAS and Jones methenamine stains).

Stages distinguished by LM, IF and EM: There are four stages of disease progression originally described by Ehrenreich-Churg[7] on electron microscopy. In actual practice, a heterogeneous

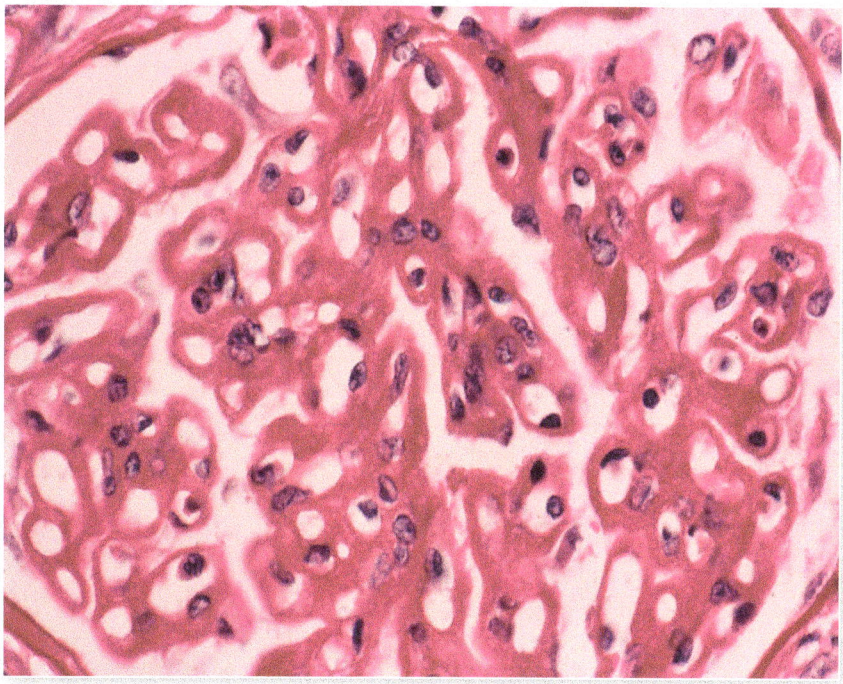

Figure 4.12: Primary membranous nephropathy (PAS × 400)

combination of these stages is seen in the glomeruli varying from one glomerulus to another in a renal biopsy.

Stage I: Features no apparent abnormality by LM with characteristic subepithelial deposits by IF and EM:

Light Microscopy:
- Normocellular glomeruli without mesangial widening and patent capillary lumina
- No apparent increase in thickness of capillary walls.

Immunofluorescence:
Finely granular contiguous deposits of IgG (2 to 3+) and less intense C3 (1 to 2+) on the glomerular capillary walls.

Electron Microscopy:
Small and sparse subepithelial deposits with focal foot process effacement of podocytes.

Stage II: Characterized by uniform thickening of glomerular capillary walls.

Light Microscopy:
- Diffuse thickening and rigidity of glomerular capillary walls on H&E and PAS stains
- "Spikes" that are perpendicular projections of capillary basement membrane on outer aspect (on the PAS and Jones Methenamine stains (Fig. 4.13A)
- Internal vacuoles or "holes" representing non- argyrophilic deposits on the capillary walls
- Seen on tangential sections of capillary walls on Jones methenamine stains.

Immunofluorescence:
Coarsely granular intense contiguous deposits of IgG (3+) and C3 (1 to 2+) on glomerular capillary walls.

Electron Microscopy:
Large aggregated immune deposits with spikes between deposits and marked hypertrophy of podocytes with foot process effacement.

Stage III: Moderate glomerular capillary wall thickening with narrowing of capillary lumina is seen.

Light Microscopy:
- Intramembranous deposits with residual spikes linked by overlying neomembrane forming a dome (Fig. 4.13B)
- Chain-like thickening of glomerular capillary walls
- Numerous internal vacuoles on special stains
- Mild mesangial sclerosis
- Foci of tubular atrophy and interstitial fibrosis.

Immunofluorescence:
Coarsely granular, less intense, capillary wall deposits of IgG (3+) and C3 (1 to 2+) (Fig. 4.14).

Electron Microscopy:
- Intramembranous electron dense to electron lucent deposits due to partial resorption of deposits (Figs 4.15A and B)

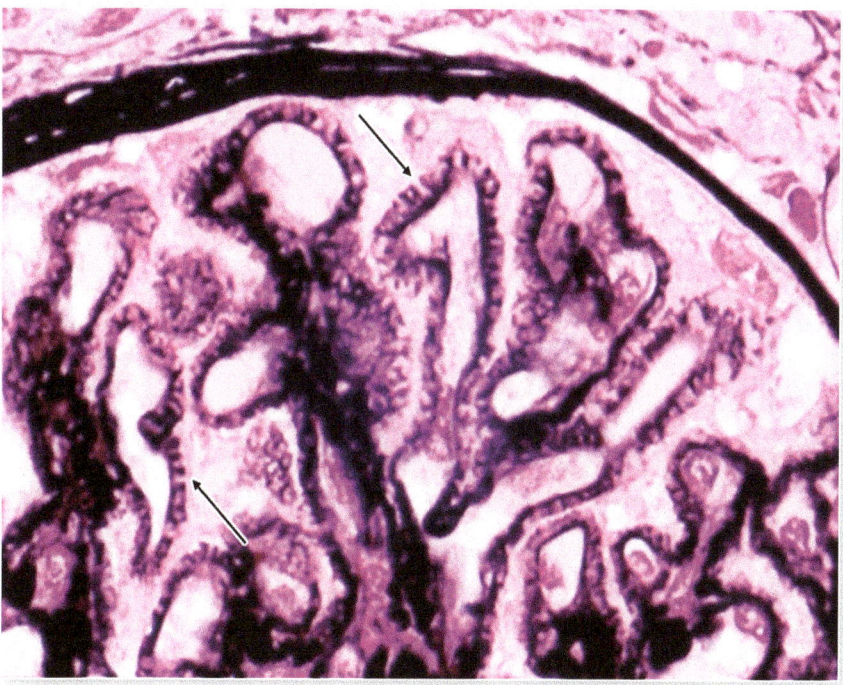

Figure 4.13A: Epimembranous spikes–arrows (JMS x 1000)

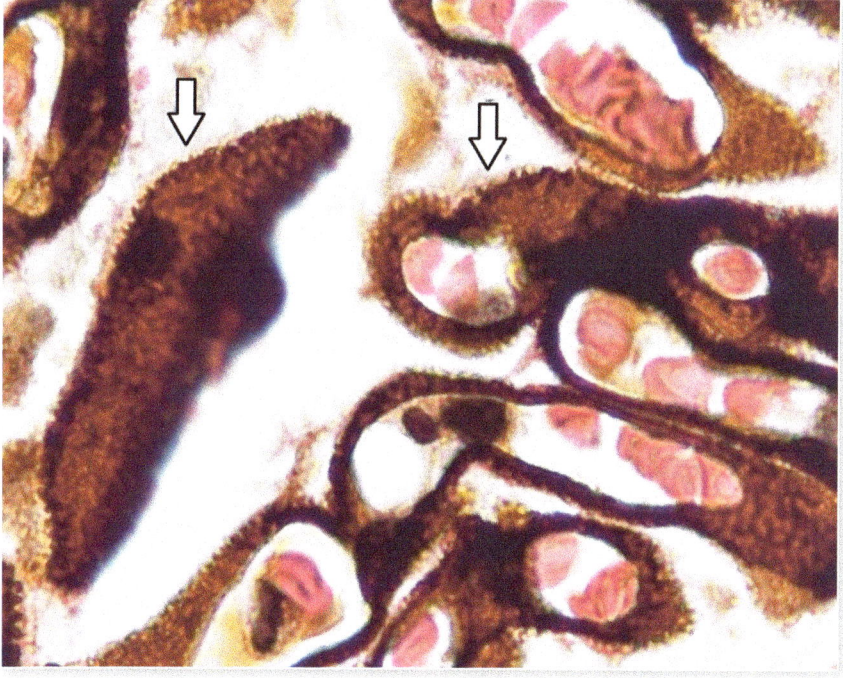

Figure 4.13B: Epimembranous spikes and domes–arrows (JMS x 1000)

Renal Biopsy Interpretation

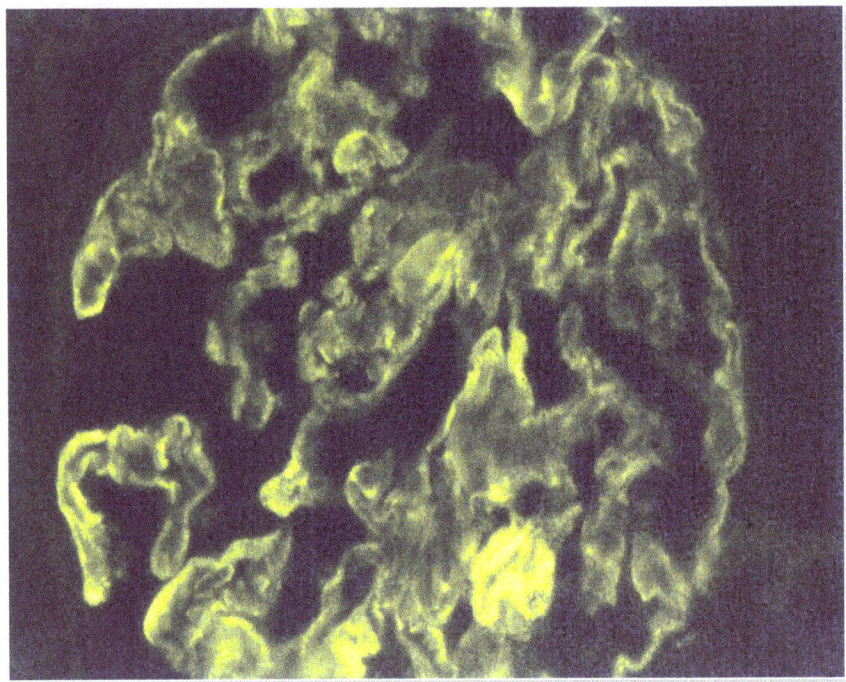

Figure 4.14: Membranous nephropathy (IF × 400)

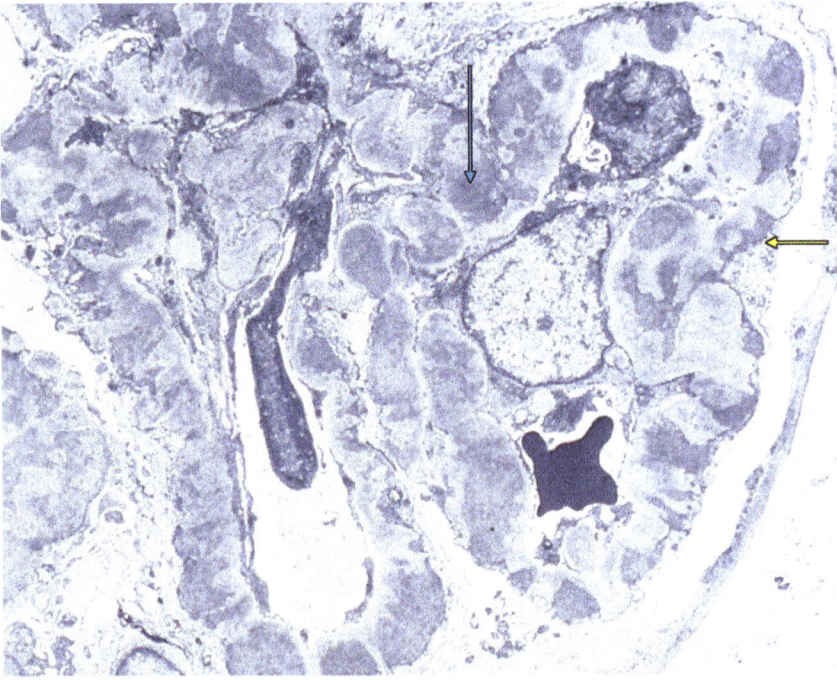

Figure 4.15A: Electron micrograph of primary membranous nephropathy—Stages II to III with subepithelial (yellow arrow) and intramembranous (blue arrow) deposits

Glomerular Diseases

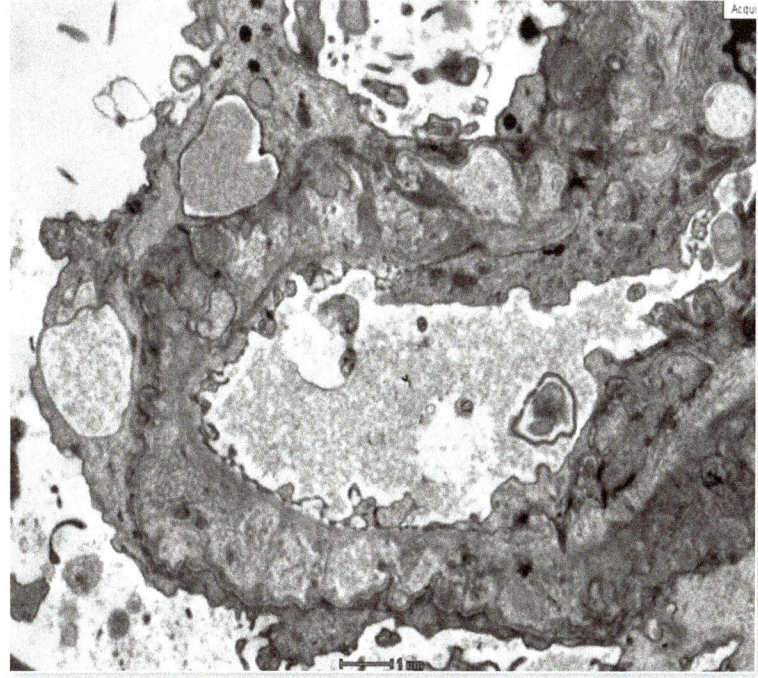

Figure 4.15B: Membranous nephropathy Stage IV with lucency of GBM (EM x 6000)

- Neomembrane formed by basement membrane material incorporating deposits
- Complex lamellated thickening of capillary walls
- Extensive foot process effacement.

Stage IV: Features marked thickening of capillary walls with resorbed deposits
- Lamellated thickening of capillary walls with foci of reduplication
- Mesangial sclerosis with segmental and global glomerulosclerosis
- Diffuse tubular atrophy with interstitial fibrosis and arteriosclerosis.

Immunofluorescence:
Nonspecific trapping of IgM and C3 in sclerotic segments.

Electron Microscopy (Fig. 4.15B):
- Marked thickening of glomerular basement membrane with lacunae and irregular lamellations
- Few residual electron dense intramembranous deposits
- Restoration of foot processes.

    Immunohistochemistry with anti-PLA2R antibodies has revealed homogeneous staining of glomerular capillary loops on formalin fixed paraffin sections of renal biopsies of primary membranous nephropathy[8] and has been currently standardized in our laboratory at CMC, Vellore for routine use. Standard immunofluorescence staining on cryostat sections and confocal fluorescent microscopy by anti-PLA2R antibody with finely granular glomerular capillary deposits, has been documented. There is a sensitivity of 75% and a specificity of 83% in this latter method, with co-localization by predominantly IgG4 deposits.[9]

Course and Prognosis

Idiopathic membranous nephropathy (IMN) has a variable prognosis and one-third of patients progress to end stage renal disease. In patients who achieve complete remission in response to immunosuppressive therapy, anti-PLA2R serum levels become undetectable months before the proteinuria resolves completely. These findings are probably a sequelae of residual structural deficits in the absence of immunologic activity. In addition, GBM remodeling and sclerotic changes that occur in the glomerulus with longstanding MN can also cause persistent proteinuria.[3] Partial or complete disappearance of subepithelial deposits against PLA2R has also been noted in serial biopsies on follow up, after treatment.

Secondary membranous nephropathy has to be differentiated from Primary Membranous Nephropathy and accounts for about 25% of cases and the known common causes include Systemic lupus erythematosus (Class V lupus nephritis), Hepatitis B viral infection, Non-steroidal anti-inflammatory drugs, Malignancy and sarcoidosis.[3] In our experience in CMC, class V lupus nephritis is the most frequent biopsy proven cause. The direct causal association with Hepatitis B viral antigenemia and other factors (Box 4.1) can also be concurrently present.

Box 4.1: Causes of secondary membranous nephropathy.[3]

Autoimmune diseases
- Systemic lupus erythematosus (class V lupus nephritis)
- Rheumatoid arthritis
- Autoimmune thyroid disease
- Sjögren syndrome
- IgG4-related systemic disease

Infectious agents
- Viral: Hepatitis B, human immunodeficiency virus
- Bacterial: Syphilis
- Parasitic: Schistosomiasis, malaria

Iatrogenic
- Nonsteroidal anti-inflammatory agents
- Anti-rheumatic drugs: D-penicillamine, gold salts
- Mercury-containing skin-lightening creams

Malignancy
- Solid tumors (colon, stomach, lung, prostate)
- Non-Hodgkin lymphoma
- Chronic lymphocytic leukemia

Microscopic Features[10]

- Non-uniform glomerular capillary wall thickening
- Mesangial matrix expansion
- Mesangial and subepithelial immune deposits
- "Full house" pattern of IgG, IgA IgM and C3 with C1q and C4 (in class V lupus nephritis)
- IgG1, IgG2 and IgG3 subclasses predominate in immune complexes
- Negative PLA2R immunostaining (on I. F. and IHC)
- Tubuloreticular endothelial inclusions in lupus nephritis (on EM).

REFERENCES

1. Narasimhan B, Chacko B, John GT, Korula A, Kirubakaran MG, Jacob CK. Characterization of kidney lesions in Indian adults: towards a renal biopsy registry. J Nephrol. 2006;19:205-10.
2. Beck Jr LH, Bonegio RG, Lambeau G, et al. M-type phospholipase A2 receptor as target antigen in idiopathic membranous nephropathy. N Engl J Med. 2009;361:11-21.
3. Hong Ma, Dana G. Sandor, Laurence H Beck Jr. The role of complement in membranous nephropathy. Seminars in Nephrology. 2013;33(6):531-42.
4. Beck Jr LH, Salant DJ. Membranous nephropathy: recent travels and new roads ahead. Kidney Int. 2010;77:765-70.
5. Jennette JC, Olson JL, Silva FG, D'Agati VD. Heptinstall's Pathology of the Kidney, UK: Wolters Kluwer; 2015.
6. D'Agati VD, Jennette JC, Silva FG. Non-Neoplastic Kidney Diseases. Atlas of Nontumor Pathology, first series, fascicle 4. American Registry of Pathology and Armed Forces Institute of Pathology Washington. 2005.
7. Ehrenreich T, Churg J. Pathology of membranous nephropathy. In: Sommers SC, Rosen P (eds). Pathology Annual. New York; Appleton-Century-crofts.1968;3:145.
8. Hoxha E, Kneißler U, Stege G, et al. Enhanced expression of the M-type phospholipase A2 receptor in glomeruli correlates with serum receptor antibodies in primary membranous nephropathy. Kidney Int. 2012;82:797-804.
9. Larsen CP, Messias NC, et al. Determination of primary versus secondary membranous glomerulopathy utilizing phospholipase A2 receptor staining in renal biopsies Mod Pathol. 2013;26(5);709-15.
10. Jennette JC, Iskandar SS, Dalldorf FG. Pathologic differentiation between lupus and non lupus membranous glomerulopathy. Kidney Int. 1983;24:377-85.

Proliferative Glomerulonephritis

This subtype of glomerulonephritis is defined by the proliferation of intrinsic glomerular cells, as a reaction to immune mediated injury. The extent of proliferation can be focal or diffuse involving less than or greater than 50% of glomeruli respectively, in a renal biopsy.

Diffuse proliferative glomerulonephritis can be classified, based on the pattern of glomerular cell proliferation and the site of immune complex and/or complement deposition, as follows:
1. Endocapillary proliferative glomerulonephritis
2. Mesangial proliferative glomerulonephritis (IgA and non-IgA subtypes)
3. Crescentic glomerulonephritis
4. Membranoproliferative glomerulonephritis
5. C3 glomerulopathy
6. C1q glomerulopathy.

DIFFUSE PREDOMINANTLY ENDOCAPILLARY PROLIFERATIVE GLOMERULONEPHRITIS

It can be idiopathic but is usually caused by nephritogenic group A beta hemolytic streptococcal infection (PSGN), commonly in developing countries with an incidence of 8.8% in our case series,[1] occurring in children 5 to 12 years of age, 1 to 3 weeks after an episode of pharyngitis or skin infection. There has been an increase in the incidence of post-infectious glomerulonephritis in adults, ranging from 12.20–19.20% in the age groups 15 to 55 years respectively.[2] Other associated bacterial infections in adults include; visceral abscess, bacterial endocarditis and pneumonia. The primary or idiopathic and postinfectious forms of glomerular immune complex disease (PIGN) lead to complement activation and inflammation with influx of neutrophils and release of proteolytic enzymes and oxidants that can degrade the capillary basement membranes. The nephritis associated plasmin receptor, glyceraldehyde-3 phospate dehydrogenase and a cationic proteinase, streptococcal pyrogenic exotoxin-B, activate the alternate pathway of the complement system.[3-6] *Staphylococcus aureus* infection (methicillin sensitive and resistant) can lead to IgA dominant PIGN and renal failure.[7]

Microscopic Features[8]

Light Microscopy (Fig. 4.16)

- Enlargement of glomeruli with lobular expansion
- Marked endothelial cell proliferation (increase in size and number)
- Occlusion of capillary lumina and neutrophilic infiltration
- Variable increase in mesangial matrix and mesangial hypercellularity in resolving PIGN.

Immunofluorescence

Granular and clumped IgG (3+) and C3 (2 to 3+) deposits on glomerular capillary walls (Fig. 4.17).

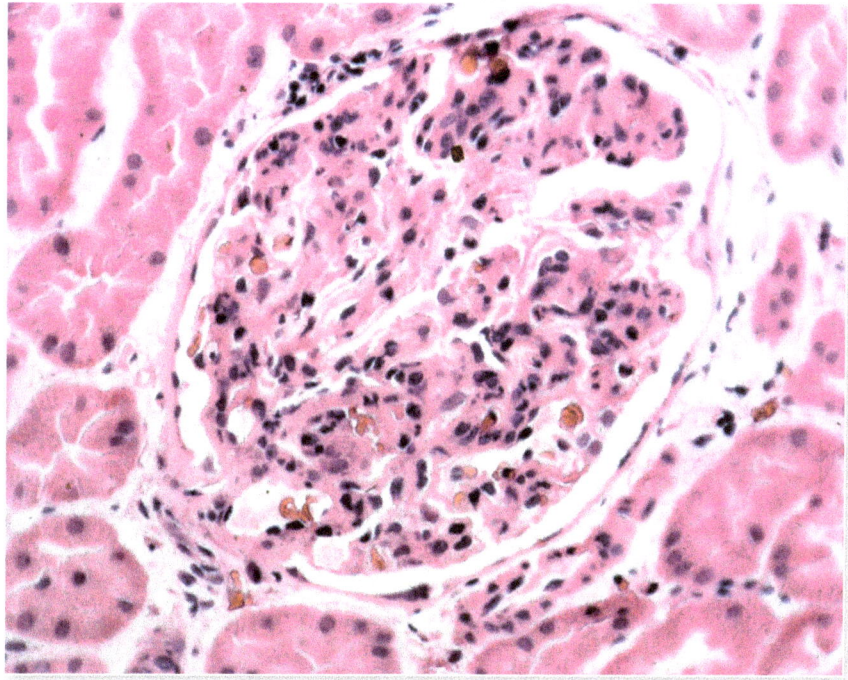

Figure 4.16: Diffuse proliferative glomerulonephritis (H&E x 400)

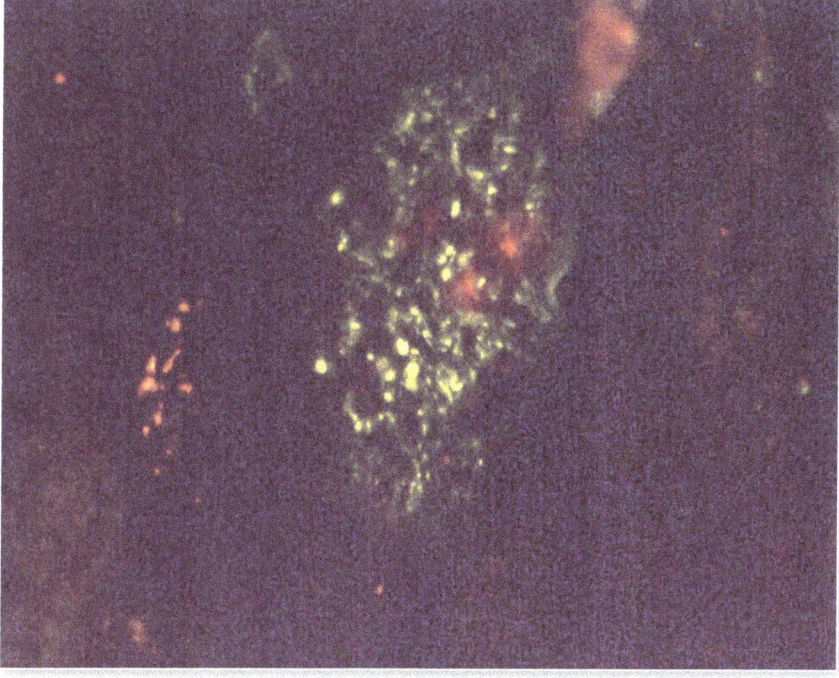

Figure 4.17: Immunofluorescent micrograph of PIGN—granular and clumped C3 deposits on glomerular capillary walls

34 Renal Biopsy Interpretation

Variant features:
- Confluent and coarsely granular or band like ("garland pattern") deposits on capillary walls
- Discrete granular deposits on capillary walls and mesangium ("Starry sky pattern")
- Predominantly mesangial deposits seen in resolving PIGN.

Electron Microscopy

Large electron dense subepithelial deposits under foot processes of podocytes (Fig. 4.18).

Course and Prognosis

Post infectious glomerulonephritis (PIGN) with acute nephritic syndrome usually resolves 2-6 weeks after the onset with symptomatic treatment with excellent outcome in children and renal biopsy is not required as a routine. Renal biopsy is indicated for complications including formation of parietal cellular crescents that can regress with immunosuppressive therapy and dialysis if required. Foci of mesangial sclerosis with reduplication of glomerular capillary walls are noted in adults with unresolved PIGN and progressive rise in serum creatinine.

Differential Diagnosis

Renal biopsy is usually done in atypical or unresolved cases of PIGN to exclude the following probabilities:
1. **Membranoproliferative glomerulonephritis (Type I)** that displays marked centrilobular matrix expansion with circumferential reduplication of glomerular capillary walls (on

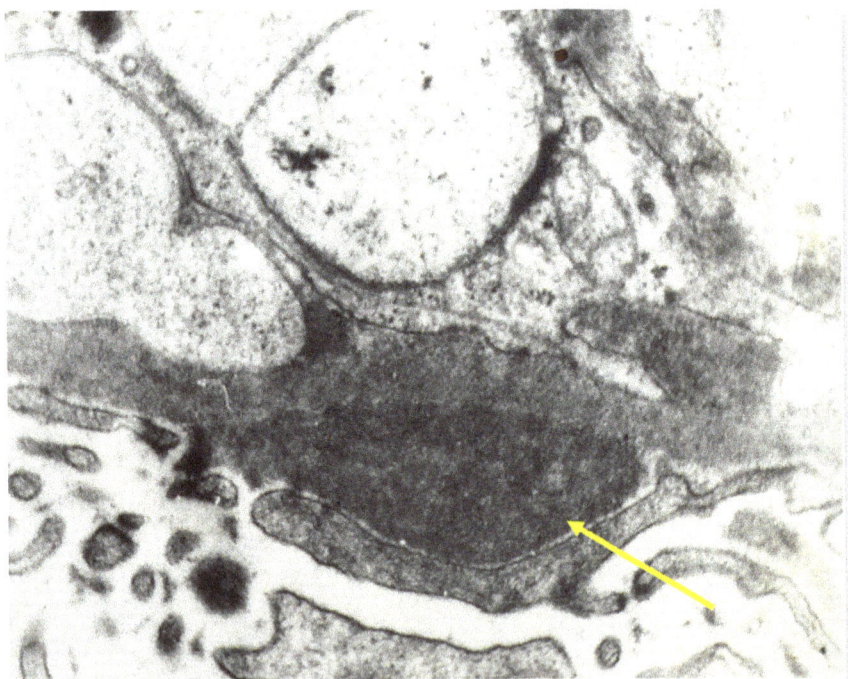

Figure 4.18: Electron micrograph of subepithelial deposits in DPGN (arrow)

PAS and Jones methenamine stains) and perilobular capillary wall deposits of C3 on immunofluorescence with subendothelial deposits and mesangial interposition on electron microscopy.[6]

2. **IgA nephropathy:** In biopsies associated with synpharyngitic macro hematuria and recurrent microscopic hematuria with diffuse endocapillary proliferation, dominant or codominant IgA deposits in the mesangium and/or capillary walls with C3 deposits are noted on immunofluorescence. IgA dominant PIGN (post-staphylococcal infection) also requires exclusion in some cases.[7]

3. **Diffuse proliferative lupus nephritis class IV** with typical features including diffuse endocapillary proliferation with marked capillary wall thickening forming "wire loops" and hyaline thrombi can be differentiated from PIGN. Immunofluorescent features with a full house pattern of glomerular capillary wall deposition of IgG, IgA, IgM, C3, C1q and C4 are confirmatory together with subendothelial deposits on the E M. These typical features are however modified or absent in cases of lupus nephritis on steroids and can closely mimic PIGN. Hence careful scrutiny of the renal biopsy, correlation with lupus serology and follow-up are required to differentiate these entities.

4. **C3 glomerulopathy:** It is a recently categorized entity that has membranoproliferative features by light microscopy with isolated C3 deposits and no immunoglobulins with mesangial and subendothelial deposits in 75% of cases on electron microscopy. This is associated with dysregulation of the alternate pathway of complement activation with genetic mutations (CFHR5) and familial forms of the disease. Subepithelial deposits can occur with acute exacerbation by concomitant streptococcal infection, in a minority of cases that are associated with persistent hypocomplementemia but lacks membranoproliferative features.[9,10]

REFERENCES

1. Balakrisnan N, John GT, Korula A, Visalakshi J, Talauikar GS, Thomas PP, et al. Spectrum of biopsy proven renal disease and changing trends at a tropical tertiary care centre, 1990-2001. Indian J Nephrol. 2003;13:29-35.
2. Narasimhan B, Chacko B, John GT, Korula A, Kirubakaran MG, Jacob CK. Characterization of kidney lesions in Indian adults: towards a renal biopsy registry. J Nephrol. 2006;19:205-10.
3. Rodriguez-Iturbe B, Musser JM. The current state of poststreptococcal glomerulonephritis. J Am Soc Nephrol. 2008; 19:1855-64.
4. Nasr SH, Markowitz GS, Stoks MB, Said SM, Valeri AM, D'Agati VD. Acute postinfectious glomerulonephritis in the modern era. Experience with 86 adults and review of literature. Medicine. 2008;87:21-32.
5. Kanjanabuch T, Kittikowit W, Elam-Ong S. An update on acute postinfectious glomerulonephritis worldwide. Nat Rev Nephrol. 2009;5:259-69.
6. Yoshizawa N, Yamakami K, Fujino M, Oda T, Tamura K, Matsumoto K, et al. Nephritis-associated plasmin receptor and acute poststreptococcal glomerulonephritis: characterization of the antigen and associated immune response. J Am Soc Nephrol. 2004;15:1785-93.
7. Koyama A, Sharmin S, Sakurai H, Shimizu Y, Hirayama K, Usui J, et al. Staphylococcus aureus cell envelope antigen is new candidate for the Induction of IgA nephropathy. Kidney Int. 2004;66:121-31.
8. D'Agati VD, Jennette JC, Silva FG. Non-neoplastic kidney diseases. Atlas of Nontumor Pathology, first series, fascicle 4. American Registry of Pathology and Armed Forces Institute of Pathology Washington, DC; 2005.
9. Fakhouri F, et al. C3 glomerulopathy: a new classification. Nat Review Nephrol. 2010;6(8):494-9.
10. Sandhu G, Bansal A, Ranade A, Jones J, Cortell S, Markowitz GS. C3 glomerulopathy masquerading as postinfectious glomerulonephritis. Am J Kidney Dis. 2012;60(6):1039-43.

IgA NEPHROPATHY

IgA nephropathy is accounted for 8.6% of primary glomerulonephritis in our case series occurring predominantly in the age group 15-34 years[1] and is the most common type of primary glomerular disease, worldwide, with an overall prevalence of 40% in Asians[2-4] and 4-15% in Indians.[5-10] Aberrant glycosylation of the IgA1 immunoglobulin hinge region with truncated o-glycans formation leads to antibody production to epitopes of the hinge region and mesangial deposition of IgA-immune complexes with activation of mesangial cells and release of pro-inflammatory mediators, podocyte loss and glomerular scarring.[11-14] The mesangiopathic form of glomerulonephritis is associated with predominantly mesangial immune complex deposits of IgA.

Microscopic Features

Light Microscopy

There are various morphological classifications including the Haas[15] and Modified WHO classification.[2] The former has been applied previously in the IgA nephropathy study from our medical center.[5]

The modified WHO classification categorizes the range and actual progression of lesions as follows:

Class I: Normal glomeruli with normal cellularity of the mesangium of 1 to 2 cells in mesangial area and no increase in mesangial matrix.

Class II: Mesangial proliferative glomerulonephritis: Mesangial hypercellularity >3 cells/mesangial area with associated mesangial matrix expansion.

Class III: Focal segmental glomerulonephritis with segmental endocapillary hypercellularity, of endothelial cells and leukocytes, involving <50% of glomeruli.

Class IV: Diffuse proliferative glomerulonephritis with endocapillary cell proliferation in >50% of glomeruli in a biopsy, associated with neutrophilic infiltration and focal crescents in a quarter of cases.

Class V: Diffuse sclerosing glomerulonephritis with residual endocapillary cellularity, segmental and diffuse global sclerosis of > 90% of glomeruli with obliteration of the lumina.

Extraglomerular compartments show tubular atrophy with interstitial fibrosis, mononuclear cell infiltrates and arteriolar sclerosis.

Immunofluorescence (Fig. 4.19)

Arborizing mesangial and/or capillary wall deposits of dominant or codominant IgA are noted with C3 deposits.

Electron Microscopy

- Mesangial electron dense deposits are seen subjacent to the paramesangial basement membrane

Glomerular Diseases

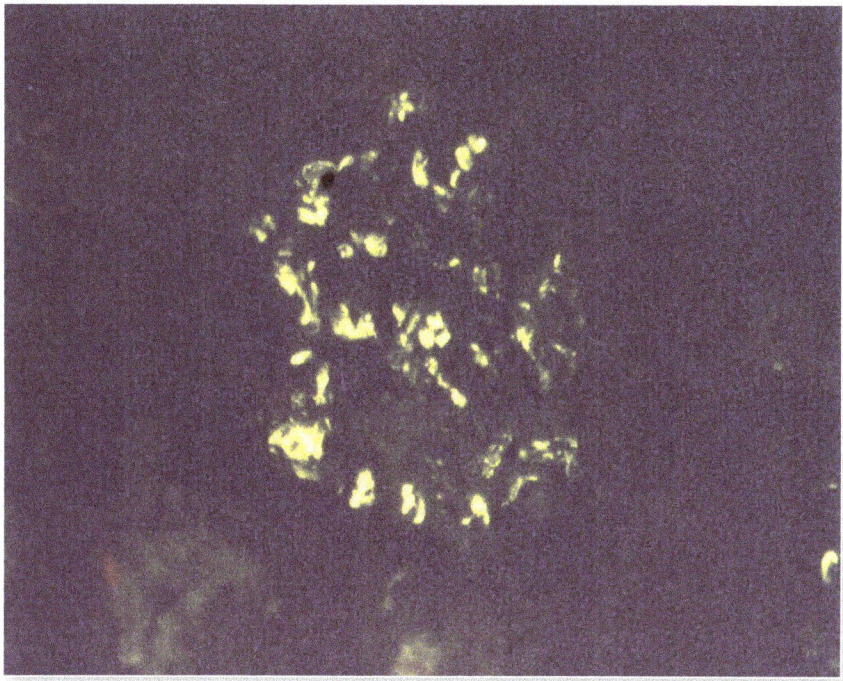

Figure 4.19: Arborizing mesangial IgA deposits 3 + (IF × 400)

- Increase in mesangial cells and mesangial matrix and/or endothelial cell proliferation
- Capillary wall deposits are present usually in the subepithelial region.

The Oxford Classification[16,17] utilizes a scoring system that has prognostic implications and has been recently validated in our center. The "MEST" score includes four pathologic variables.

These variables were divided into categories without significantly losing prognostic information as follows:
- *Mesangial hypercellularity score*: ≤0.5 (M0) or >0.5 (M1) (M1 corresponds to >50% of glomeruli with mesangial hypercellularity) (Figs 4.20 and 4.21)
- *Endocapillary hypercellularity*: Present or absent (E0 or E1) (Fig. 4.22)
- *Segmental sclerosis*: Present or absent (S0 or S1). Sclerosis is defined as obliteration of capillary lumina by increased extracellular matrix (Fig. 4.23)
- *Tubular atrophy/Interstitial fibrosis*: <25%, 26–50% and >50% of the renal cortex (T0, T1 and T3) (Fig. 4.24).

Mesangial hypercellularity is subclassified as:
- <4 mesangial cells/mesangial area = normal
- 4–5 mesangial cells/mesangial area = mild mesangial hypercellularity
- 6–7 mesangial cells/mesangial area = moderate mesangial hypercellularity
- 8 or more mesangial cells/mesangial area = severe mesangial hypercellularity.

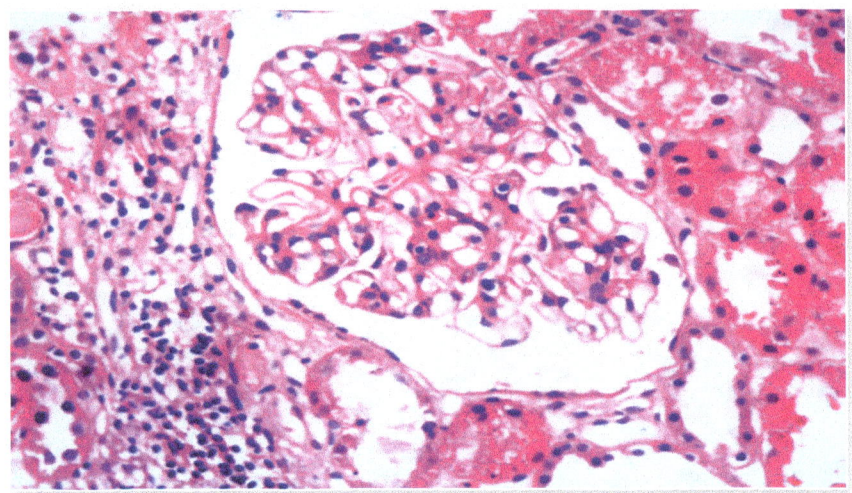

Figure 4.20: Mesangial cellularity less than 4 cells per mesangial area (M0) (PAS x 400)

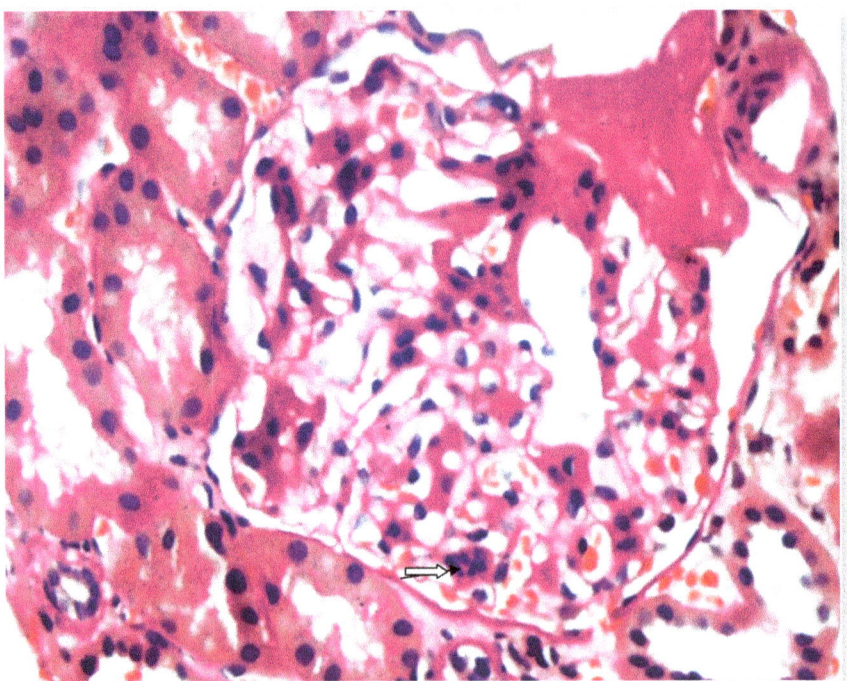

Figure 4.21: Mesangial cellularity 4–5 cells per mesangial area (M1) (arrow) (PAS x 400)

Glomerular Diseases

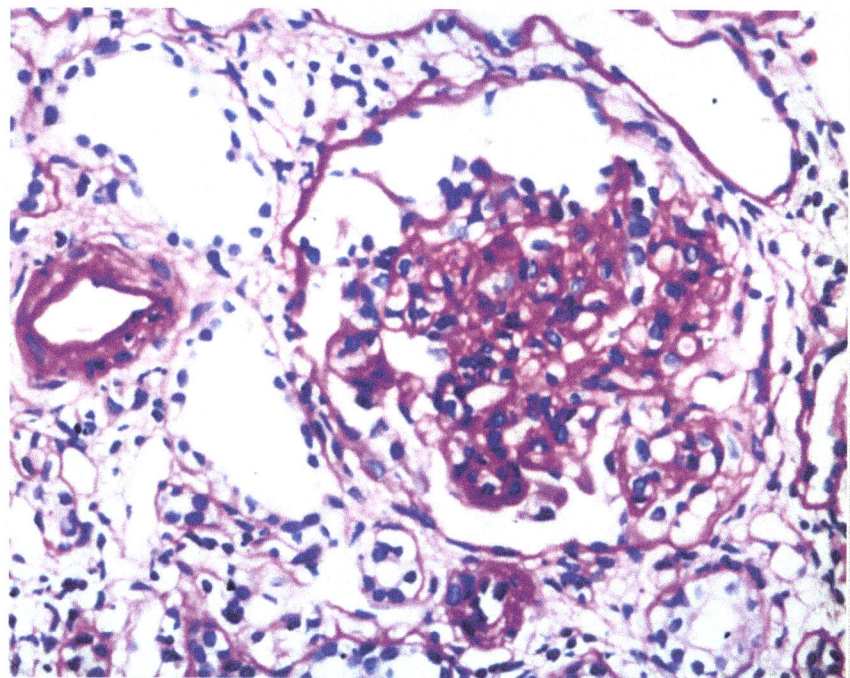

Figure 4.22: Endocapillary hypercellularity (E1) (PAS x 400)

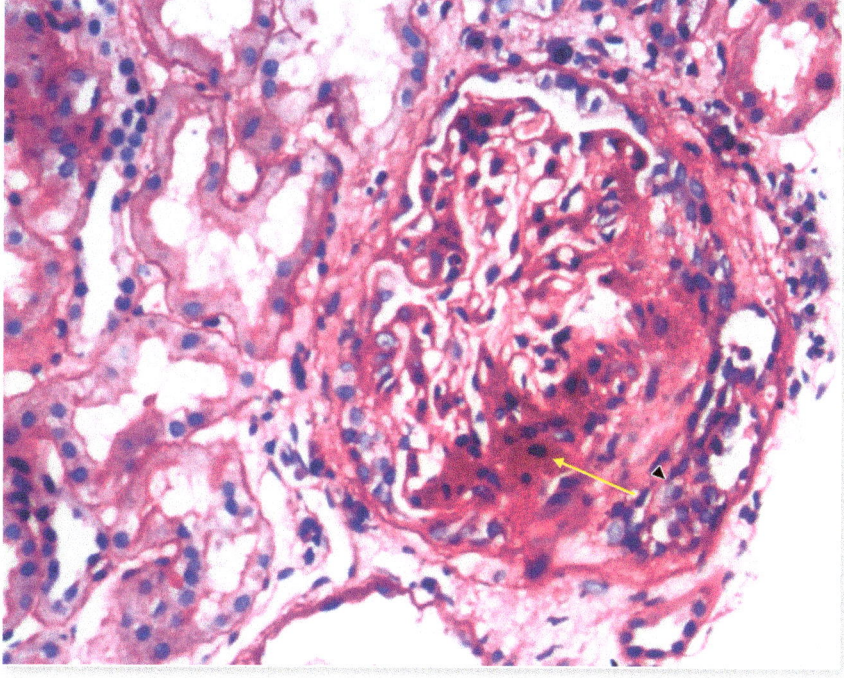

Figure 4.23: Segmental sclerosis (S1)(arrow) (PAS x 400)

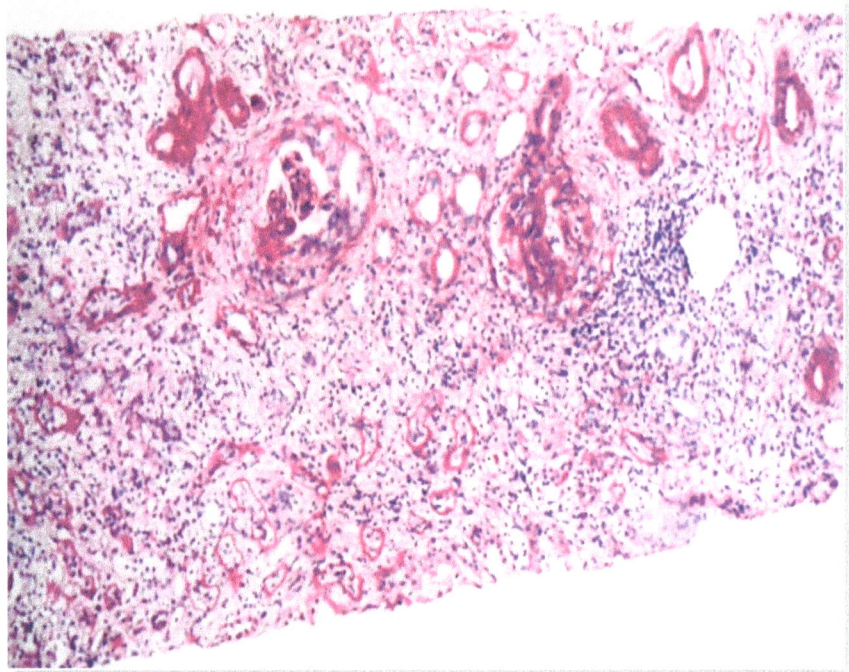

Figure 4.24: Diffuse interstitial fibrosis and tubular atrophy (>50% = T2), PAS × 200

Differential Diagnosis

IgA dominant postinfectious glomerulonephritis: Associated with staphylococcal infections[18] (*Staphylococcus aureus* and methicillin resistant *Staphylococcus aureus*): Complicating diabetic nephropathy shows diffuse endocapillary proliferation or mild mesangial proliferation, coarse mesangial and capillary wall IgA deposits on IF and large subepithelial humps on EM. There is associated hypocomplementemia, in contrast to IgA nephropathy. Mesangial IgA deposits can persist, while the subepithelial deposits display partial resorption on EM in the resolving phase, in the paramesangial region. In resolving PIGN, C3 deposits are found in the mesangium, on IF.

Secondary IgA nephropathy occurs with chronic liver disease, inflammatory bowel disease, rheumatologic diseases, systemic vasculitis, as in Henoch Schonlein purpura and HIV nephropathy.[19]

Course and Prognosis

IgA nephropathy usually has a benign course, 15-20% of cases progress to end stage renal failure. Indian cohorts as in previous studies from CMC, Vellore[7-9] have a malignant profile with a rapidly progressive clinical course requiring immunosuppression and renin-angiotensin system blockade. Renal survival at 10 years was 35%, when compared to 80-85% among Caucasians.[4,6] In western cohorts, the Oxford "MEST" scores were shown to have independent prognostic value in predicting outcome.[16] In our center from a recent study of 286 cases done to validate the MEST scoring system, endocapillary hypercellularity (E1), segmental sclerosis (S1) and tubulointerstitial lesions (T1 and T2) correlated with reduced eGFR at the time of the biopsy. Segmental sclerosis (S1) and tubular atrophy/interstitial fibrosis (T score) were significantly associated with reduced eGFR at the follow up of one year, whereas endocapillary hypercellularity (E1) was associated with high ranges of proteinuria. In comparison to the Oxford study[16,17] tubular atrophy/interstitial fibrosis was the only factor found to influence renal survival when either end stage renal failure or 50% reduction of eGFR was taken as the outcome.

REFERENCES

1. Narasimhan B, Chacko B, John GT, Korula A, Kirubakaran MG, Jacob CK. Characterization of kidney lesions in Indian adults: towards a renal biopsy registry. J Nephrol. 2006;19:205-10.
2. D'Agati VD, Jennette JC, Silva FG. Non-Neoplastic Kidney Diseases. Atlas of Nontumor Pathology, first series, fascicle 4. American Registry of Pathology and Armed Forces Institute of Pathology, Washington: DC; 2005.
3. Ibels LS, Györy AZ. IgA nephropathy: analysis of the natural history, important factors in the progression of renal disease, and a review of the literature. Medicine (Baltimore) 1994;73(2):79-102.
4. D'Amico G. Natural history of idiopathic IgA nephropathy and factors predictive of disease outcome. Semin Nephrol. 2004;24(3):179-96.
5. George J, Ninan VT, Thomas PP, Jacob CK, Shastry JCM, Primary IgA nephropathy in adults. J Assoc Physicians India. 1993;41(8):489-91.
6. Chacko B, John G.T, Neelakantan N, Korula A, et al. Presentation, prognosis and outcome of IgA nephropathy in Indian adults. Nephrology. 2005;10:496-503.
7. Date A, Raghavan R, John TJ, Richard J, Kirubakaran MG, Shastry JC. Renal disease in adult Indians: a clinicopathological study of 2, 827 patients. Q J Med. 1987;64(245):729-37.
8. Bhuyan UN, Dash SC, Srivastava RN, Tiwari SC, Malhotra KK. IgA associatedglomerulonephritis. J Assoc Physicians India. 1992;40(5):310-3.
9. Sehgal S, Datta BN, Sakhuja V, Chugh KS. Primary IgA nephropathy: a preliminary report. Indian J Pathol Microbiol. 1995;38(3):233-7.
10. Chandrika BK. IgA nephropathy in Kerala, India: a retrospective study. Indian J Pathol Microbiol. 2009;52(1):14-6.
11. Coppo R, Amore A. Aberrant glycosylation in IgA nephropathy (IgAN). Kidney Int. 2004;65(5):1544-7.
12. Tomana M, Novak J, Julian BA, Matousovic K, Konecny K, Mestecky J. Circulating immune complexes in IgA nephropathy consist of IgA1 with galactose-deficient hingeregion and antiglycan antibodies. J Clin Invest. 1999;104(1):73-81.
13. Suzuki H, Fan R, Zhang Z, Brown R, Hall S, Julian BA, et al. Aberrantly glycosylated IgA1 in IgA nephropathy patients is recognized by IgG antibodies with restricted heterogeneity. J Clin Invest. 2009;119(6):1668-77.
14. Barratt J, Feehally J. Primary IgA nephropathy: new insights into pathogenesis. Semin Nephrol. 2011;31(4):349-60.
15. Haas M. Histologic subclassification of IgA nephropathy: a clinicopathologic study of 244 cases. Am J Kidney Dis. 1997;29(6):829-42.
16. Roberts ISD, Cook HT, Troyanov S, Alpers CE, Amore A, Barratt J, et al. The Oxford classification of IgA nephropathy: pathology definitions, correlations, and reproducibility. Kidney Int. 2009;76(5):546-56.
17. Cattran DC, Coppo R, Cook HT, Feehally J, Roberts ISD, Troyanov S, et al. The Oxford classification of IgA nephropathy: rationale, clinicopathological correlations, and classification. Kidney Int. 2009;76(5):534-45.
18. Nasr SH, Markowitz GS, Whelan JD, et al. IgA-dominant acute poststaphylococcal glomerulonephritis complicating diabetic nephropathy. Hum Pathol. 2003;34:1235.
19. Donadio JV, Grande JP. IgA nephropathy. N Engl J Med. 2002;347(10):738-48.

NON-IgA MESANGIAL PROLIFERATIVE GLOMERULONEPHRITIS

Non-IgA mesangial proliferative glomerulonephritis has been the predominant subtype of primary glomerulonephritis in our case series of biopsy proven renal disease in adults[1] with a varying incidence of 7.3–20.2% in adults and 11.3% in children[2] respectively, presenting mainly with nephrotic syndrome and less often with hematuria.

Microscopic Features

Diffuse mesangial hypercellularity of varying degree (>4 cells per mesangial area) with matrix expansion (Fig. 4.25).

Immunofluorescence

Negative in the majority and mesangial C3 deposits rarely.

Electron Microscopy

- Mesangial cell proliferation with mesangial matrix expansion
- Mesangial sclerosis with capsular synechiae and fibrous crescents present with steroid resistance
- Immune deposits are rare.

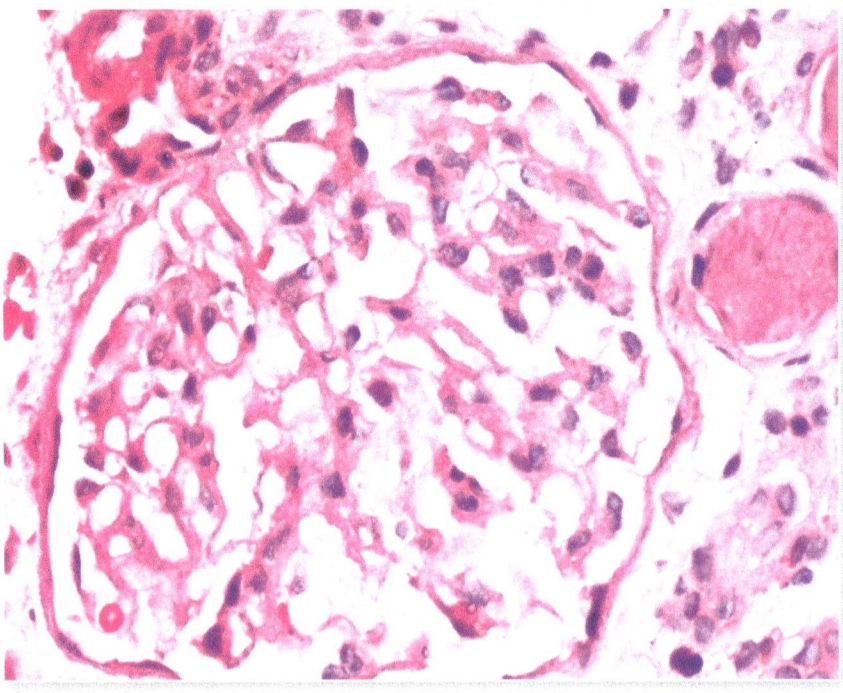

Figure 4.25: Non-IgA mesangial proliferative glomerulonephritis (PAS x 400)

Course and Prognosis

This entity has been mainly reported in developing countries[3] and has a variable course responding to steroids in the majority with steroid dependence and resistance in the remaining cases.

REFERENCES

1. Narasimhan B, Chacko B, John GT, Korula A, Kirubakaran MG, Jacob CK. Characterization of kidney lesions in Indian adults: towards a renal biopsy registry. J Nephrol. 19:20:205-10.
2. Balakrisnan N, JohnGT, Korula A, Visalakshi J, Talauikar GS, Thomas PP, et al. Spectrum of biopsy proven renal disease and changing trends at a tropical tertiary care centre, 1990-2001. Indian J Nephrol. 2003;13;29-35.
3. Waikhom R, et al. Non-IgA mesangioproliferative glomerulonephritis: a benign entity. Nephrol Dial Transplant. 2011; 0:1–6. doi: 10. 1093/ndt/gfr653.

CRESCENTIC GLOMERULONEPHRITIS

Crescentic glomerulonephritis is associated with disruption of glomerular capillary walls leading to macrophage, T cell and plasma protein infiltration into the Bowman's space and reactive parietal epithelial cell proliferation.[1] The idiopathic or primary renal limited form comprised 3.5% of Primary Glomerulonephritis in our case series, presenting with rapidly progressive renal failure. This is classified into the following categories with distinctive immunofluorescent features[2] as follows:

Type I: Anti-GBM disease with linear IgG deposits on the glomerular capillary walls (in 15% of cases of RPGN).

Type II: Immune complex mediated type with granular capillary wall deposits of immunoglobulins and complement (in 25% of cases of RPGN).

Type III: Pauci-immune type with few or no immune deposits (associated with ANCA-mediated small vessel vasculitis in 60% of cases of RPGN).

The pauci-immune subtype is the most common, in western[2,3] and Indian cohorts,[4] occurring more frequently in adults. Aberrant T cell response and T cell regulatory function are implicated in the pathogenesis of ANCA-associated crescentic glomerulonephritis.[1] Release of proinflammatory cytokines from infiltrating macrophages in crescents cause upregulation of leukocyte cell adhesion molecules and glomerular necrosis.[5] In children, the immune complex subtype is secondary to post-streptococcal and other forms of immune complex glomerulonephritis.[2,6]

Microscopic Features[2,3]

Light Microscopy

- Crescentic proliferation composed of 2 or more layers of parietal epithelial cells with macrophages in >50% of glomeruli (Fig. 4.26)
- Compression of hypercellular to sclerotic glomerular tufts by circumferential cellular crescents
- Fibrocellular crescents form with disruption of Bowman's capsule
- Entry of periglomerular fibroblasts with collagen deposition and formation of fibrous crescents
- Foci of glomerular tuft fibrinoid necrosis seen in types I and III with rupture of glomerular capillary walls.

Electron Microscopy

Extensive disruption of glomerular basement membrane (GBM) and Bowman's capsule with segmental necrosis in types I and III. Immune deposits are found in type II.

Differential Diagnosis

1. *Goodpasture's syndrome*: Anti-GBM disease is associated with pulmonary hemorrhage and the pulmonary renal vasculitic syndrome in more than 50% of cases and ANCA positivity in a third to quarter cases.

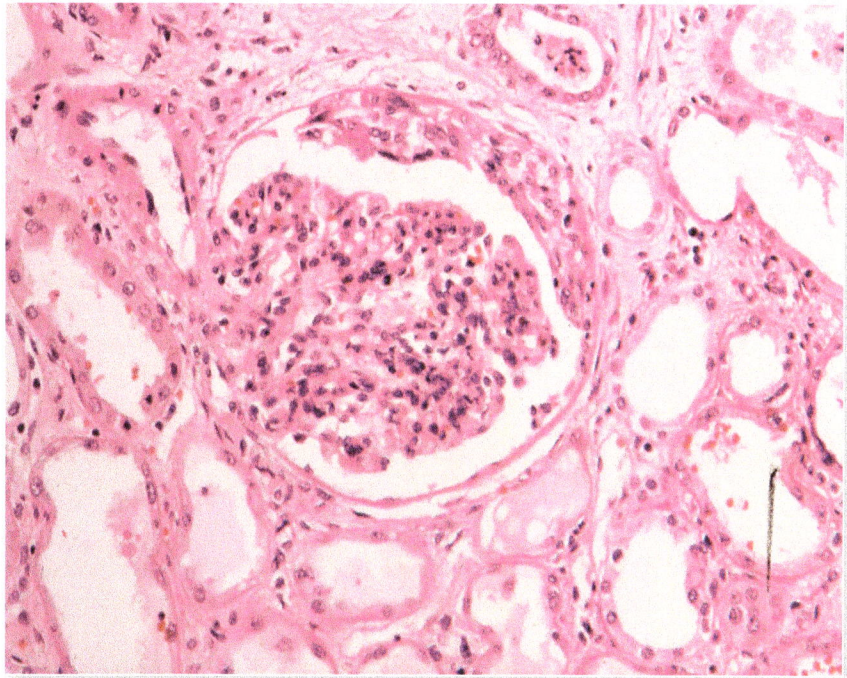

Figure 4.26: Diffuse proliferative glomerulonephritis with cellular crescent (H&Ex 200)

2. *Immune complex associated secondary systemic renal diseases* include Post-infectious glomerulonephritis, IgA nephropathy, Henoch-Schonlein purpura nephritis, Lupus nephritis, membranoproliferative glomerulonephritis, Membranous glomerulonephritis and fibrillary glomerulonephritis.
3. *Systemic ANCA–associated small vessel vasculitis* include granulomatous polyangiitis (Wegener's granulomatosis), microscopic polyangiitis and Churg-Strauss syndrome.

Prognosis

The percentage of crescents (>80%) and type of crescents (fibrocellular to fibrous) with glomerulosclerosis and extent of tubulointerstitial fibrosis correlate with adverse outcome and decreased survival rates. Anti-GBM type of crescentic GN is most aggressive with the highest frequency of crescents, followed by the pauci-immune subtype at diagnosis.[3] ANCA negative pauci-immune variant has a higher rate of disease progression[6] and worse outcome.

REFERENCES

1. Tarzi RM, Cook TH, Pusey CD. Crescentic glomerulonephritis: new aspects of pathogenesis. Seminars in Nephrology. 2001;31(4):361-8.
2. Jennette JC, Thomas DB. Crescentic glomerulonephritis. Nephrol Dial Transplant. 2001;16(Suppl 6):80-2.
3. Jennette JC. Rapidly progressive glomerulonephritis. Kidney Int. 2003;63(3):1164-7.
4. Gupta R, Singh L, Sharma A, Bagga A, Agarwal SK, Dinda AK. Crescentic glomerulonephritis: a clinical and histomorphological analysis of 46 cases. Indian J Pathol Microbiol. 2011;54(3):497-500.
5. Atkins RC, et al. Modulators of crescentic glomerulonephritis. JASN. 1996;7(11):2271-8.
6. Sinha A, et al. Aetiology and outcome of crescentic glomerulonephritis. Indian Pediatr. 2013;50:283-8.

MEMBRANOPROLIFERATIVE GLOMERULONEPHRITIS

Membranoproliferative glomerulonephritis (MPGN) is a lesion characterized by glomerular capillary wall thickening with circumferential duplication, combined with mesangial and endocapillary hypercellularity, caused by persistent antigenemia and deposition of immune complexes. This accounted for 3.7% of biopsy proven cases of primary glomerulonephritis in our experience, presenting with nephrotic syndrome, a male preponderance and a higher incidence in the age group of 15 to 34 years.

The traditional classification of primary (idiopathic) MPGN of types I, II, and III is based on ultrastructural features and location of electron dense immune deposits.[1] As many of the cases of Types I and III do not contain immunoglobulins by immunofluorescence, a new pathogenetic classification of MPGN has been proposed, comprising two major categories; immunoglobulin-mediated and complement mediated, based on immunofluorescence features.[2,3]

Immune complex mediated MPGN is associated with IgG, C3 and C4 deposition along glomerular capillary walls and activation of the classical and terminal complement pathway, caused by chronic infections, autoimmune diseases and dysproteinemias.

Complement mediated MPGN is characterized by predominant C3 deposition due to dysregulation of the alternate complement pathway and absence of immunoglobulins, known as "C3 glomerulopathy". The latter includes two major entities known as "dense deposit disease" and "C3 glomerulonephritis". C3 glomerulonephritis is heterogeneous and can have morphological features of MPGN type I or type III of the traditional classification and are associated with genetic or acquired dysregulation of the alternate complement pathway. Electron microscopy cannot differentiate immune complex mediated from predominantly complement mediated categories of MPGN, except for dense deposit disease, that has distinctive features.[4]

There are complex mechanisms involved in the etiopathogenesis of MPGN, including genetic and acquired, aberrant regulation of the complement pathway[5] with superimposed autoimmune phenomena and uncontrolled activation of C3 convertase, that have not been fully resolved to date, to direct exact evaluation and treatment.

Membranoproliferative Glomerulonephritis Type I

It is an immune complex glomerulonephritis associated with activation of the classical complement pathway and decreased serum C3 and C4 levels. The immune complexes and activated complement fragments C3a and C5a cause leukocytic infiltration in the acute phase. A reparative phase with the classical features[1,2,4] is seen as follows:

Microscopic Features

Light Microscopy (Fig. 4.27)
- Marked glomerular enlargement with uniform centrilobular mesangial matrix expansion
- Accentuated lobulation of the tufts with mesangial cell proliferation
- Variable degree of endocapillary hypercellularity and neutrophilic infiltration
- Marked capillary wall thickening with **circumferential reduplication** (**tram track** or **double contour**)
- Mesangial sclerosis with segmental or nodular sclerosis in advanced lesions
- Extraglomerular compartment shows foci of tubulointerstitial scarring and arteriosclerosis.

Glomerular Diseases

Immunofluorescence
- Fine to coarsely granular peripheral capillary wall deposits of C3 (2 to 3+) and less intense IgG deposits with perilobular accentuation (Fig. 4.28).

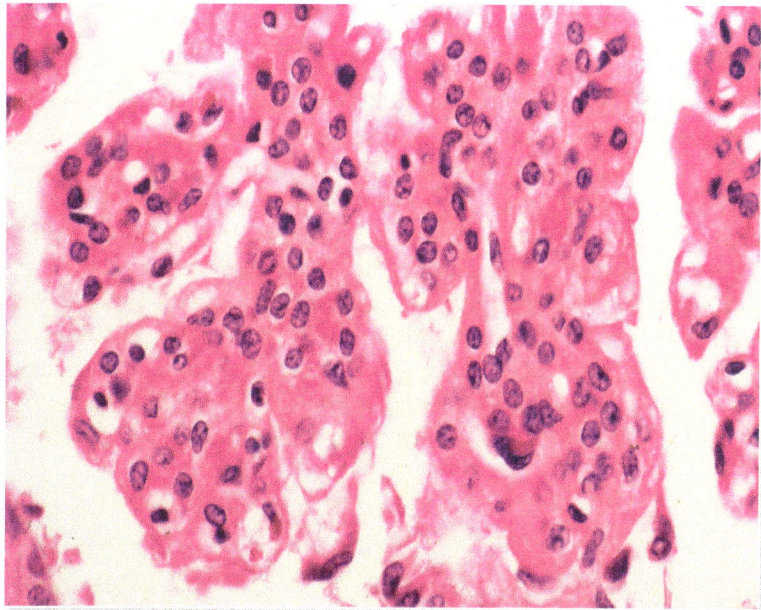

Figure 4.27: MPGN type I with reduplication of capillary walls (H & E x 400)

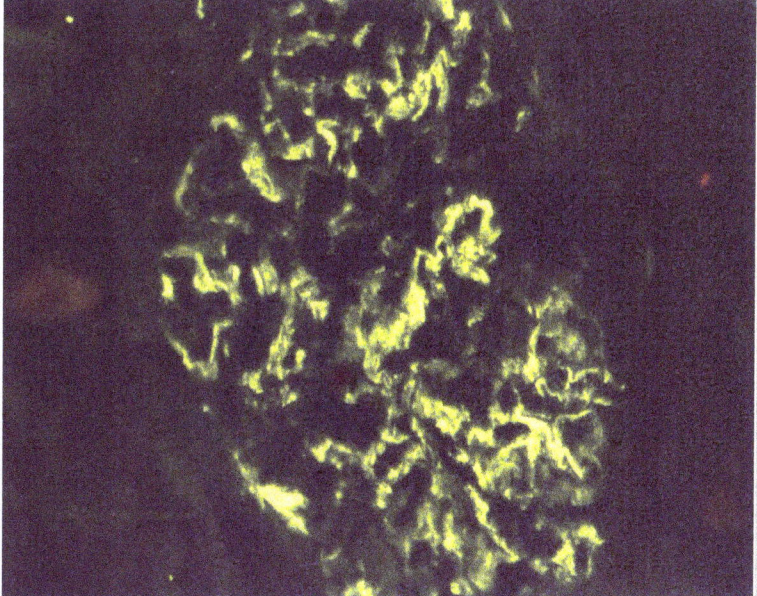

Figure 4.28: Granular perilobular capillary wall deposits of C3 on immunofluorescence (400X)

48 Renal Biopsy Interpretation

Electron Microscopy

- Mesangial matrix expansion with mesangial cell interposition in subendothelial region (Fig. 4.29)
- Large discrete subendothelial deposits with thickening of GBM by mesangial matrix or layers of new basement membrane material formed by mesangial or endothelial cells.

Differential Diagnosis

The majority of cases of MPGN-Type I are secondary to known causes[6] such as chronic bacterial (including abscesses, infective endocarditis and shunt nephritis) and fungal infections, Hepatitis B or Hepatitis C viral antigenemia, cryoglobulinemia, autoimmune diseases (SLE, Sjogren syndrome and rheumatoid arthritis, mixed connective tissue disease), parasitic infections (schistosomiasis), malignancy and monoclonal gammopathy/dysproteinemias, that have to be excluded by appropriate investigations and clinical correlation.[4]

Membranoproliferative features with a similar morphological pattern can be found in non-immunoglobulin mediated lesions of chronic thrombotic microangiopathy (TMA), associated with HUS/TTP, atypical HUS, drug-induced TMA, malignant hypertension, collagen vascular diseases, transplant glomerulopathy, bone marrow transplantation and radiation-induced nephropathy.[2,3] These lesions are distinguished by immunofluorescence and electron microscopy.

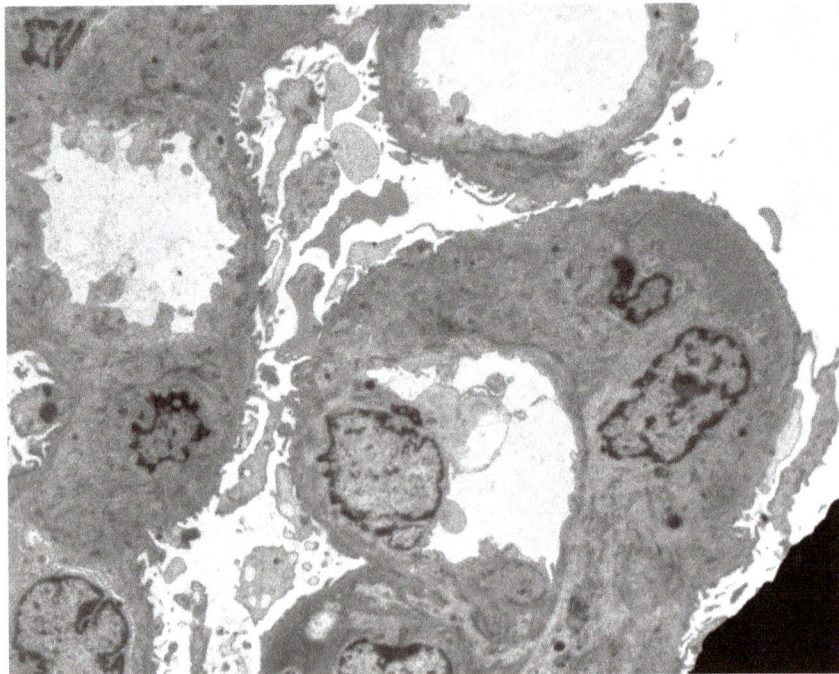

Figure 4.29: Membranoproliferative glomerulonephritis type I with subendothelial immune deposits and mesangial interposition with marked capillary wall thickening (EM x 4200)

Membranoproliferative Glomerulonephritis Type II or Dense Deposit Disease (DDD)

It is defined by electron dense deposits in the lamina densa of GBM, associated with uncontrolled systemic activation of the alternate complement pathway and C3 deposition due to autoantibodies to C3 convertase (C3bBb) in >80% cases and in some cases by complement regulator factor H gene mutations or its autoantibodies.[5,7,8] This entity has a varied morphology, an equal gender predilection and classically presents with nephritic-nephrotic syndrome, primarily in children, 5 to 15 years of age and young adults.

Microscopic Features

Light microscopy-typical features[7,9]

- Non-uniform glomerular capillary wall thickening, alternating with relatively attenuated segments or capillary walls of normal thickness (Fig. 4.30)
- Mesangial expansion with variable increase in mesangial cellularity
- Membranoproliferative features are infrequently present
- Endocapillary cell proliferation is uncommon
- Nodular mesangial sclerosis with capsular synechiae and parietal cell proliferation or crescents in advanced lesions
- Intramembranous deposits are eosinophilic on the H & E stain and fuschinophilic on Masson trichrome (Fig. 4.31)
- Non-argyrophilic deposits are noted on the Jones methenamine stain[8]
- On paraffin sections, deposits stain positive with the thioflavin stain under the fluorescent microscope.[10]

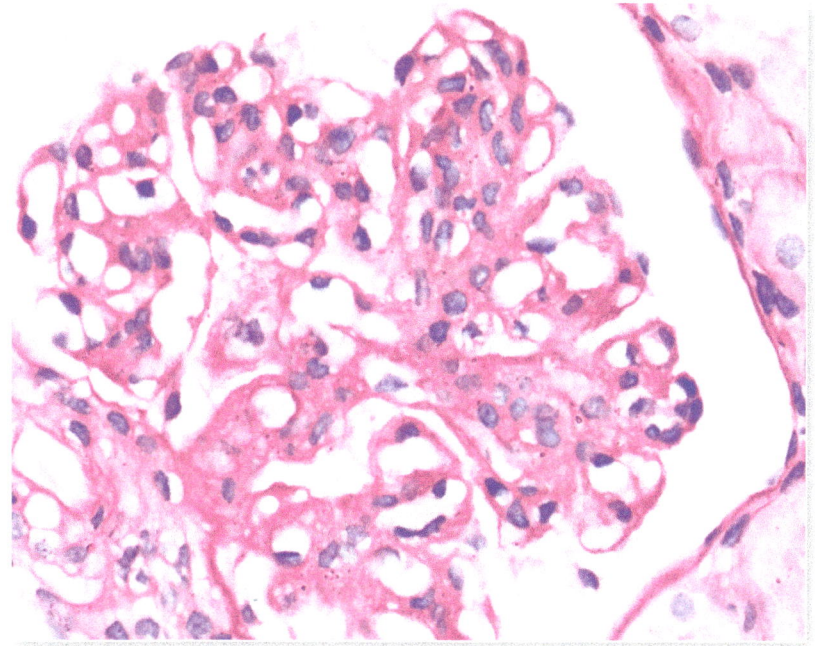

Figure 4.30: MPGN-II (Dense deposit disease/C3 glomerulopathy) (PAS x 400)

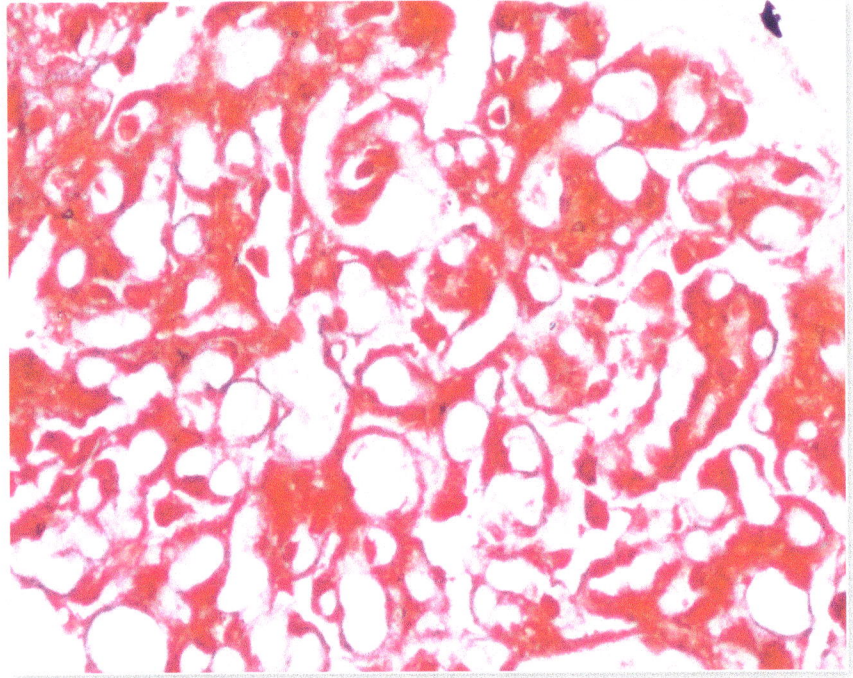

Figure 4.31: Dense deposit disease (Masson trichrome x 400)

Immunofluorescence[7]
- Interrupted granular deposits to linear bands of C3 (2 to 3+) +/- IgM deposits on the glomerular capillary walls
- Scattered to coarse spherical mesangial granules of C3 (mesangial rings)
- Capillary walls are negative for IgG.

Electron Microscopy[7]
- Classical elongated ribbon-like densely osmophilic extensive or segmental deposits in lamina densa of GBM (Fig. 4.32)
- Intervening normal segments of lamina densa are usually present
- Electron dense deposits are also present on the basal lamina of Bowman's capsule and tubular basement membranes.

Associated Features

There is hypocomplementemia associated with serum C3 nephritic factor (C3NeFa), an autoantibody to C3 convertase (C3bBb) in >80% of cases, stabilizing it against complement factor H decay with prolonged C3 activation. Acquired partial lipodystrophy has been reported in some cases of DDD, with deposition of complement components and destruction of subcutaneous adipocytes in the face and upper half of the body. Ocular drusen can develop with lipoproteinaceous deposits, seen on fundoscopy, in Bruch's basement membrane, that demarcates the retina from choroidal blood vessels. Long-term visual complications occur in 10% of these cases.[8]

Glomerular Diseases

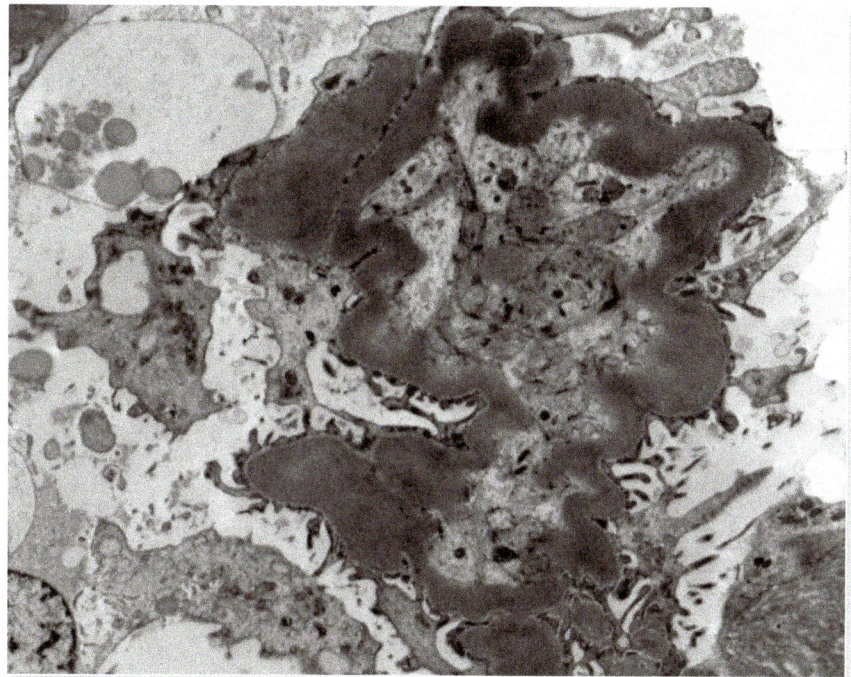

Figure 4.32: Dense deposit disease/C3 glomerulopathy (EM x 4200)

Differential Diagnosis

C3 glomerulonephritis: As detailed under complement mediated C3 glomerulopathy.

Membranoproliferative Glomerulonephritis Type III

It is a rare variant of MPGN with two distinctive subtypes described by Burkholder, Strife and Anders respectively.[11,12] There are subtle differences in light microscopic and immunofluorescent features from MPGN type I and distinctive features by electron microscopy.

Light Microscopic Features (Figs 4.33 and 4.34)

- Markedly enlarged glomeruli with lobular accentuation
- Diffuse capillary wall thickening with global hypercellularity
- Subepithelial spikes focally present on the silver stain.

Immunofluorescence

- Intense, finely granular to band—like C3 (3+) deposits on the glomerular capillary walls
- Mesangial staining by C3 can be present.

Electron Microscopy

Burkholder variant displays combined features of MPGN type I and membranous nephropathy with subendothelial and discrete subepithelial deposits with epimembranous spikes.

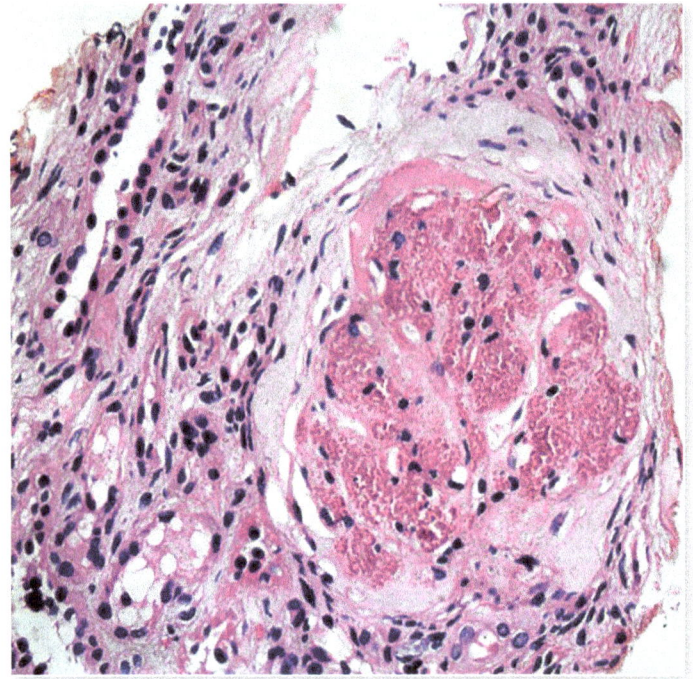

Figure 4.33: MPGN type III (PAS x 200)

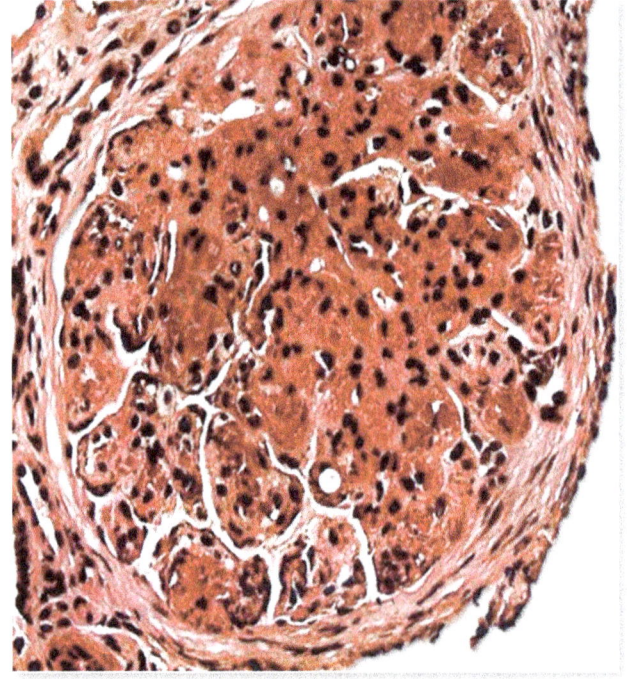

Figure 4.34: MPGN type III (JMS x 400)

Strife and Anders subtypes display subendothelial deposits in conjunction with layered intramembranous deposits in the lamina densa and contiguous subepithelial deposits associated with disruption and lamination of the GBM (Figs 4.35 and 4.36). The deposits are partially confluent due to interruption or breaks of the lamina densa and are covered over by layers of newly formed lamina densa type basement membrane material. The latter are silver negative on ultrathin silver impregnated plastic embedded sections, studied by electron microscopy.

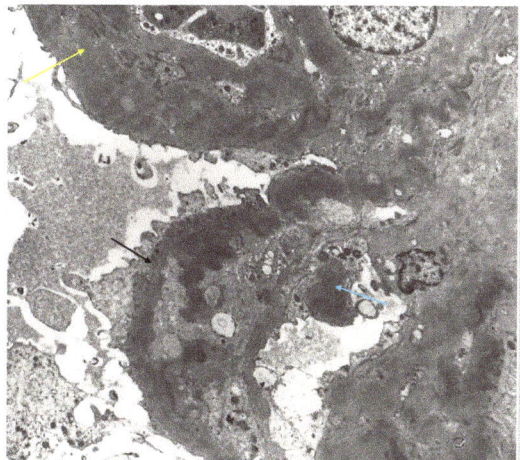

Figure 4.35: MPGN type III with subepithelial (black), intramembranous (yellow arrow) and subendothelial (blue arrow) deposits (EM x 3900)

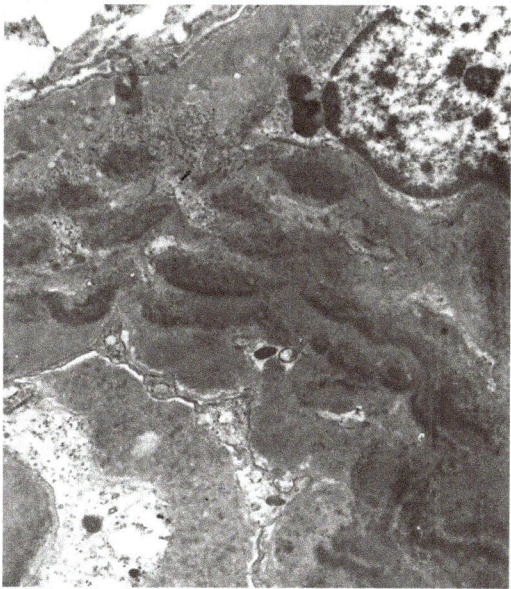

Figure 4.36: MPGN type III with layered intramembranous deposits in disrupted, GBM (EM x 6720)

Course and Prognosis

MPGN type I has an indolent course, undergoes remission in 15–20% cases with immunosuppression and progresses to end-stage renal disease in 40% cases. MPGN type II (DDD) has an aggressive course with 10-year progression to ESRD in 36.5–50%of cases and a higher rate of recurrence in renal transplants. MPGN type III has a guarded long-term prognosis with persistent hypocomplementemia, proteinuria, hypertension and renal failure with frequent relapses and greater decline of GFR. The extent of tubulointerstitial fibrosis, tubular atrophy, crescent formation and global glomerulosclerosis are prognostic indicators in a renal biopsy.[5,8,13,14]

C3 GLOMERULOPATHY

C3 glomerulopathy is a recently categorized type of primary glomerular disease caused by genetic or acquired dysregulation of the alternate complement system with isolated C3 deposition and absence of or scanty immunoglobulins:[15]

The following entities are actually forms of C3 glomerulopathy by the original defining criteria:
- Dense deposit disease
- Idiopathic C3 glomerulonephritis
- Familial membranoproliferative glomerulonephritis, type III
- *CFHR5* nephropathy (familial C3 glomerulonephritis associated with heterozygous mutation in complement factor H related protein-5 gene)
- Membranoproliferative glomerulonephritis type I with isolated subendothelial deposition of C3.

In the consensus report, the term C3 glomerulopathy is used for a disease process caused by abnormal control of complement activation, deposition and degradation with predominant glomerular C3 deposits and electron dense deposits on EM.[16] In practice, "glomerulonephritis with dominant C3" is the preferred morphological term used for lesions with dominant C3c staining*, that excludes immune complex diseases and identifies the C3 glomerulopathies, requiring alternate complement pathway (AP) evaluation.

Idiopathic C3 glomerulonephritis is heterogeneous by light microscopy with intermediate features between immune complex mediated MPGN and dense deposit disease.[3] This differs from dense deposit disease by the presence of mesangial and subendothelial deposits and membranoproliferative features by light microscopy in typical cases and absence of intensely electron dense deposits replacing the lamina densa. In a minority, there is mesangial proliferation with mesangial and additional subepithelial immune deposits.

Dense deposit disease has been associated with the presence of autoantibodies against complement factor H, C3 nephritic factor and genetic deficiency of complement factor H; whereas both C3 nephritic factor and mutations in regulatory proteins of the alternative complement pathway have been detected in patients with C3 glomerulonephritis. These diseases can be part of a continuum as is evident in some cases of MPGN with extensive C3 deposits, which show intramembranous dense deposits in some capillary tufts and other foci with subendothelial and subepithelial deposits.[17] There are excellent comprehensive reviews of

---

* C3 glomerulopathy consensus criteria16 defines, dominant C3 staining as an intensity of C3c of 2 orders magnitude or greater than any other immune reactants on a scale of 0 to 3 (including 0, trace, 1+, 2+, 3+).

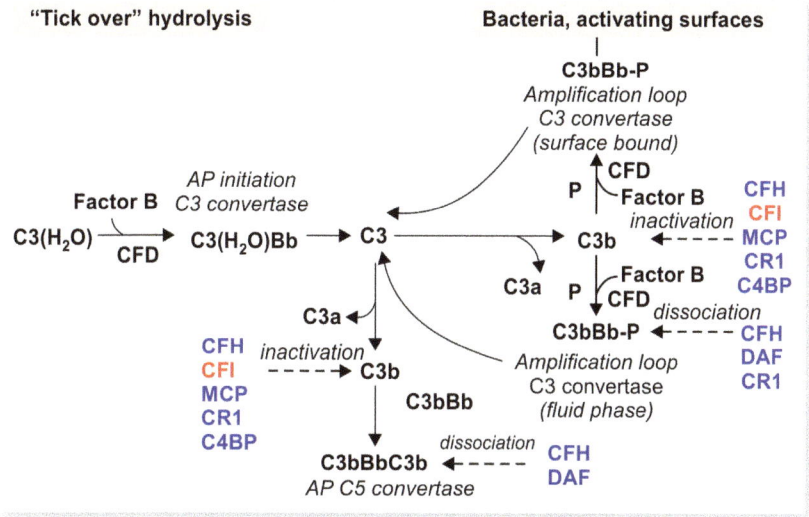

Figure 4.37: Alternative pathway of complement

Source: Noris M, Remuzzi G. Complement-mediated kidney Diseases: Overview of complement activation and regulation. Seminars in Nephrology. 2013;33(6):479-492 DOI: 10. 1016/j. semnephrol. 2013. 08. 001-OPEN ACCESS ARTICLE

complement mediated renal diseases and the classical alternate and lectin pathways with the solid and liquid phase regulators and role of complement factors and related proteins involved in the amplification loop of C3 (Fig. 4.37).[18,19] The alternate complement pathway is activated and usually maintained at a low level by the "tick-over" mechanism of spontaneous hydrolysis of C3 to C3b, that binds complement factor B (CFB) to form C3bBb, the fluid phase C3 convertase, that amplifies C3 cleavage to C3a and C3b. The latter process is modulated by regulatory proteins, complement factors H and I (CFH and I) and membrane cofactor protein (MCP). A genetic or acquired defect (including autoantibodies to regulatory proteins and complement factors) in the activation or inhibition of C3 convertase, leads to unrestrained hyperactivity of C3 due to "dysregulation" and the C3 glomerulopathies. An infection, at the onset could trigger this process, with persistent, uncontrolled alternate complement pathway activation, leading to chronicity, in the later stages.[16]

Laser microdissection of glomeruli from paraffin sections and liquid chromatography followed by mass spectroscopy (LCMS) has shown components of alternate complement pathway and soluble terminal membrane attack complex proteins with fluid phase regulators, clusterin and vitronectin, in the dense deposit form of C3 glomerulopathy.[20] In contrast, glomeruli from immune complex-mediated MPGN contained C3 and C4 complement proteins and factor H-related protein (FHR-1). In C3 glomerulonephritis, a proteomic profile similar to that of DDD was reported in a recent case series of 12 cases. Factor H autoantibodies and mutations in complement factor H, factor I and complement factor H-related protein genes were also detected.[21]

Microscopic Features

These are varied, ranging from mesangial to membranoproliferative or endocapillary patterns as follows:[21-24]

Light Microscopy

- Enlargement of glomerular tufts
- Mesangial and variable endocapillary proliferation
- Focal neutrophilic infiltrate
- Mesangial matrix expansion with capillary wall thickening and foci of reduplication
- Membranoproliferative features, simulating MPGN, types I or III.

Immunofluorescence[25]

- Mesangial and capillary wall deposits of C3 (2 to 3+) in the majority (>50%)
- Capillary wall C3 deposits in 26% cases and mesangial only in <10% cases.

Electron Microscopy[15,16]

- Features of MPGN with electron dense mesangial and focal subendothelial deposits in about 75% of cases
- Less electron dense (than DDD), more confluent, intramembranous, with fraying of lamina densa (as in MPGN III)
- Mesangial cell and matrix proliferation with mesangial and subepithelial immune deposits in a minority of biopsies.

Familial MPGN type III is associated with subepithelial and subendothelial deposits and a genetic mutation encoding the alternate pathway regulator, complement factor H, linked to chromosome-1.[15,19]

CFHR5 nephropathy was originally reported in Greek Cypriot families with autosomal dominant inheritance and is associated with predominantly subendothelial deposits and focal transmembranous deposits of C3.

Complement factor-H related protein-5 gene mutation leads to enhanced competitive inhibition or deregulation of complement factor H by complement factor H-related protein-5 and excessive C3 activation (Figs 4.38A and B).[15,26,27]

MPGN type I can also be concomitantly associated with dysregulation of the alternate complement pathway (due to mutations in genes that encode the regulatory proteins) and presence of C3 Nephritic factor with uncontrolled amplification of C3.[15,19]

Investigations to Assess AP Dysfunction[15,16]

- Serum complement level, factors H, I and B level
- Alternate pathway functional assay (APFA) including immunosorbent assay for C3 nephritic factor, anti-factor H autoantibodies
- CD46 (membrane cofactor protein) expression of peripheral blood mononuclear cells
- Screening for genetic mutations encoding alternate complement pathway regulators: Complement factor H, complement factor I, CD46, complement factor H-related proteins: 1 to 5.
- AP activators: Complement factor B and C3 are indicated to confirm a diagnosis of C3 glomerulopathy.

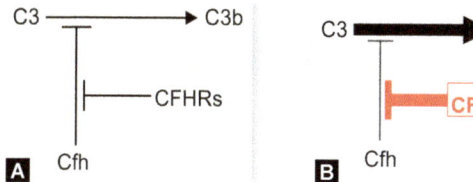

Figures 4.38A and B: Complement factor H deregulation. (A) Competitive inhibition (deregulation) of complement factor H by CFHRs; (B) CFHR gene mutation leads to enhanced Cfh deregulation and excessive C3 activation

Source: Barbour TD, Pickering MC, Cook HT. Dense deposit disease and C3 glomerulopathy. Seminars in Nephrology. 2013;33 (6):493-507 – OPEN ACCESS ARTICLE

Differential Diagnosis

Atypical proliferative (post-infectious) glomerulonephritis: with persistent renal dysfunction after 8 weeks has to be investigated to exclude C3 glomerulopathy by the careful integration of light microscopic, immunofluorescent and electron microscopic features. Subepithelial "humps" can be present in cases of C3 glomerulonephritis and can follow an episode of streptococcal infection. Careful follow up is required, with further investigations, if normalization of C3 levels does not occur in 8 to 12 weeks after infection-associated C3 dominant glomerulonephritis.[16]

Course and Prognosis

The renal function is maintained in 50% of patients with C3 glomerulonephritis and 15% of cases progress to end-stage renal disease.[15,25] A recent case series has shown no decline of renal function on early and long-term follow-up and on treatment with ACE inhibitors and renin-angiotensin blockade, steroids and mycophenolate mofetil/cyclophosphamide.[21] The experience with anti-C5 targeted therapy in C3 glomerulopathies and recurrent C3 glomerulonephritis, after transplantation is limited.[16]

REFERENCES

1. Heptinstall RH, Jennette JC. Heptinstall's Pathology of the Kidney [Internet]. Lippincott Williams and Wilkins; 2007 [cited 2014 Aug 13]. Available from: http://books. google. co. in/books?hl=enandlr=andid=oWymx 2hp1OoCandoi=fndandpg=PA843anddq=Heptinstall+6th+editionandots=kuqylzCHrnandsig=WheVH_wCsHVnsIFNRmc1Ej0258s
2. Sethi S, Fervenza FC. Membranoproliferative glomerulonephritis—a new look at an old entity. N Engl J Med. 2012;366(12):1119-31.
3. Sethi S, Fervenza FC. Membranoproliferative glomerulonephritis: pathogenetic heterogeneity and proposal for a new classification. Seminars in nephrology [Internet]. Elsevier; 2011 [cited 2014 Aug 4]. p. 341–8. Available from: http://www. sciencedirect. com/science/article/pii/S0270929511000660.
4. Fervenza FC, Sethi S, Glassock RJ. Idiopathic membranoproliferative glomerulonephritis: does it exist? Nephrol Dial Transplant. 2012;27(12):4288-94.
5. Servais A, Noël L-H, Roumenina LT, Le Quintrec M, Ngo S, Dragon-Durey M-A, et al. Acquired and genetic complement abnormalities play a critical role in dense deposit disease and other C3 glomerulopathies. Kidney Int. 2012;82(4):454-64.
6. Rennke HG. Secondary membranoproliferative glomerulonephritis. Kidney Int. 1995;47(2):643-56.

7. Appel GB, Cook HT, Hageman G, Jennette JC, Kashgarian M, Kirschfink M, et al. Membranoproliferative glomerulonephritis type II (Dense Deposit Disease): An Update. J Am Soc Nephrol. 2005;16(5):1392-403.
8. Barbour TD, Pickering MC, Terence Cook H. Dense deposit disease and C3 glomerulopathy. Semin Nephrol. 2013;33(6):493-507.
9. Walker PD, Ferrario F, Joh K, Bonsib SM. Dense deposit disease is not a membranoproliferative glomerulonephritis. Mod Pathol. 2007;20(6):605-16.
10. Date A, Neela P, Shastry JCM. Thioflavin T fluorescence in membranoproliferative glomerulonephritis. Nephron. 1982;32(1):90-2.
11. Burkholder PM, Marchand A, Krueger RP. Mixed membranous and proliferative glomerulonephritis. A correlative light, immunofluorescence, and electron microscopic study. Lab Investig J Tech Methods Pathol. 1970;23(5):459-79.
12. Strife CF, McEnery PT, McAdams AJ, West CD. Membranoproliferative glomerulonephritis with disruption of the glomerular basement membrane. Clin Nephrol. 1977;7(2):65-72.
13. Bennett WM, Fassett RG, Walker RG, Fairley KF, d'Apice AJ, Kincaid-Smith P. Mesangiocapillary glomerulonephritis type II (dense-deposit disease): clinical features of progressive disease. Am J Kidney Dis. 1989;13(6):469–76.
14. Strife CF, Jackson EC, McAdams AJ. Type III membranoproliferative glomerulonephritis: long-term clinical and morphologic evaluation. Clin Nephrol. 1984;21(6):323-34.
15. Fakhouri F, Frémeaux-Bacchi V, Noël L-H, Cook HT, Pickering MC. C3 glomerulopathy: a new classification. Nat Rev Nephrol. 2010;6(8):494-9.
16. Pickering MC, D'Agati VD, Nester CM, Smith RJ, Haas M, Appel GB, et al. C3 glomerulopathy: consensus report. Kidney Int. 2013;84(6):1079-89.
17. Sethi S, Fervenza FC, Zhang Y, Nasr SH, Leung N, Vrana J, et al. Proliferative Glomerulonephritis Secondary to Dysfunction of the Alternative Pathway of Complement. Clin J Am Soc Nephrol. 2011;6(5):1009-17.
18. Noris M, Remuzzi G. Overview of complement activation and regulation. Semin Nephrol. 2013;33(6):479-92.
19. Bomback AS, Appel GB. Pathogenesis of the C3 glomerulopathies and reclassification of MPGN. Nat Rev Nephrol. 2012;8(11):634-42.
20. Sethi S, Gamez JD, Vrana JA, Theis JD, Bergen HR, Zipfel PF, et al. Glomeruli of Dense Deposit Disease contain components of the alternative and terminal complement pathway. Kidney Int. 2009;75(9):952-60.
21. Sethi S, Fervenza FC, Zhang Y, Zand L, Vrana JA, Nasr SH, et al. C3 glomerulonephritis: clinicopathological findings, complement abnormalities, glomerular proteomic profile, treatment, and follow-up. Kidney Int. 2012;82(4):465-73.
22. Servais A, Fremeaux-Bacchi V, Lequintrec M, Salomon R, Blouin J, Knebelmann B, et al. Primary glomerulonephritis with isolated C3 deposits: a new entity which shares common genetic risk factors with haemolytic uraemic syndrome. J Med Genet. 2007;44(3):193-9.
23. Barbour TD, Pickering MC, Cook HT. Recent insights into C3 glomerulopathy. Nephrol Dial Transplant. 2013;28(7):1685-93.
24. Rabasco-Ruiz C, Huerta-Arroyo A, Caro-Espada J, Gutiérrez-Martínez E, Praga-Terente M. C3 glomerulopathies. A new perspective on glomerular diseases. Nefrol Publ Of Soc Esp Nefrol. 2013;33(2):164-70.
25. Medjeral-Thomas NR, O'Shaughnessy MM, O'Regan JA, Traynor C, Flanagan M, Wong L, et al. C3 Glomerulopathy: Clinicopathologic Features and Predictors of Outcome. Clin J Am Soc Nephrol. 2014;9(1):46-53.
26. Gale DP, de Jorge EG, Cook HT, Martinez-Barricarte R, Hadjisavvas A, McLean AG, et al. Identification of a mutation in complement factor H-related protein 5 in patients of Cypriot origin with glomerulonephritis. The Lancet. 2010;376(9743):794-801.
27. Gale DP, Maxwell PH. C3 glomerulonephritis and CFHR5 nephropathy. Nephrol Dial Transplant. 2013;28(2):282-8.

C1Q GLOMERULOPATHY

C1q glomerulopathy is a type of proliferative glomerulonephritis with mesangial deposits of predominant C1q with less intense deposits of immunoglobulins and C3, reported originally by Jennette and Hipp CG,[1] with variable clinical manifestations,[2] including severe proteinuria and nephrotic syndrome, occurring mainly in children with an incidence of 1.4–16.3%[3,4] and seronegative for lupus nephritis.[5]

Microscopic Features

It includes the following in varying combination[1,6-8]
- Normal to minimal mesangial alterations by light microscopy
- Variable mesangial hypercellularity
- Foci of segmental sclerosis with obliteration of capillary lumina
- Focal segmental proliferation with crescents in a minority.

Immunofluorescence

- Paramesangial comma shaped C1q deposits (2 to 3+), IgG (1+), IgM (1+)
- C3 (1+), C4 trace to minimal.

Electron Microscopy

- Electron dense deposits in mesangium subjacent to paramesangial GBM
- Prominent but variable extent of foot process effacement.

Course and Prognosis

Steroid resistant nephrotic syndrome is the usual mode of presentation with frequent recurrence and full remission has been reported in some cases. It is uncertain, whether C1q deposition represents an immune complex disease or a nonspecific trapping in the mesangium. Current reviews of this entity have questioned the validity and significance of the C1q deposits and that has no impact in steroid responsiveness or long-term survival.[4,9,10]

REFERENCES

1. Jennette JC, Hipp CG. C1q nephropathy: a distinct pathologic entity usually causing the nephrotic syndrome. Am J Kidney Dis .1985;6:103.
2. Jennette JC, Wilkman AS, Hogan SL, et al. Clinical and pathologic features of C1q nephropathy. J Am Soc Nephrol 1993; 4:681.
3. Iskandar SS, Browning MC, Lorentz WB. C1q nephropathy: a pediatric clinicopathologic study. Am J Kidney Dis 1991;18:459.
4. Wenderfer SE, Swinford RD, Braun MC. C1q nephropathy in the pediatric population: pathology and pathogenesis. Pediatr Nephrol. 2010;25(8):1385-96.
5. Levart TK, et al. C1q nephropathy in childrenPediatr Nephrol. 2005;20(12):1751-61.
6. Markowitz GS, Schwimmer JA, Stokes MB, et al. C1q nephropathy. A variant of focal segmental glomerulosclerosis. Kidney Int. 2003;64:1232.
7. Muorah M, et al. C1q nephropathy: a true immune complex disease or an immunologic epiphenomenon. NephrolDial Transplant. 2009;2(4):285-91.
8. Mii A, et al. Current status and issues of C1q nephropathy Clinical and experimental. Nephrology. 2009;13(4):263-74.
9. Lau KK, et al. C1q nephropathy: features at presentation and outcome. Pediatr Nephrol. 2005;20(6):744-9.
10. Vizjak A, et al. Pathology, clinical presentations and outcomes of C1q nephropathy. JASN. 2008;19(11):2234-7.

FOCAL (SEGMENTAL) PROLIFERATIVE GLOMERULONEPHRITIS

Focal (segmental) proliferative glomerulonephritis is a less common form of proliferative glomerulonephritis. The primary or an idiopathic form of focal immune complex glomerulonephritis had an incidence of 1.8% in our case series[1] and presented with proteinuria/hematuria or nephrotic syndrome.

Light Microscopy

- Focal and segmental endocapillary proliferation of less than half of the circumference of <50% of glomeruli
- Focal cellular, fibrocellular and fibrous crescents in <50% of glomeruli
- Segmental scars with adhesions, merging with fibrous crescents
- Focal and segmental sclerosis with capsular synechiae.

Immunofluorescence

- Granular deposits of IgG and C3 in the mesangium and/or capillary walls (idiopathic form). The secondary forms of Focal Proliferative Glomerulonephritis are more frequent and occur in association with the following renal diseases (and detailed under systemic glomerular diseases):
  - Resolving Post infectious glomerulonephritis
  - IgA nephropathy and Henoch-Schonlein purpura
  - Systemic lupus erythematosus
  - Vasculitis (ANCA mediated)
  - Antiglomerular basement membrane disease
  - Infective endocarditis (Focal embolic GN).

Course and Prognosis

It is variable and progression depends on the severity of underlying secondary systemic disease.

REFERENCE

1. Balakrisnan N, John GT, Korula A, Visalakshi J, Talauikar GS, Thomas PP, et al. Spectrum of biopsy proven renal disease and changing trends at a tropical tertiary care centre, 1990-2001. Indian J Nephrol. 2003;13;29-35.

CHAPTER 5

Systemic Glomerular Diseases

ABSTRACT

The classification and pathognomonic features of lupus nephritis with individual classes and their differential diagnosis are comprehensively detailed together with the presentation, course and prognosis. The variants of class IV lupus nephritis frequently reported in a renal biopsy are highlighted. The importance of active and chronic glomerular lesions and their indices in the evaluation and final diagnosis is ascertained. The associated vascular lesions are clearly delineated with illustrations to differentiate lupus vasculopathy and thrombotic microangiopathy with the phospholipid antibody syndrome from true lupus vasculitis.

This chapter also includes details of renal involvement by other collagen vascular diseases, such as mixed connective tissue disease, systemic sclerosis, Sjögren syndrome, rheumatoid arthritis and the spectrum of lesions reported in a renal biopsy with their interpretation. The defining serologic criteria and autoantibodies detected are also mentioned as supportive evidence. The vascular complications of these autoimmune diseases including the scleroderma renal crisis and features of malignant hypertension are elucidated.

Collagen Vascular Diseases

These are multisystem diseases with glomerular involvement as a major manifestation including: **Collagen vascular diseases**, comprising **Lupus nephritis (LN), Mixed connective tissue disease, Systemic sclerosis, Sjogren syndrome** and **Rheumatoid arthritis.**

SYSTEMIC LUPUS ERYTHEMATOSUS

Systemic lupus erythematosus (SLE) is an autoimmune chronic inflammatory multisystem disease with involvement of various organs and protean manifestations. The renal disease is known as lupus nephritis and is characterized by exacerbations and remissions leading eventually to chronic renal failure. Lupus nephritis constituted 6.5% of the secondary renal diseases in our case series.[1] The diverse morphologic complexities of lupus nephritis are categorized into distinct classes designated under the modified International Society of Nephrology/Renal Pathology Society (ISN/RPS) Classification of 2003.[2,3] This classification incorporates and provides for the semiquantitative assessment of the features of disease activity and chronicity that are important for prognostication and are predictors of response to immunosuppression. There is a greater degree of uniformity of reporting and reproducibility, among different pathologists, utilizing this classification.

ISN/RPS CLASSIFICATION OF LUPUS NEPHRITIS (2003)

Class I: **Minimal mesangial LN:** Normal glomeruli by LM, but mesangial immune deposits by IF

Class II: **Mesangial proliferative LN:** Purely mesangial hypercellularity of any degree or mesangial matrix expansion by LM, with mesangial immune deposits. There may be a few isolated subepithelial or subendothelial deposits visible by IF or EM but not by LM.

Class III: **Focal LN**[a] Active* or inactive focal, segmental, and/or global endocapillary and/or extracapillary GN involving <50% of all glomeruli, typically with focal subendothelial immune deposits, with or without mesangialalterations.

III (A): Purely active lesions: focal proliferative LN.
III (A/C): Active and chronic lesions: focal proliferative and sclerosing LN.
III (C): Chronic* inactive with glomerular scars: focal sclerosing LN.

Class IV: **Diffuse LN**[a] Active or inactive diffuse, segmental, and/or global endocapillary and/or extracapillary GN involving >50% of all glomeruli, typically with diffuse subendothelial immune deposits, with or without mesangial alterations.This class is divided into diffuse segmental (IV-S) when >50% of the involved glomeruli have segmental lesions and diffuse global (IV-G) when >50% of the involved glomeruli have global lesions. *Segmental* is defined as a lesion that involves less than half of the glomerular tuft.

IV-S (A) or IV-G (A): Purely active lesions: diffuse segmental or global proliferative LN.
IV-S (A/C) or IV-G (A/C): Active and chronic lesions: diffuse segmental or global proliferative and sclerosing LN.
IV-S (C) or IV-G (C): Inactive with glomerular scars: diffuse segmental or global sclerosing LN.

Class V: **Membranous LN**[b] Global or segmental subepithelial immune deposits or their morphologic sequelae by LM and by IF or EM, with or without mesangial alterations.

Class VI: **Advanced sclerosing LN:**
About 90% or more of glomeruli globally sclerosed without residual activity.

Abbreviations: LM, light microscopy; IF, immunofluorescence; EM, electron microscopy; GN, glomerulonephritis.
[a]Indicate the proportion of glomeruli with active and with sclerotic lesions. Indicate the proportion of glomeruli with fibrinoid necrosis and with cellular crescents.

Indicate and grade (mild, moderate, severe) tubular atrophy, interstitial inflammation, and fibrosis, severity of arteriosclerosis or other vascular lesions.

[b]May occur in combination with III or IV, in which case both will be diagnosed; may show advanced sclerosis.

Adapted from: Weening, JJ, D'Agati, VD, et al. Classification of glomerulonephritis in systemic lupus erythematosus revisited. Kidney International. 2004;(65):521-30.

*Active Glomerular Lesions[2]
- Endocapillary hypercellularity+/- leukocytic infiltration
- Karyorrhexis and/or Fibrinoid necrosis/Rupture of GBM
- Cellular or Fibrocellular crescents
- "Wireloops" and or hyaline thrombi (Intraluminal immune aggregates).

*Chronic Glomerular Lesions[2]
- Segmental or global glomerulosclerosis
- Fibrous adhesions and/or fibrous crescents.

Class-I Minimal Mesangial Lupus Nephritis

It is associated with very mild clinical renal manifestations with microhematuria and subnephrotic proteinuria and rarely presents for a biopsy in about 5–10% cases of SLE. American College of Rheumatology (ACR) criteria may be present and lupus serology may be positive.

Microscopic Features[5]

Normocellular glomeruli by light microscopy is the usual feature (Fig. 5.1).

Immunofluorescence
Sparse segmental or global mesangial immune deposits are present.

Electron Microscopy
Small electron dense deposits in the mesangium are noted.

Class-II Mesangial Proliferative Lupus Nephritis

It has an incidence of 10–20% and is associated with mild hematuria and subnephrotic proteinuria with positive ANA, dsDNA and decreased C3 and C4. About 15% of cases show a mild decrease in glomerular filtration rate.

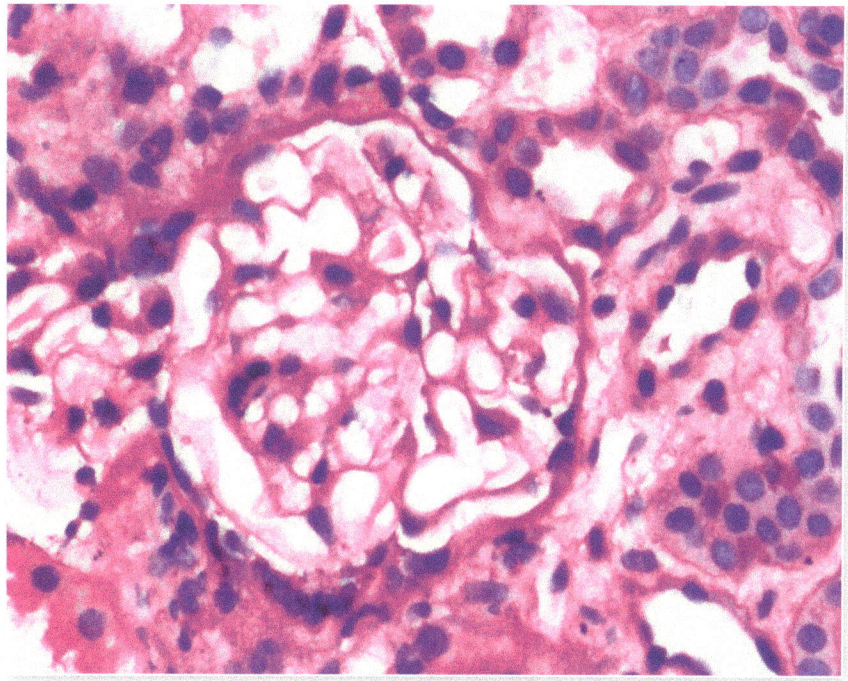

Figure 5.1: Class I: Minimal mesangial lupus nephritis (PAS × 400)

Microscopic Features[2,5]

Light Microscopy
- Segmental or global mesangial hypercellularity (3 or more mesangial cells per mesangial area) and/or variable mesangial matrix expansion with patent capillary lumina (Fig. 5.2)
- Capillary walls are of normal thickness with mild to moderate mesangial proliferation
- Thickening of paramesangial capillary walls noted with severe mesangial proliferation
- Associated narrowing of capillary lumina is noted in the latter type.

Immunofluorescence
Mesangial deposits of IgG, IgA, IgM, C3 with C1q and C4 (2 to 3+) intensity.

Electron Microscopy
- Mesangial electron dense immune deposits in the majority of cases
- Occasional minute subendothelial or subepithelial deposits can be present.

Prognosis[5]

Mesangial proliferative lupus nephritis has an excellent prognosis with a 5 years renal survival of >90%. Transformation to diffuse proliferative or focal proliferative lupus nephritis can occur with increase in proteinuria, active urine sediment and reduction of GFR in some cases spontaneously or with immunosuppressive therapy.

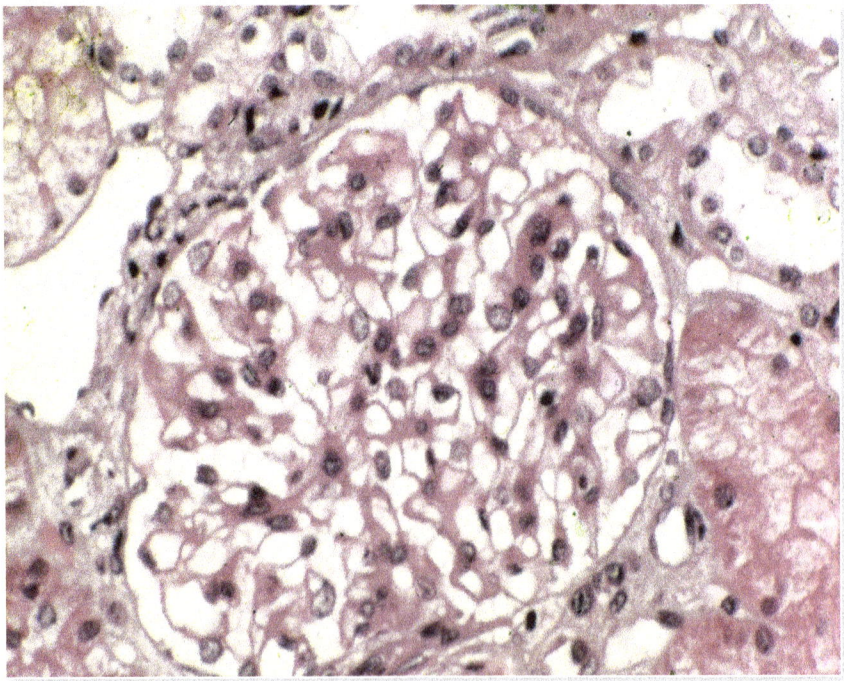

Figure 5.2: Class II: Mesangial proliferative lupus nephritis (H & E X 400)

Class III Focal (Proliferative) Lupus Nephritis

It has an incidence of 20-35% and is characterized by hematuria with active urinary sediment in 25-50% and proteinuria in 50% with nephrotic syndrome in 30% cases. Hypertension and rise in serum creatinine are noted in 10-30% of patients with positive ANA, elevated dsDNA and reduced serum complement in >50% of cases.

Microscopic Features

Light Microscopy [(Class III (A) Lupus Nephritis)][2,5]

- Focal and segmental endocapillary cell proliferation in <50% of glomeruli involving <50% of the glomerular tuft (Fig. 5.3)
- Segmental occlusion of capillary lumina
- Neutrophilic infiltrates with incipient focal necrosis of capillary walls and karyorrhectic nuclear fragments
- Overt segmental fibrinoid necrosis of glomerular tufts seen on H & E (Fig. 5.4) and fibrin stains (Masson trichrome and MSB stains)
- Rupture of capillary walls on the PAS and Jones methenamine stains
- Diffuse mesangial cell and matrix proliferation in the remainder of the glomerular tufts
- Overlying cellular crescents with segmental scars (Masson trichrome positive, PAS negative) and fibrous crescents in **Class IIIA/C lupus nephritis**
- Foci of segmental sclerosis (PAS positive) and capsular synechiae in **Class III (C) lupus nephritis**

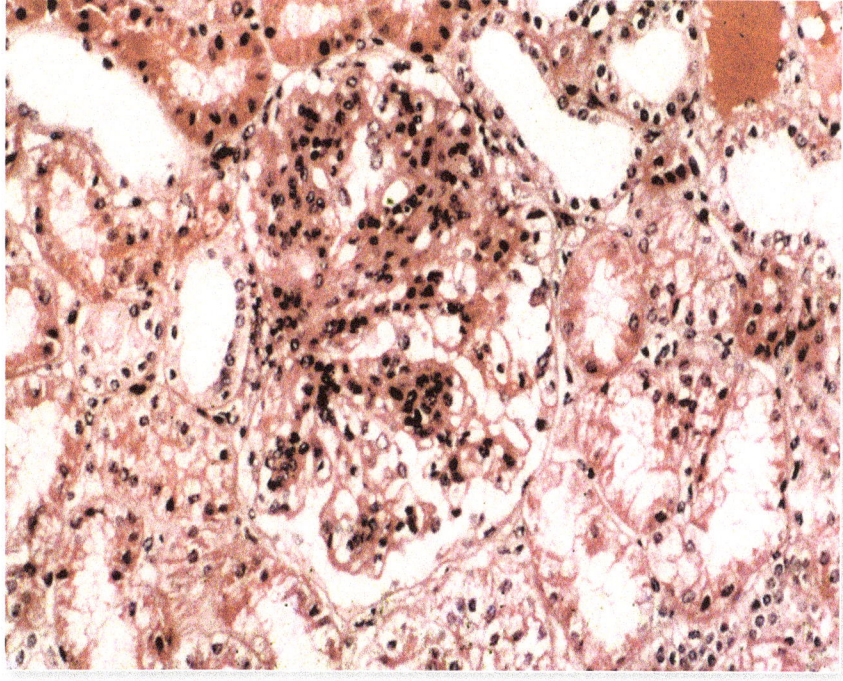

Figure 5.3: Class III: Focal segmental proliferative lupus nephritis (H & E X 400)

66 Renal Biopsy Interpretation

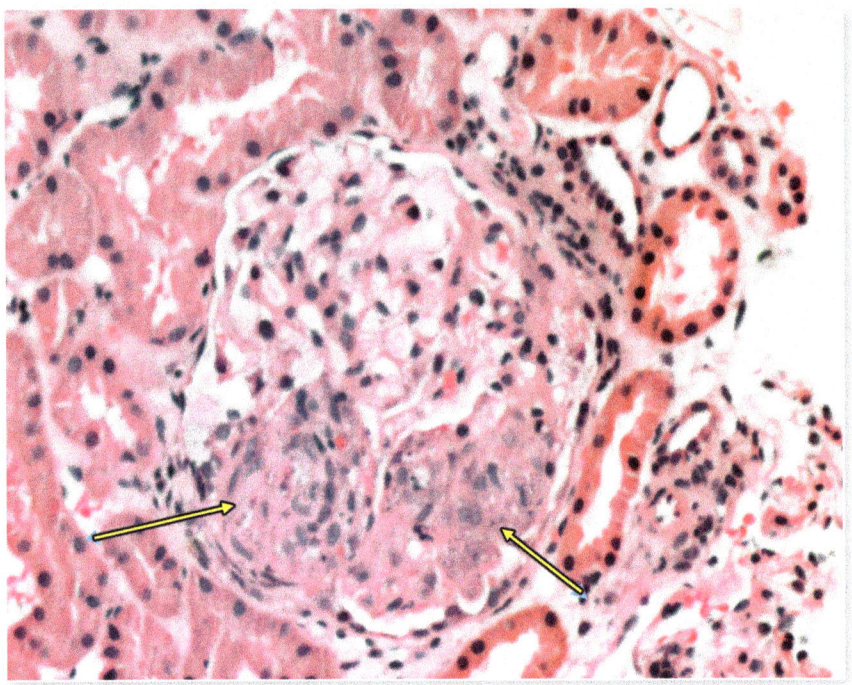

Figure 5.4: Class III: Focal segmental proliferative and necrotizing lupus nephritis (arrows) (H & E × 200)

- Segmental wire loop lesions and capillary hyaline thrombi are rarely present in our experience.

Extraglomerular Compartment
- Interstitial edema and inflammatory cell infiltrates with tubular dilatation and necrosis in the active phase
- Foci of interstitial fibrosis and tubular atrophy with arteriosclerosis are seen in chronic phase.

Immunofluorescence
- Granular mesangial and capillary wall deposits of IgG (3+) with IgA (2 to 3+), IgM (2 to 3+) C3 (2 to 3+), C1q and C4 (2 to 3+) (Fig. 5.5)
- Wire loop type accentuated capillary wall deposits with smooth outer contour are rare.

Electron microscopy
Mesangial and focal segmental subendothelial electron dense capillary wall deposits are typical features.

Differential Diagnosis

Focal and segmental necrotizing glomerular lesions of ANCA mediated vasculitis can be distinguished by immunofluorescence with the pauci-immune deposits of C3 (1 to 2+) on focal capillary walls.

Systemic Glomerular Diseases

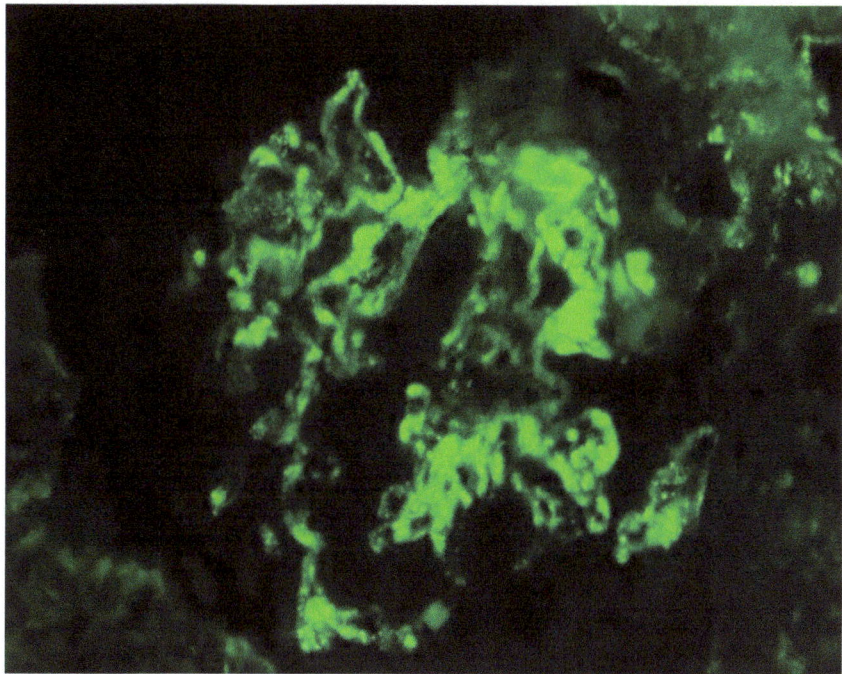

Figure 5.5: Mesangial and focal IgG (3+) deposits in Class III LN (IF × 200)

Course and Prognosis[5]

Class III lupus nephritis has a variable course with a 5-year survival rate of 70-85% and progression to irreversible renal failure in the minority. Class transformation occurs in some cases mainly in continuum to class IV and less commonly to class V lupus nephritis and regression to class II lupus nephritis, reported on repeat biopsies after treatment with steroids.

Class IV Diffuse (Proliferative) Lupus Nephritis

It has an incidence of 35-65% of biopsy proven lupus nephritis presenting with severe proteinuria in the nephrotic range, hematuria, active urine sediment and reduced glomerular filtration rate with positive lupus serological markers.

Microscopic Features

Light Microscopy
Classical pathognomonic features:[5]
- Diffuse and global endocapillary cell proliferation of ≥ 50% of glomeruli involving more than 50% of the tufts (Fig. 5.6)
- Marked lobular expansion and occlusion of capillary lumina
- Neutrophilic infiltration and karyorrhectic punctate nuclear debris
- Diffuse capillary wall thickening with marked segmental accentuation and *"wire loops"*
- Rigid refractile eosinophilic thickening of peripheral circumference of capillary walls (Fig. 5.7)
- Associated with massive subendothelial deposits seen on the PAS and Masson trichrome stains

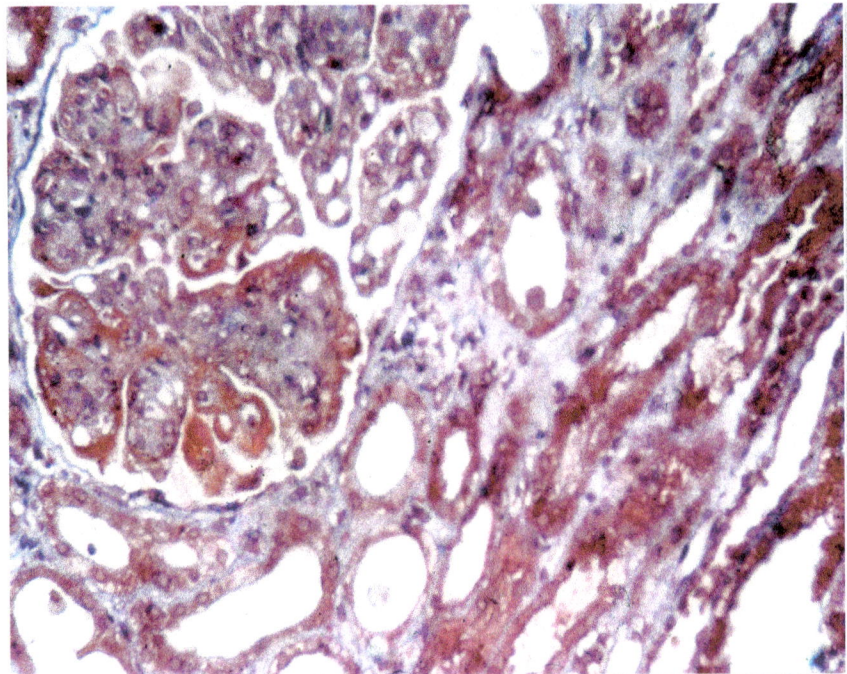

Figure 5.6: Class IV: Diffuse proliferative lupus nephritis with wire loop lesion (Masson trichrome 400)

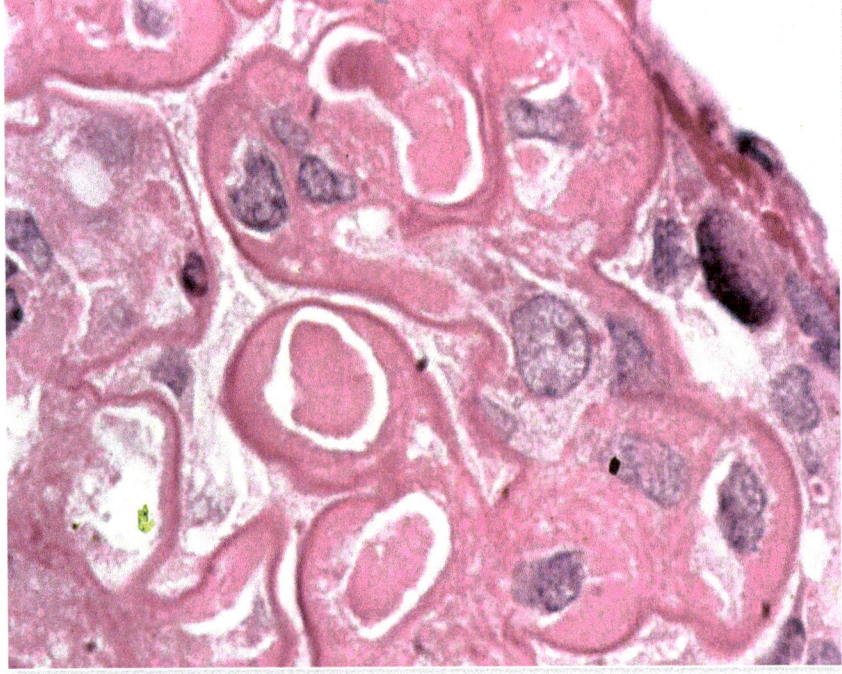

Figure 5.7: Class IV: Diffuse proliferative lupus nephritis with "wire loops" and hyaline thrombi (H & E x 1000)

Systemic Glomerular Diseases

- Large globular intraluminal immune deposits known as *"hyaline thrombi"* seen in continuity (Fig. 5.7)
- Hematoxylin bodies: Smudged, clumped lilac-staining structures of altered nuclear chromatin merge with surrounding flecks of hematoxyphilic nuclear material in the capillary wall (on exposure to ANA in ambient serum and are found in 2% of cases in this category) (Fig. 5.8).

Subtypes and Variants of Class IV Lupus Nephritis[2,5]

- *Diffuse global proliferative lupus nephritis class IV-G:* More than 50% of glomeruli with global lesions [(active (A), active and sclerosing (A/C) and sclerosing (C) lesions respectively)]
- *Diffuse segmental proliferative lupus nephritis class IV-S:* More than 50% of glomeruli with segmental lesions (as above), involving less than half their circumference
- *Diffuse crescentic variant:* More than 50% of glomeruli with crescents (cellular to fibrocellular and fibrous)
- *Membranoproliferative variant:* With circumferential reduplication of capillary walls due to subendothelial neomembrane formation and mesangial interposition similar to MPGN type I
- *Diffuse lupus nephritis with diffuse massive subendothelial deposits* with minimal glomerular hypercellularity or diffuse mesangial hypercellularity.

Extraglomerular compartments show diffuse tubulointerstitial scarring and arteriosclerosis.

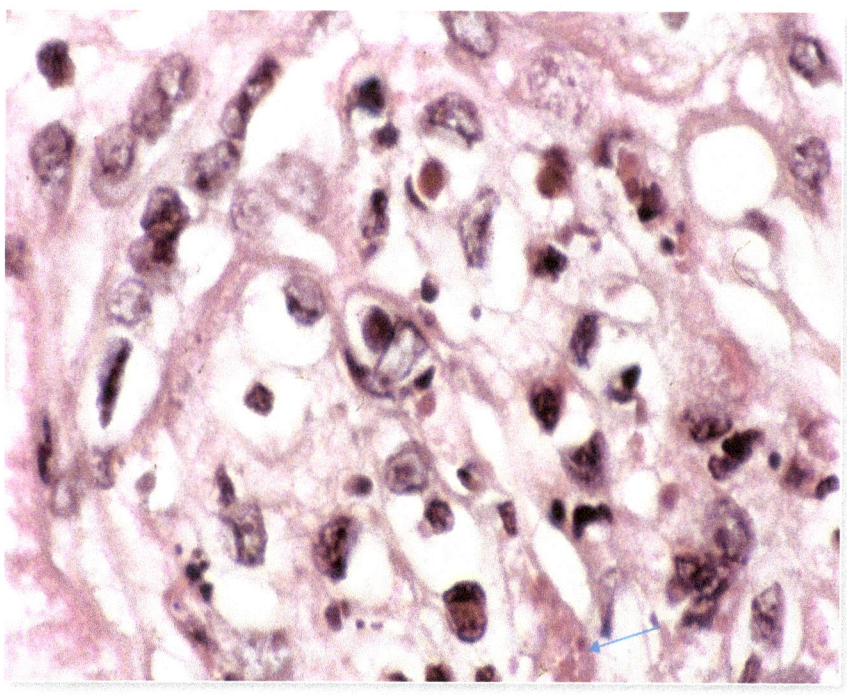

Figure 5.8: Hematoxylin bodies (arrow) in class IV lupus nephritis (H & E x 400)

Immunofluorescence (Figs 5.9 and 5.10)

- Coarsely granular global capillary wall deposits of IgG, IgA, IgM and C3 with C1q and C4 of 3+ intensity
- Segmental accentuation of capillary wire loops with smooth outer contour (Fig. 5.9).

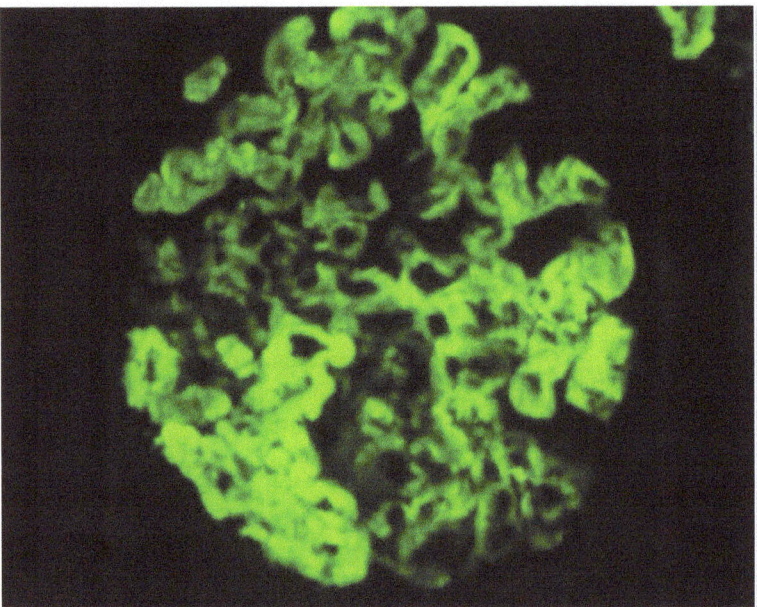

Figure 5.9: C1q (3+) glomerular capillary wall deposits with segmental accentuation in class IV LN (IF x 400)

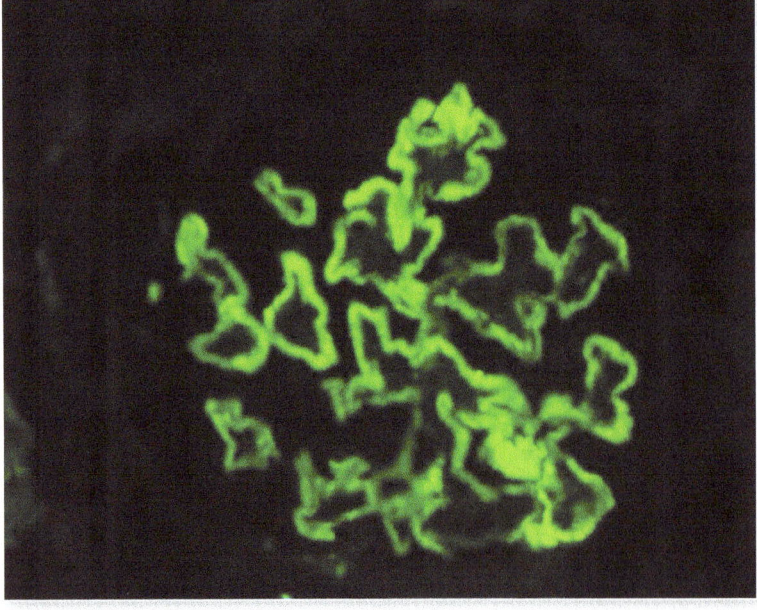

Figure 5.10: Perilobular IgG (3+) deposits in MPGN variant of class IV LN (IF x 200)

Electron Microscopy[5]

- Large subendothelial and intraluminal electron dense deposits in glomerular capillary lobules (Fig. 5.11)
- "Finger print" whorled, lamellated substructure with thin curvilinear bands, 10–15 nm in thickness and cross-striations with a periodicity, are seen in 5–10% cases, around the GBM
- Intracellular tubuloreticular inclusions in dilated cisternae of endoplasmic reticulum of endothelial cell and infiltrating lymphocytes
- Known as "interferon footprints" (due to interferon-alpha produced by activated T lymphocytes)
- Frequently present with confronting cylindrical cisternae in minimally treated and active disease
- Parallel linear arrays and tubulofibrillar structures, 50–100 nm thickness, in the deposits
- Associated with circulating cryoglobulins, particularly in untreated cases of lupus nephritis
- Dense rounded core of altered nuclear material with degenerate cytoplasmic organelles and delimiting membrane representing hematoxylin bodies are rarely seen.

Differential Diagnosis

1. **Diffuse proliferative glomerulonephritis (post-infectious type)** does not have the pathognomonic features of class IV lupus nephritis. The classical light microscopic, immunofluorescent and lupus serological features are often altered, diminished or absent in the latter on renal biopsies after steroid therapy.

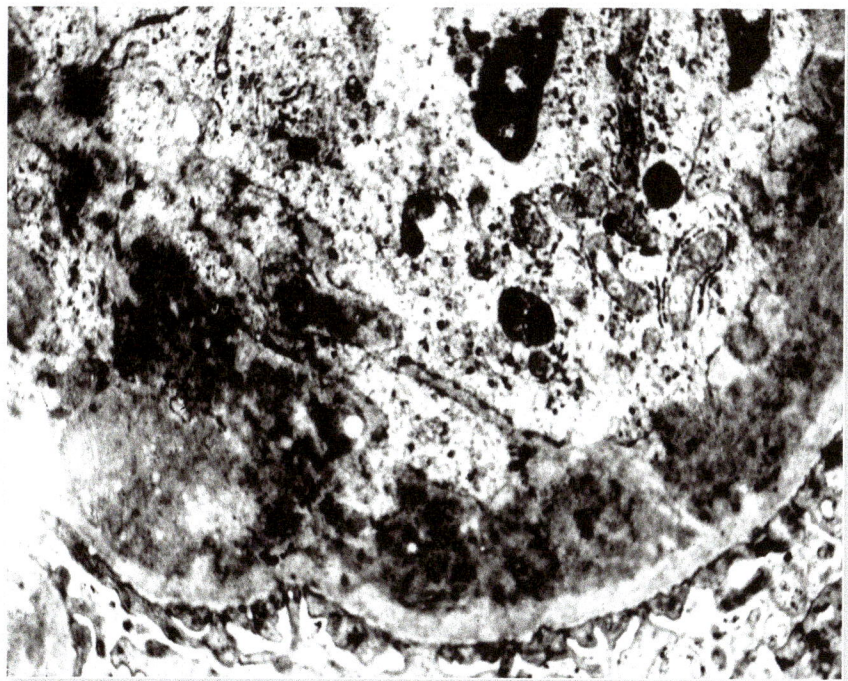

Figure 5.11: Electron micrograph with subendothelial deposits in class IV lupus nephritis

2. **Membranoproliferative glomerulonephritis type I** can be differentiated from the membranoproliferative variant of class IV lupus nephritis by the full house pattern of immunofluorescence including C1q deposits in the latter and positive lupus serological markers. In biopsies done after immunosuppressive therapy, these features are modified or absent.
3. **Cryoglobulinemic glomerulonephritis** with diffuse proliferative or membranoproliferative features, intracapillary hyaline thrombi and similar organized substructure of immune deposits can be distinguished by the predominant monoclonal IgM deposits on the capillary walls and in the luminal thrombi on immunofluorescence. Mixed polyclonal cryoglobulins can concomitantly be present in association with lupus nephritis, class IV.

Course and Prognosis[5]

Diffuse proliferative lupus nephritis class IV-G has a relentless course with remissions and relapse and a 10-year survival rate of 50–75%. The segmental form (class IV-S) is less common and has been reported to have a varying and comparatively worse prognosis when severe necrotizing lesions are present in cases from some centers.[6,7] Class transformation to class V is more frequent than regression to class III or class II on treatment with steroids and cyclophosphamide. In our experience, hypertension, nephrotic proteinuria and high activity index were predictive prognostic factors in the progression to end-stage renal failure in DPLN-IV.[8]

Class V Membranous Lupus Nephritis

It has an incidence of 10–15% and the majority present with nephrotic syndrome and hematuria with hypertension in a minority with normal renal function.

Microscopic Features[5]

Light Microscopy
- Marked diffuse glomerular capillary wall thickening of >50% of the circumference of >50% of glomeruli
- Mesangial matrix expansion with variable mesangial hypercellularity
- Stages of progression are similar to primary membranous nephropathy.

Immnofluorescence
- Fine to coarsely granular contiguous capillary wall deposits of IgG, IgA, IgM, C3 with C1q and C4 (2 to 3+)
- Mesangial deposits also present to varying extent.

Electron Microscopy
- Diffuse subepithelial electron dense deposits with epimembranous spikes of GBM
- Resorption of intramembranous deposits with neomembrane formation in advanced stages
- Mesangial and few scattered subendothelial deposits can be present.

Mixed subtypes in the ISN/RPS classification[2] include Class V+ Class III and ClassV+ Class IV. The additional designation of Class V in a background of Class III or Class IV requires capillary wall thickening of at least 50% of the glomerular capillary surface area in at least 50% of glomeruli in a renal biopsy. Active lesions of Class III or IV when combined with a diffuse membranous lupus nephritis have to be mentioned in the final diagnosis.

Differential Diagnosis

Primary membranous nephropathy is not associated with mesangial immune complexes or a fullhouse pattern on immunofluorescence and is positive for PLA2R antibody on standard and confocal fluorescent microscopy and validated in our experience on IHC on formalin fixed paraffin embedded sections in contrast to class V lupus nephritis.

Course and Prognosis[5]

Pure class V is associated with preservation or gradual reduction of GFR with the onset of segmental or global glomerular sclerosis. Combined class V and class IV has a worse prognosis than isolated class V lupus nephritis. Class transformation to class IV or combined class V and class III occur with increased renal insufficiency and reduction in GFR. Renal vein thrombosis can occur as a complication of class V membranous nephropathy associated with marked glomerular capillary congestion with intraluminal fibrin strands, margination of leukocytes and interstitial edema with microhemorrhage.

Class VI Advanced Sclerosing Lupus Nephritis[2,5]

It involves ≥90% glomeruli with global sclerosis and there is no residual active glomerular disease present attributable to lupus nephritis. Class III, class IV or class V can progress to class VI, which can be confirmed on sequential renal biopsies. There is associated diffuse tubulointerstitial scarring with mononuclear cell infiltrates and vascular sclerosis. These are irreversible end-stage lesions and associated with a poor prognosis and outcome.

Immunofluorescence and Electron Microscopy

Focal granular immune deposits are identified in sclerotic glomeruli and walls of blood vessels.
These are irreversible end-stage lesions and associated with a poor prognosis and outcome.
Activity and chronicity scores[9,10] (Table 5.1) are an adjunct to the classification of lupus nephritis as a guide to treatment and prognosis in a given biopsy. There is no uniformity of agreement regarding the predictability and reproducibility of these indices.[11] The percentage of glomeruli with severe active lesions such as fibrinoid necrosis and crescents and other active and chronic lesions have to be included in the final diagnostic report.[2,5]

Vascular Lesions in Systemic Lupus Erythematosus (SLE)[5,12]

The pathogenetic mechanisms leading to vascular lesions in SLE primarily cause endothelial injury due to one or more factors such as immune complexes, cell mediated mechanisms, antiphospholipid antibodies, anti-endothelial antibodies, superimposed anti-neutrophil cytoplasmic antibodies, host/genetic factors and concomitant activation of coagulation factors. The type, extent and severity of these lesions have considerable prognostic and therapeutic value.

Table 5.1: Activity and chronicity indices: Semiquantitative

Index of activity (Total score = 24)	
Endocapillary hypercellularity	(0–3 +)
Leukocyte infiltration	(0–3 +)
Subendothelial hyaline deposits	(0–3 +)
Fibrinoid necrosis/karyorrhexis	(0–3 +) x 2
Cellular crescents	(0–3 +) x 2
Interstitial inflammation	(0–3 +)
Index of chronicity (Total score = 12)	
Glomerular sclerosis	(0–3 +)
Fibrous crescents	(0–3 +)
Tubular atrophy	(0–3 +)
Interstitial fibrosis	(0–3 +)

1. **Uncomplicated vascular immune deposits:** It is characterized by immune deposits of IgG, IgA, IgM, C3 and C1q in the walls of arterioles, interlobular arteries and veins, less often.

Microscopic features:
- Mild thickening of intimal basal lamina
- Electron deposits in subendothelial basement membrane are seen.

2. **Non-inflammatory necrotizing vasculopathy (Lupus vasculopathy):** Occurs in class IV lupus nephritis.

It is involving preglomerular arterioles and interlobular arteries associated with hypertension and rapid progression to renal failure with active urinary sediment and positive lupus serology.

Microscopic features:
- Intraluminal and mural deposits of glassy eosinophilic material, devoid of inflammatory cell infiltrates (Fig. 5.12)
- Positive for fibrin with MSB and fuchsinophilic on Masson trichrome stain
- Associated endothelial swelling and medial degeneration are noted
- Immune deposits on IF and EM with insudation of plasma proteins and fibrin.

3. **Thrombotic microangiopathy:** It involves preglomerular arterioles, interlobular arteries and glomeruli.

Microscopic features:
- Fibrinthrombi and glomerular mesangiolysis (Fig. 5.13)
- Subendothelial floccular fibrin tactoids
- Endothelial necrosis with double contours of capillary walls
- Entrapped fragmented erythrocytes are seen.

Immunofluorescence shows IgM with C3 deposits and fibrin in glomerular capillary walls.

Systemic Glomerular Diseases

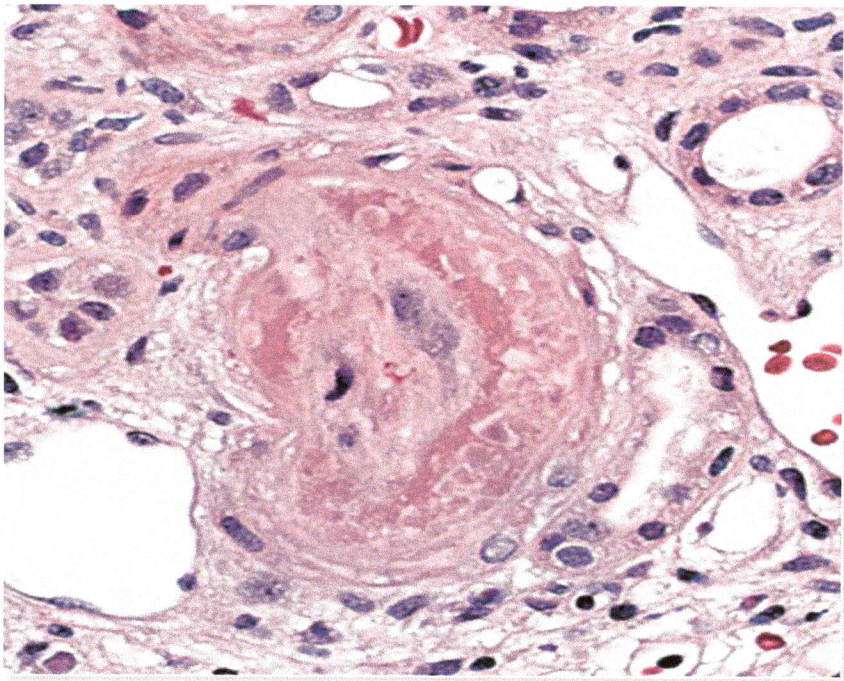

Figure 5.12: Lupus vasculopathy (H & E x 200)

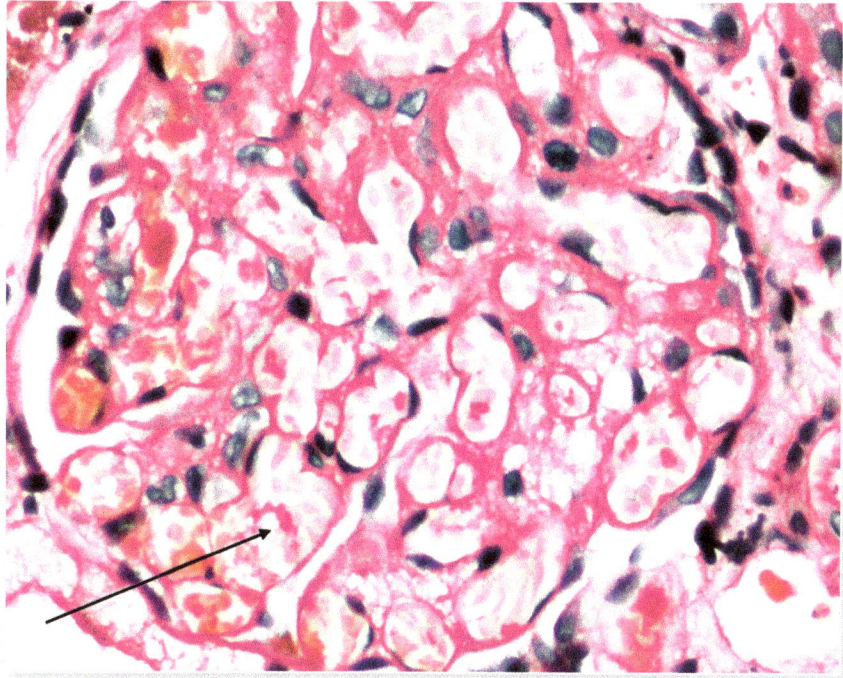

Figure 5.13: Class IV lupus nephritis and concomitant thrombotic microangiopathy with mesangiolysis (arrow) (H & E x 400)

Associated syndromes: Hemolytic uremic syndrome/thrombotic Thrombocytopenic Purpura with microangiopathic hemolyticanemia and thrombocytopenia can precede, occur concurrently with or follow the onset of SLE and is linked to an autoantibody to Von Willebrand cleaving protease.

Antiphospholipid antibody syndrome can be superimposed secondarily on all classes of lupus nephritis or occur primarily, independently associated with antibodies to naturally occurring phospholipids including cardiolipin. The plasma inhibitor known as "lupus anticoagulant" prolongs phospholipid dependent coagulation tests including activated partial thromboplastin time in vitro that is not reversed by dilution with normal platelet free plasma. The lupus anticoagulant promotes coagulation in vivo probably by platelet and endothelial activation with glomerular capillary arteriolar and venous thrombosis leading to renal infarction and cortical necrosis with rapidly progressive renal failure.

4. **True inflammatory vasculitis:** It can occur with active or inactive forms of any class of lupus nephritis associated with pANCA positivity in more than one-third of patients and requiring aggressive immunosuppression.

Microscopic features:
- Mural inflammatory cell infiltration of the intima and media of medium sized or large arteries
- Fibrinoid mural necrosis is seen with rupture of elastic lamellae (Fig. 5.14)

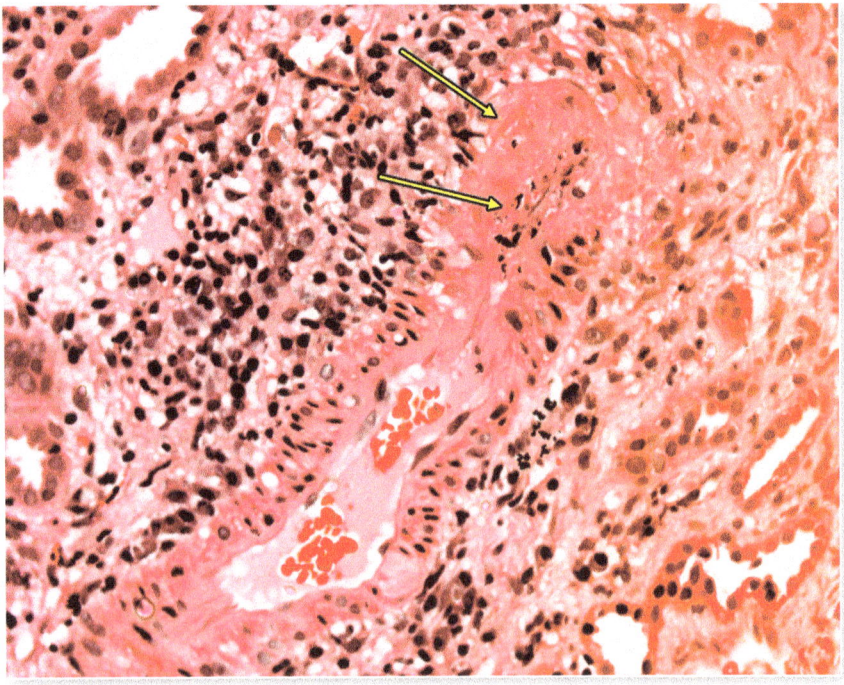

Figure 5.14: Concomitant acute necrotizing vasculitis (arrows) in DPLN class IV (H & E x 200)

- Focal and segmental glomerular capillary fibrinoid necrosis, devoid of endocapillary proliferation
- Remainder of glomerular tuft is unremarkable.

Immunofluorescence is negative for immunoglobulins and complement.

REFERENCES

1. Narasimhan B, Chacko B, John GT, Korula A, Kirubakaran MG, Jacob CK. Characterization of kidney lesions in Indian adults: towards a renal biopsy registry.J Nephrol. 2006;19(2):205-10.
2. Weening JJ, D'agati VD, Schwartz MM, Seshan SV, Alpers CE, Appel GB, et al. The classification of glomerulonephritis in systemic lupus erythematosus revisited.Kidney Int. 2004;65(2):521-30.
3. Weening JJ, D'Agati VD, Schwartz MM, Seshan SV, Alpers CE, Appel GB, et al. The classification of glomerulonephritis in systemic lupus erythematosus revisited. J Am Soc Nephrol. 2004;15(2):241-50.
4. Tan EM, Cohen AS, Fries JF, Masi AT, Mcshane DJ, Rothfield NF, et al. The 1982 revised criteria for the classification of systemic lupus erythematosus. Arthritis Rheum.1982;25(11):1271-7.
5. Seshan SV, Jennette JC. Renal disease in systemic lupus erythematosus with emphasis on classification of lupus glomerulonephritis: advances and implications. Arch Pathol Lab Med. 2009;133(2):233-48.
6. Hill GS, Delahousse M, Nochy D, Bariéty J. Class IV-S versus class IV-G lupus nephritis: clinical and morphologic differences suggesting different pathogenesis. Kidney Int. 2005;68(5):2288-97.
7. Markowitz GS, D'Agati VD. The ISN/RPS 2003 classification of lupus nephritis: an assessment at 3 years. Kidney Int. 2007;71(6):491-5.
8. Abraham MA, Korula A, Jayakrishnan K, John GT, Thomas PP, Jacob CK. Prognostic factors in diffuse proliferative lupus nephritis. J Assoc Physicians India.1999;47(9):862-5.
9. Austin III HA, Muenz LR, Joyce KM, Antonovych TA, Kullick ME, Klippel JH, et al. Prognostic factors in lupus nephritis: contribution of renal histologic data.Am J Med.1983;75(3):382-91.
10. Austin HA, Muenz LR, Joyce KM, Antonovych TT, Balow JE. Diffuse proliferative lupus nephritis: identification of specific pathologic features affecting renal outcome. Kidney Int.1984;25(4):689-95.
11. Schwartz MM, Lan S, Bernstein J, Hill GS, Holley K, Lewis EJ. Irreproducibility of the activity and chronicity indices limits their utility in the management of lupus nephritis. Am J Kidney Dis. 1993;21(4):374-7.
12. Appel GB, Pirani CL, D'Agati V. Renal vascular complications of systemic lupus erythematosus. J Am Soc Nephrol.1994;4(8):1499-515.

MIXED CONNECTIVE TISSUE DISEASE

Mixed connective tissue disease (MCTD) is an overlap syndrome, originally reported by Sharp,[1] et al. characterized by two or more features of defined autoimmune diseases including systemic lupus erythematosus, systemic sclerosis (Scleroderma), rheumatoid arthritis, polymyositis or dermatomyositis and Sjogren syndrome and high titers of circulating antibody to nuclear ribonuclear protein antigen (anti-U1 RNP) and U1-70 kd small nuclear ribonuclear protein (snRNP) occurring in women with a peak age of onset at 20 to 30 years.[2] Renal involvement[3] is noted in 25% of cases by:

- Membranous nephropathy or mesangial proliferative glomerulonephritis or combined sclerosing features
- Focal proliferative crescentic glomerulonephritis with necrotizing arteritis in occasional cases
- Renovascular intimal proliferation and medial hypertrophy.

Immunofluorescence

Immunofluorescence shows predominantly IgG and and less intense C3 glomerular deposits.

Concomitant involvement of lungs is reported in 75% (primary pulmonary hypertension and interstitial lung disease), with vasculopathy including Raynaud phenomenon, severe arthritis in 60%, cardiac disease (pericarditis) in 10-30%, inflammatory myopathy, variable gastrointestinal disease (esophageal dysfunction), nonspecific serologic (positive high titer speckled ANA and rheumatoid factor) and hematologic abnormalities.[4,5]

Course and Prognosis[6-8]

Mixed connective tissue disease has a variable prognosis with morbidity and mortality associated with steroid unresponsive complications of pulmonary hypertension, scleroderma, renovascular hypertension, myocarditis and cerebral hemorrhage.

REFERENCES

1. Sharp GC, Irvin WS, Tan EM, et al. Mixed connective tissue disease—an apparently distinct rheumatic disease syndrome associated with a specific antibody to an extractable nuclear antigen (ENA). Am J Med. 1972;52:148.
2. Tani S, Carli I, Vagnani S, Tolarico R, Baldini C, Mosca M, et al. The diagnosis and classification of mixed connective tissue disease. Journal of Autoimmun. 2014;48-49(Feb-March):46-9.
3. Kitridou RC, Akmal M, Turkel SB, et al. Renal involvement in mixed connective tissue: a longitudinal Clinicopathologic study. Semin Arthritis Rheum. 1986;16:135.
4. Pope JE. Other manifestations of connective tissue disease. Rheum Dis Clin North Am. 2005;31(3):519.
5. Szodoray P, Hajas A, Kardos L, et al. Distinct phenotypes in mixed connective tissue disease: subgroups and survival. Lupus. 2012;21(13):1412-22.
6. Celikbilek M, Elsurer R, Afsar B, et al. Mixed connective tissue disease: a case with scleroderma renal crisis following abortion. Clin Rheumatol. 2007;26:1545.
7. Yamaguchi T, Ohshima S, Tanaka T, et al. Renal crisis due to intimal hyperplasia in a patient with mixed connective tissue disease (MCTD) accompanied by pulmonary hypertension. Intern Med. 2001;40:1250.
8. Lundberg IE. The prognosis of mixed connective tissue disease. Rheum Dis Clin North Am. 2005;31:535.

SYSTEMIC SCLEROSIS

Systemic sclerosis is a multisystem autoimmune disease, characterized by accumulation of collagen and diffuse thickening of walls of blood vessels with intimal proliferation and luminal narrowing associated with localized or diffuse cutaneous sclerosis. Renal vascular involvement due to vascular endothelial injury occurs in 60-80% of cases of systemic sclerosis with clinical evidence in 50% of cases presenting with mild proteinuria, elevated serum creatinine and hypertension.[1] Scleroderma renal crisis occurs in 5-20% of diffuse cutaneous systemic sclerosis.[2-4]

Microscopic Features

Light Microscopy

- Concentric "onion-skin" intimal fibrosis of arcuate and interlobular arteries with luminal obliteration
- Ischemic glomerular retraction with dilatation of Bowman's space and capsular fibrosis

- Intercapillary matrix expansion and mesangial sclerosis with secondary focal segmental glomerulosclerosis.

Immunofluorescence

Negative or nonspecific trapping of IgM and C3 in sclerotic tufts.

Complications

Scleroderma renal crisis is associated with increased vascular permeability, activation of coagulation cascade and vascular thrombosis. Vascular hypoperfusion results in juxtaglomerular apparatus hyperplasia with renin secretion and accelerated hypertension leading to acute onset of oligoanuric renal failure. Features of malignant hypertension can develop with hypertensive retinopathy and encephalopathy, microangiopathic hemolytic anemia and thrombocytopenia. Autoantibodies including speckled ANA and anti-polymerase III are also detected.

Microscopic Features[2-5]

- Predominant involvement of extraglomerular small blood vessels
- Thrombotic microangiopathy with fibrinoid necrosis of preglomerular arterioles, interlobular and sub-arcuate arteries
- Ischemic necrosis and glomerular capillary thrombosis less frequent
- Acute tubular necrosis or cortical parenchymal necrosis
- Myxoid intimal thickening and concentric intimal fibrosis of intraparenchymal arteries and periadventitial fibrosis with tubulointerstitial fibrosis are seen as sequelae in the healing and chronic phase
- C4d staining of peritubular capillary walls is seen in a subset of cases on IF or IHC due to antibody mediated vascular injury.

Electron Microscopy

- Endothelial swelling and detachment of glomerular capillaries
- Subendothelial expansion by fluffy electron lucent or hyaline material in lamina rara interna
- Mesangial interposition in chronic phase with reduplication of GBM and glomerulosclerosis.

Differential Diagnosis[2]

Malignant hypertensive nephrosclerosis, HUS/TTP, chronic transplant rejection and primary antiphospholipid antibody syndrome have the underlying features of a thrombotic microangiopathy. Hence the renal biopsy cannot distinguish these lesions from scleroderma-associated renal crisis, but can predict outcome and irreversibility of renal failure from the degree and extent of parenchymal lesions present.

Prognosis

End-stage renal disease with dialysis dependent chronic renal failure occurs despite long-term use of antihypertensive angiotensin-convertase inhibitors, requiring renal transplantation.[6]

REFERENCES

1. Donohoe JF. Scleroderma and the kidney. Kidney Int. 1992;41:462-77.
2. Batal I, Domsic RT, Shafer A, et al. Renal biopsy findings predicting outcome in scleroderma renal crisis. Hum Pathol. 2009;40:332-40.
3. Gouge SF, Wilder K, Welch P, et al. Scleroderma renal crisis prior to scleroderma. Am J Kidney Dis. 1989;14:236.
4. Zwettlwer U, Andrassy K, Waldherr R, Ritz E. Scleroderma renal crisis as a presenting feature in the absence of skin involvement. Am J Kidney Dis. 1993;22:53.
5. Batal I, Domsic RT, Medsger TA Jr, Bastacky S. Scleroderma renal crisis: a pathology perspective. Int J Rheumatol. 2010;7:1-7 doi:10.1155/2010/543704.
6. Poormoghim H, Lucas M, Fertig N, Medsger TA Jr. Systemic sclerosis sine scleroderma: demographic, clinical and serological features and survival in forty-eight patients. Arthritis Rheum. 2000;43:444.

SJOGREN'S SYNDROME

Sjogren's syndrome is a systemic autoimmune chronic inflammatory disease primarily involving exocrine salivary and lacrimal glands with "xerostomia" and "keratoconjunctivitis sicca" as the predominant manifestations and less frequently, other organs including the kidneys.[1] The secondary form occurs in association with other collagen vascular/autoimmune diseases including rheumatoid arthritis and systemic lupus erythematosus, MCTD, polymyositis, chronic, active, hepatitis (Hepatitis C), primary biliary cirrhosis and Crohn's disease. The associated serological markers include ANA (homogeneous or speckled) and hypergammaglobulinemia with rheumatoid factor (IgG and IgM classes), mixed cryoglobulinemia, anti-Ro SSA and anti-La SSB and organ specific antibodies (anti-thyroid microsomal and thyroglobulin). Renal involvement includes tubulointerstitial nephritis in the initial phase and glomerulonephritis later.

Microscopic Features[2-4]

Tubulointerstitial Lesions

- Dense lymphoplasmacytic infiltrates with tubulitis and tubular atrophy
- CD4 positive T lymphocytes predominate
- Interstitial fibrosis with secondary mesangial sclerosis and glomerular tuft atrophy with capsular fibrosis.

Immunofluorescence

Tubulointerstitial IgG and C3 deposits.

Glomerular Lesions

- Mesangial to focal or diffuse proliferative, membranoproliferative or membranous and crescentic glomerulonephritis
- Mesangial, subendothelial or subepithelial immune complex deposits containing IgG and/or C3
- IgM deposits are noted in association with cryoglobulinemic membranoproliferative glomerulonephritis

Systemic Glomerular Diseases

- Renal vasculitis has been rarely reported with necrotizing glomerulonephritis in a minority of cases.

Course and Prognosis[5,6]

The tubulointerstitial lesions present with distal renal tubular acidosis (type I) in 15–50% of cases and are commonly associated with metabolic acidosis and reduced urinary titrable acidity complicated by hypercalciuria and nephrocalcinosis.[5] Proximal renal tubular acidosis (Type II or Fanconi syndrome) is less frequent leading to chronic renal failure in severe cases. The glomerular lesions usually respond to immunosuppression and cytotoxic drugs.[6]

REFERENCES

1. Bossini N, et al. Clinical and morphological features of Primary Sjogren's syndrome. Nephrol Dial Transplant. 2001;16(12);2328-36.
2. Maripuri S, et al. Renal involvement in primary Sjogren's syndrome: a clinicopathologic study. CJASN. 2009;4(9):1423-31.
3. Kronbichler A, et al. Renal involvement in Autoimmune connective tissue diseases. BMC Medicine. 2013;11:95.
4. Goules A, Masouridi S, Tzioufas AG, Ioannidis JP, Skopouli FN, Moutsopoulos HM. Clinically significant and biopsy-documented renal involvement in primary Sjogren syndrome. Medicine (Baltimore). 2000;79:241-9.
5. Pessler F, Emery H, Dai L, Wu YM, Monash B, Cron RQ, et al. The spectrum of renal tubular acidosis in paediatric Sjogren syndrome. Rheumatology (Oxford). 2006;45:85-91.
6. Ren H, Wang WM, Chen XN, Zhang W, Pan XX, Wang XL, et al. Renal involvement and followup of 130 patients with primary Sjogren's syndrome. J Rheumatol. 2008;35:278-84.

RHEUMATOID ARTHRITIS

An immune mediated chronic inflammatory disease is characterized by deforming arthritis with destruction of articular cartilage and bone erosions, involving multiple joints. The extra-articular manifestations include rheumatoid nodules, systemic vasculitis and seropositivity for rheumatoid factor.[1] The associated reported renal lesions with a variable occurrence are as follows:

Glomerular Lesions[2,3]

Light Microscopy

- Mesangial proliferative glomerulonephritis is the most common feature
- Membranous nephropathy
- Minimal change nephropathy
- Focal proliferative glomerulonephritis
- Focal and segmental glomerulosclerosis
- Focal necrotizing and crescentic glomerulonephritis (pauci-immune ANCA associated)
- Secondary IgA nephropathy
- Acute interstitial nephritis
- Rheumatoid vasculitis involving large renal arteries with aneurysm formation is uncommon.

Drug-induced Nephrotoxicity[4,5]

Analgesic nephropathy with papillary necrosis and chronic interstitial nephritis.

Nonsteroidal anti-inflammatory drugs with acute interstitial nephritis, minimal change disease and membranous nephropathy.

Penicillamine and gold toxicity with membranous glomerulopathy.

Cytotoxic and disease modifying anti-rheumatic drugs (DMARD) with tubulointerstitial and vascular toxicity.[5]

Amyloidosis[2,6]

Secondary amyloidosis with strong reactivity to serum amyloid A protein on immunohistochemical or immunofluorescent stains is associated with pale eosinophilic deposits in glomerular and extraglomerular compartments by light microscopy. These deposits are Thioflavine-T positive and congophilic with apple green birefringence on polarized light. Immunofluorescence is negative for kappa and lambda light chains.

REFERENCES

1. Scott DL, Wolfe F, Huizinga TW. Rheumatoid arthritis. Lancet. 2010;376:1094-108.
2. Kronbichler A, Mayer G. Renal involvement in connective tissue diseases. BMC-Medicine. 2013;11:95.
3. Helin HJ, Korpela MM, Mustonen JT, Pasternack AI. Renal biopsy findings and clinicopathologic correlations in rheumatoid arthritis. Arthritis Rheum.1995;38(2):242-7.
4. Schiff MH, Whelton A. Renal toxicity associated with disease-modifying antirheumatic drugs used for the treatment of rheumatoid arthritis. Semin Arthritis Rheum. 2000;30:196-208.
5. Stokes MB, Foster K, Markowitz GS, Ebrahimi F, Hines W, Kaufman D, et al. Development of glomerulonephritis during anti-TNF-alpha therapy for rheumatoid arthritis. Nephrol Dial Transplant. 2005;20:1400-6.
6. Kuroda T, Tanabe N, Kobayashi D, Wada Y, Murakami S, Nakano M, et al. Significant association between renal function and area of amyloid deposition in kidney biopsy specimens in reactive Amyloidosis associated with rheumatoid arthritis. Rheumatol Int. 2012;32:3155-62.

CHAPTER 6

Diabetic Nephropathy

> **ABSTRACT**
>
> The incidence of diabetic nephropathy and non-diabetic renal glomerular lesions in our medical center is documented. The current Renal Pathology Society classification of diabetic nephropathy has been applied here for routine diagnostic renal biopsies and for validation in the Indian cohort, based on the grading of mesangial expansion and glomerular capillary wall involvement. The scoring system utilized for assessment of severity of associated tubulointerstitial lesions is linked to prognosis. The vascular lesions have been shown to correlate with urinary albumin secretion and hypertension.
>
> Non-diabetic glomerular lesions prevalent in our center and comparison to multicenter western cohorts are included as important features occurring concomitantly or independently with differing clinical presentation, course and prognosis. Other parenchymal lesions referred for a renal biopsy in the diabetic are also mentioned.
>
> The differential diagnosis of diabetic glomerulosclerosis and their interpretation include other forms of nodular glomerulosclerosis as seen in, light chain deposition disease, nodular amyloidosis and idiopathic nodular glomerulosclerosis.

INTRODUCTION

Diabetic nephropathy (DN) is characterized by persistent albuminuria (>300 mg/24 hours), reduction in glomerular filtration rate, hypertension and progression to renal failure in about 60% of cases. Type I diabetes comprises 5–10% and type II about 90% of patients with diabetes mellitus. In the preclinical phase, microalbuminuria of 30–300 mg/24 hours is a predictor of the risk of development of diabetic nephropathy and renal function deterioration.[1] The incidence of biopsy proven diabetic nephropathy in our case series has been 2.5%.[2] Renal biopsies are also done for non-diabetic renal lesions accounting for 72% in our series of 288 biopsies from non-insulin dependent diabetic patients,[2] and a wider range of 12–81% in a comparative Asian cohort.[3]

MICROSCOPIC FEATURES[1,4]

Light Microscopy

- Enlarged glomeruli with diffuse increase in mesangial matrix and thickening of capillary walls
- Diffuse intercapillary mesangial expansion with sclerosis and narrowing of lumina (Figs 6.1 and 6.2)
- Nodular expansion of matrix rimmed by mesangial cells
- Asymmetric ovoid or spherical laminated varied size nodules, Kimmelstiel-Wilson's lesions (KIW lesion) (Fig. 6.1)

- Intensely periodic acid-Schiff (PAS) positive and Jones methenamine silver stain (JMS positive)
- Associated dissolution and fraying of mesangial matrix with mesangiolysis
- Ectasia of peripheral glomerular capillary lumina due to loss of anchorage of glomerular basement membrane (GBM)
- Formation of glomerular capillary microaneurysms with compaction of fibrillar matrix and increased nodularity (Fig. 6.1)
- Insudation of hyaline material between endothelial cells and GBM, forming "fibrin caps" in capillary lumina
- "Capsular drops" formed between parietal epithelial cells and Bowman's capsule are specific for DN (Fig. 6.2)
- Capsular fibrosis with synechiae associated with mesangial sclerotic lesions and global glomerulosclerosis
- Hyaline afferent and efferent arteriolosclerosis, the latter is specific for DN (Fig. 6.2).

Immunofluorescence

Nonspecific linear staining of glomerular capillary walls and trapping of IgM and C3 in sclerotic tufts.

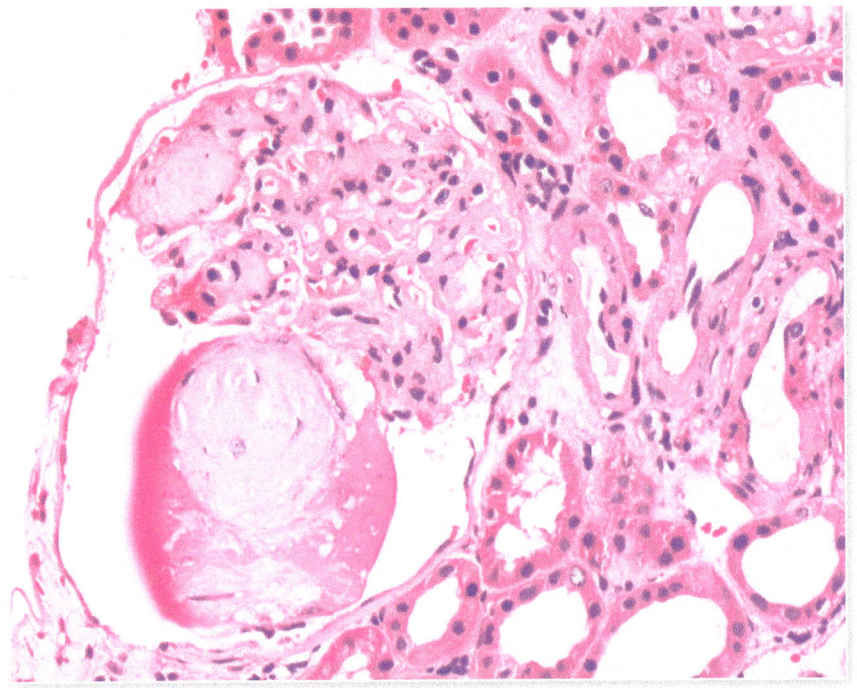

Figure 6.1: Diabetic diffuse intercapillary and nodular glomerulosclerosis with capillary microaneurysm (H & E x 200)

Diabetic Nephropathy

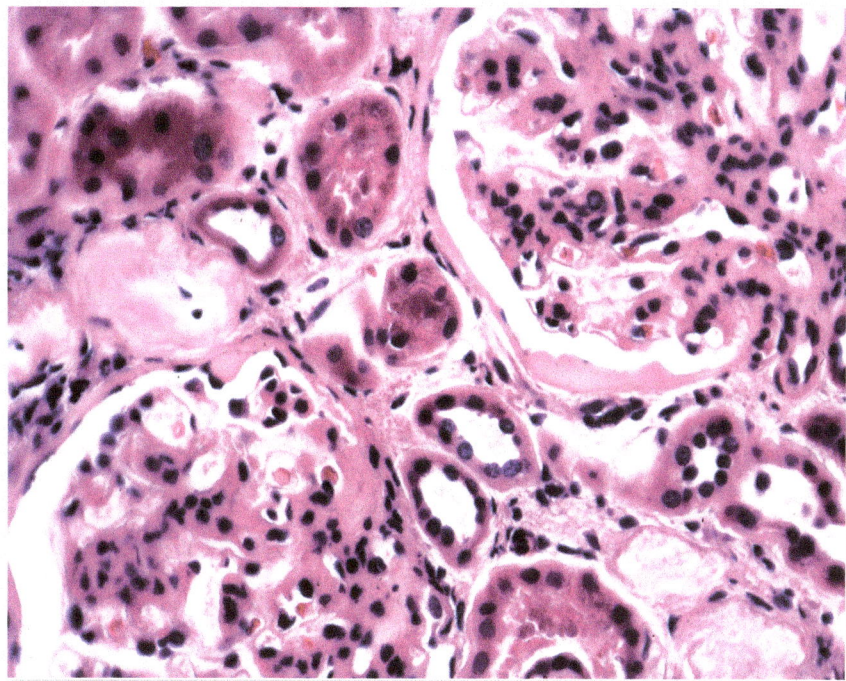

Figure 6.2: Diffuse intercapillary diabetic glomerulosclerosis with capsular drop and hyaline afferent and efferent arteriolosclerosis (H & E x 200)

Electron Microscopy

Diffuse thickening of GBM including the lamina densa and increase in mesangial matrix are characteristic features.[5]

GLOMERULAR CLASSIFICATION OF DIABETIC NEPHROPATHY

Glomerular classification of diabetic nephropathy[4] is a consensus classification developed by international experts for the Renal Pathology Society (RPS) applicable to both type I and type II diabetes mellitus. This consists of four progressive classes, based on glomerular lesions with separate evaluation for interstitial and vascular lesions and good interobserver reproducibility, as follows:

- Class I: Mild or nonspecific LM changes and EM-proven GBM thickening
- Class IIa: Mild mesangial expansion (>25% of mesangial area)
- Class IIb: Severe mesangial expansion (>25% of mesangial area)
- Class III: Nodular sclerosis (with Kimmelstiel-Wilson's lesions)
- Class IV: Advanced diabetic glomerulosclerosis (with global glomerulosclerosis in >50% of glomeruli).

Class I: Isolated GBM thickening, assesed by electron microscopy (EM) as >395 nm in female and >430 nm in male individuals, 9 years of age and older is characteristic of early DN and increases with duration of disease. Direct measurements of GBM width on EM are currently computer assisted or alternatively, orthogonal grid intercepts can be placed over photomicrographs for this purpose with cut off values optimized in the laboratory for children and adults.[5,6] This feature can be associated with mild or nonspecific ischemic type changes by LM without significant mesangial matrix expansion or K-W lesions in this category.

Class II: Mesangial expansion as defined by an increase in extracellular material in the mesangium such that the width of the interspace exceeds two mesangial cell nuclei in at least two glomerular lobules.

Class IIa: Mild mesangial expansion: The expanded mesangial area is smaller than the mean area of a capillary lumen in >25% of the total mesangium in this category.

Class IIb: Severe mesangial expansion: The expanded mesangial area is larger than the mean area of a capillary lumen in >25% of the total mesangium in this class, as it restricts the glomerular capillaries and reduces the capillary filtration area. K-W lesions and >50% globally sclerosed lesions are not present in this category.

Class III: Nodular sclerosis: In this category, at least one Kimmelstiel-Wilson lesion is found, within the expanded mesangium, associated with a longer duration of diabetes and severe retinopathy[3] and higher serum creatinine level. Microvascular injury leads to detachment of endothelial cells from the GBM and mesangiolysis with disruption of its attachment to the GBM. This precedes the formation of the KW nodules consisting of compacted matrix with collagen fibrils, small lipid particles and cellular debris.[1,4]

Class IV: Advanced diabetic glomerulosclerosis: There are >50% globally sclerosed glomeruli and clinical or pathological evidence attributable to DN in this category. This is the end-stage of multifactorial factors with advanced glycation end products formed by glycosylation of collagen, mesangial matrix and GBM proteins. Extracellular matrix proteins (Collagen types I, III, IV and fibronectin) are increasingly deposited in the mesangium from class II to III onwards.[7-14] Arteriolar hyalinosis or the "capsular drop" are evidence of DN as also the presence of retinopathy as clinical evidence.

This glomerular classification of diabetic nephropathy has been tested in a study by the international RPS experts that can be validated in larger representative Indian or Asian cohorts. A recent validation study of this classification showed a 5-year renal survival rate of diabetic nephropathy as 100.0% in Classes I and IIa, 75.0% in Class IIb, 66.7% in Class III, and 38.1% in Class IV [p = 0.002].[15]

Tubulointerstitial Lesions[1] and Vascular Lesions

Tubular basement membrane thickening of non-atrophic tubules increases in severity with class III and class IV glomerular lesions and are accentuated on the PAS and JMS stains. Interstitial fibrosis and tubular atrophy (IF/TA) are scored together as a percentage of the total involved area of the renal cortex. The scoring system is based on the intensity of interstitial mononuclear cell infiltrates (T1 <25%, T2 25–50%) comprising T lymphocytes and macrophages. Severity of glomerular and interstitial lesions could be independent factors in the progression of DN and are closely inter-linked to the prognosis.[1] Multivariate analysis of glomerular and extraglomerular lesions in another cohort, utilizing the scoring system of Tervaert, et al.[4] with a mean follow-up of 59 months, has shown that interstitial fibrosis/tubular atrophy was the only significant predictor of renal survival.[16]

Vascular Lesions[17]

The extent of arterial hyalinosis correlates with urinary albumin excretion and disease progression. Increase in vascular lesions such as, arteriosclerosis with intimal fibroplasia involving larger arteries is associated with severe glomerulosclerosis. The ratio of intimal matrix to media increases with microalbuminuria.[17] The thickness of the intima of the most severely involved artery, proportionate to the media (either less than or/greater than the latter) is scored as suggested in the criteria.[4]

Differential Diagnosis

1. *Hypertensive nephropathy* is characterized by diffuse intercapillary sclerosis, associated with ischemic atrophy and hyaline afferent arteriolosclerosis and can concomitantly occur with DN K-W nodular lesions are not seen with isolated hypertensive nephrosclerosis.
2. *Light chain deposition disease* is associated with nodular glomerulosclerosis with uniformity of size of the nodules within each glomerulus, with greater glomerular cellularity and lesser degree of diffuse or marked capillary wall thickening than DN.
3. *Nodular amyloidosis*: The nodules are congophilic and stain for amyloid with ThioflavinT and are PAS/JMS negative.
4. *MPGN* with nodular sclerosis is associated with circumferential reduplication of capillary walls and immune deposits on IF and EM.

Non-diabetic Glomerular Lesions

Renal biopsy is indicated in diabetics with onset of proteinuria without retinopathy, renal failure without proteinuria, sudden onset of nephrotic syndrome, rapid decline of GFR or persistent gross and microhematuria, to confirm the presence of concomitant non-diabetic renal disease.[2,18-20] In our experience, 72% of non-diabetic renal lesions (NDRD) were associated with non-insulin dependent diabetes mellitus.[2] The commonest glomerular lesions were proliferative glomerulo nephritis (48%), FSGS (23%), membranous nephropathy (9.2%), in our case series. Membranousnephropathy (23.2%), IgA nephropathy (20.3%) and PIGN (20.9%) predominated in multi-center western cohorts.[19]

Other parenchymal lesions include concomitant acute/chronic interstitial nephritis, renal papillary necrosis associated with urinary tract obstruction and the Armanni-Ebstein lesion with glycogen deposition in the straight segment of the proximal tubule, now rarely seen with adequate glycemic control.

REFERENCES

1. Fioretto P, Mauer M. Histopathology of diabetic nephropathy. Seminars in Nephrology. 2007;27:195-207.
2. Narasimhan B, Chacko B, John GT, Korula A, Kirubakaran MG, Jacob CK. Characterization of kidney lesions in Indian adults: towards a renal biopsy registry. J Nephrol. 2006;19:205-10.
3. Mak SK, Gwi E, Chan KW, Wong PN, Lo KY, Lee KF, et al. Clinical predictors of non-diabetic renal disease in patients with non-insulin dependent diabetes mellitus. Nephrol Dial Transplant. 1997;12:2588-91.

4. Tervaert TWC, Mooyaart AL, et al. Pathological classification of diabetic nephropathy. J Am Soc Nephrol. 2010;21: 556-63.
5. Haas M. Alport syndrome and thin glomerular basement membrane nephropathy: a practical approach to diagnosis. Arch Pathol Lab Med. 2009;133:224-32.
6. Dische FE. Measurement of glomerular basement membrane thickness and its application to the diagnosis of thin-membrane nephropathy. Arch Pathol Lab Med. 1992;116:43-9.
7. Fioretto P, Mauer M, Brocco E, Velussi M, Frigato F, Muollo B, et al. Patterns of renal injury in NIDDM patients with microalbuminuria. Diabetologia. 1996;39:1569-76.
8. Najafian B, Caramori ML, Mauer M, et al. Clustering of type 1 and type 2 diabetic patients based on diabetic nephropathy structural-functional relationships. J Am Soc Nephrol. 2005;16:679A.
9. Mauer SM, Steffes MW, Ellis EN, Sutherland DE, Brown DM, Goetz FC: Structural-functional relationships in diabetic nephropathy. J Clin Invest. 1984;74:1143-55.
10. Perrin NE, Torbjornsdotter TB, Jaremko GA, Berg UB: The course of diabetic glomerulopathy in patients with type I diabetes: a 6-year follow-up with serial biopsies. Kidney Int. 2006;69:699-705.
11. Stout LC, Kumar S, Whorton EB: Focal mesangiolysis and the pathogenesis of the Kimmelstiel–Wilson nodule. Hum Pathol. 1993;24:77-89.
12. Bangstad HJ, Osterby R, Dahl-Jorgensen K, Berg KJ, Hartmann A, Hanssen KF. Improvement of blood glucose control in IDDM patients retards the progression of morphological changes in early diabetic nephropathy Diabetologia. 1994;37:483-90.
13. Nishi S, Ueno M, Hisaki S, Iino N, Iguchi S, Oyama Y, et al. Ultrastructural characteristics of diabetic nephropathy. Med Electron Microsc. 2000;33:65-73.
14. Qian Y, Feldman E, Pennathur S, Kretzler M, Brosius FC III. From fibrosis to sclerosis: mechanisms of glomerulosclerosis in diabetic nephropathy. Diabetes. 2008;57:1439-45.
15. Oh SW, Kim S, Na KY, Chae DW, Kim S, Jin DC, et al. Clinical implications of pathologic diagnosis and classification for diabetic nephropathy). Diabetes Res Clin Pract. 2012;97(3):418-24.
16. Okada T, Nagao T, Matsumoto H, Nagaoka Y, Wada T, Nakao T. Histological predictors for renal prognosis in diabetic nephropathy in diabetes mellitus type 2 patients with overt proteinuria. Nephrology (Carlton). 2012;17(1):68-75.
17. Osterby R, Asplund J, Bangstad HJ, Nyberg G, Rudberg S, Viberti GC, et al. Neovascularization at the vascular pole region in diabetic glomerulopathy. Nephrol Dial Transplant. 1999;14:348-52.
18. John GT, Date A, Korula A, Jeyaseelan L, Shastry JCM, Jacob CK. Nondiabetic renal disease in noninsulin-dependent diabetics in a South Indian Hospital. Nephron. 1994;67:441-3.
19. Mazzucco G, Bertani T, Fortunato M, Bernardi M, Leutner M, Boldorini R, et al. Different patterns of renal damage in type 2 diabetes mellitus; a multicentric study on 393 biopsies. Am J Kidney Dis. 2002;39:713-20.
20. Soni S, Gowrishankar S, et al. Non-diabetic renal disease in type 2 diabetes mellitus. Nephrology. 2006;11(6):533-7.

CHAPTER 7

Systemic and Renal Limited Vasculitides

ABSTRACT

This chapter comprehensively classifies and elucidates the various forms of ANCA-mediated renal limited and systemic vasculitis including granulomatous polyangiitis (Wegener's granulomatosis), microscopic polyangiitis, Churg-Strauss disease and pauci-immune crescentic and necrotizing glomerulonephritis.

The new histopathologic classification of pauci-immune ANCA-mediated renal vasculitis,[15] proposed by AE Berden and Ingeborg Bajema of the International Working Group of Renal Pathologists (IWGRP) comprising four morphologic categories in a renal biopsy as validated in our medical center is the major feature of this chapter. The course and prognosis and correlation of the estimated Glomerular Filtration rate (eGFR) at the onset and follow-up at 1 year with independent predictors of outcome are highlights from a recent study of 135 cases of renal vasculitis.

The large and medium vessel vasculitides are also mentioned as lesions that are rarely encountered in a renal biopsy. The former include giant cell arteritis and Takayasu arteritis and the latter, polyarteritis nodosa and kawasaki disease.

INTRODUCTION

Vasculitis is a systemic disease defined by mural inflammation with necrosis of blood vessels, that can be restricted to certain organs as in the renal limited form. The major categories of non-infectious vasculitis can involve large, medium and small caliber blood vessels.[1,2] The major forms of primary systemic renal vasculitides reported in a renal biopsy, involve small blood vessels including glomerular capillaries comprising mainly Wegener's granulomatosis (Granulomatous polyangiitis/GPA), microscopic polyangiitis and Churg-Strauss disease.[3,4] These lesions are associated with antineutrophilic cytoplasmic autoantibodies (ANCA) in 90% of cases to target antigens in the primary granules of neutrophils and lysosomal granules of monocytes. Neutrophils and monocytes that are activated by ANCA interact with endothelial cells via adhesion molecules and release toxic factors including oxidants causing apoptosis and necrosis.[5,6] Activated T cells and macrophages augment this response with granuloma formation in GPA.[7,8]

Pauci-immune crescentic and necrotizing glomerulonephritis is a renal limited form of ANCA-associated vasculitis with a paucity of staining for immunoglobulins and complement on immunofluorescence, and associated with rapidly progressive renal failure. About 10–30% of these cases are ANCA negative associated with more severe and chronic glomerular lesions.

Major Categories of Non-infectious Vasculitis[1]

LARGE VESSEL VASCULITIS

- Giant cell arteritis
- Takayasu's arteritis.

MEDIUM-SIZED VESSEL VASCULITIS

- Polyarteritis nodosa
- Kawasaki disease
- Primary granulomatous central nervous system vasculitis.

SMALL VESSEL VASCULITIS

- ANCA-associated small vessel vasculitis
  - Wegener's granulomatosis
  - Microscopic polyangiitis
  - Churg-Strauss syndrome
  - Drug-induced ANCA-associated vasculitis.
- Immune-complex small vessel vasculitis
  - Henoch-Schonlein purpura
  - Cryoglobulinemic vasculitis
  - Lupus vasculitis
  - Rheumatoid vasculitis
  - Sjogren's syndrome vasculitis
  - Hypocomplementemic vasculitis
  - Behcet's disease
  - Goodpasture's syndrome
  - Serum sickness vasculitis
  - Drug-induced immune complex vasculitis
  - Infection-induced immune complex vasculitis.
- Paraneoplastic small vessel vasculitis
- Inflammatory bowel disease vasculitis

ANCA-associated Small Vessel Vasculitis

Wegener's Granulomatosis (Granulomatous Polyangiitis—GPA) involves the upper and lower respiratory tracts in 95% of cases with granulomatous inflammation and necrotizing vasculitis with focal segmental necrotizing glomerulonephritis in 70–80% cases. The majority are associated with cytoplasmic anti-PR3 ANCA (c ANCA) on indirect immunofluorescence.[9,10]

Microscopic Features[11,12]

Light Microscopy (Figs 7.1 to 7.8)

- Focal segmental fibrinoid necrosis with lysis of mesangial cells and matrix/glomerular capillary walls with eosinophilic, fibrin-rich material

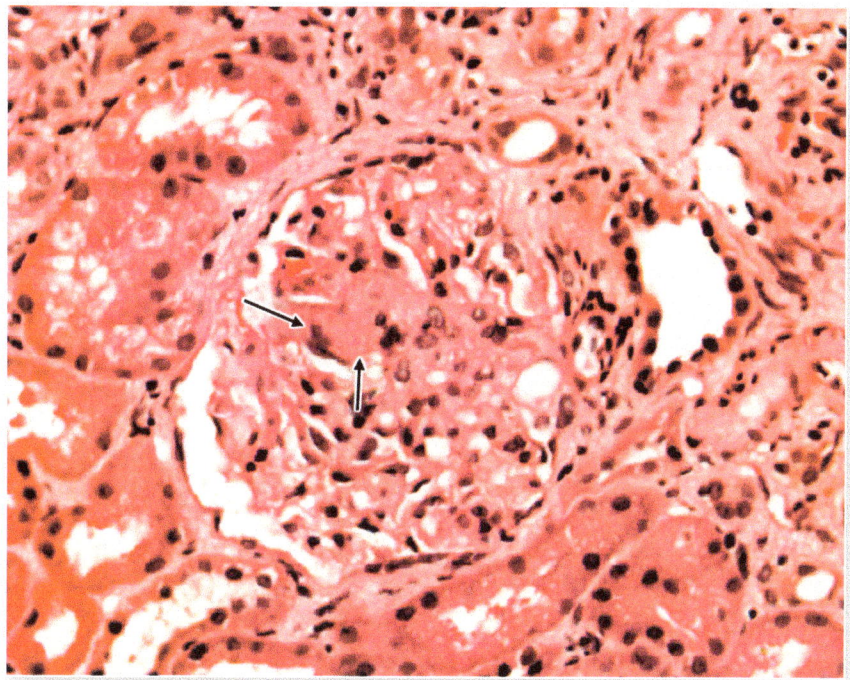
Figure 7.1: Focal segmental necrotizing glomerulonephritis (arrow) (H & E x 400)

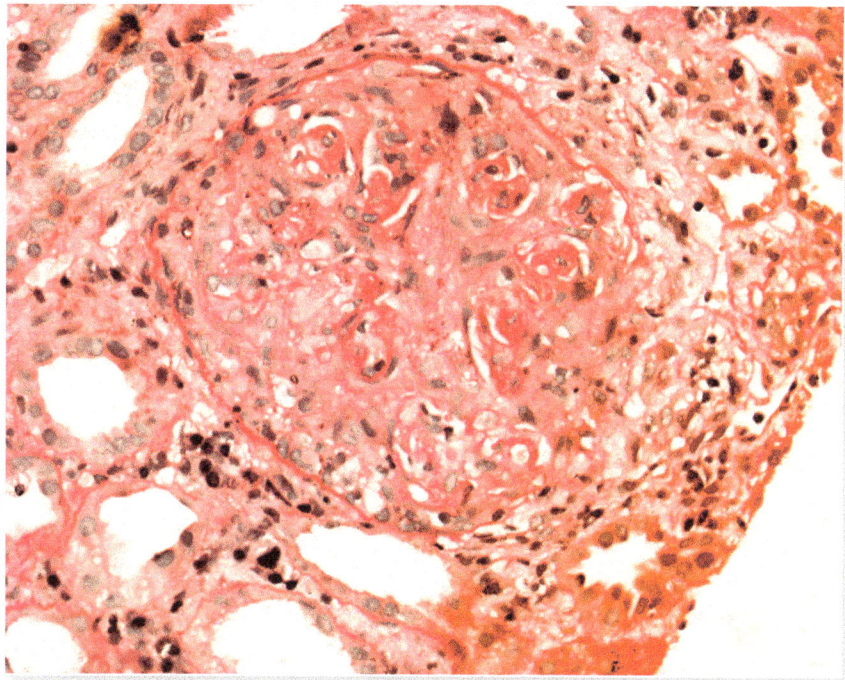
Figure 7.2: Fibrocellular crescent (PAS x 400)

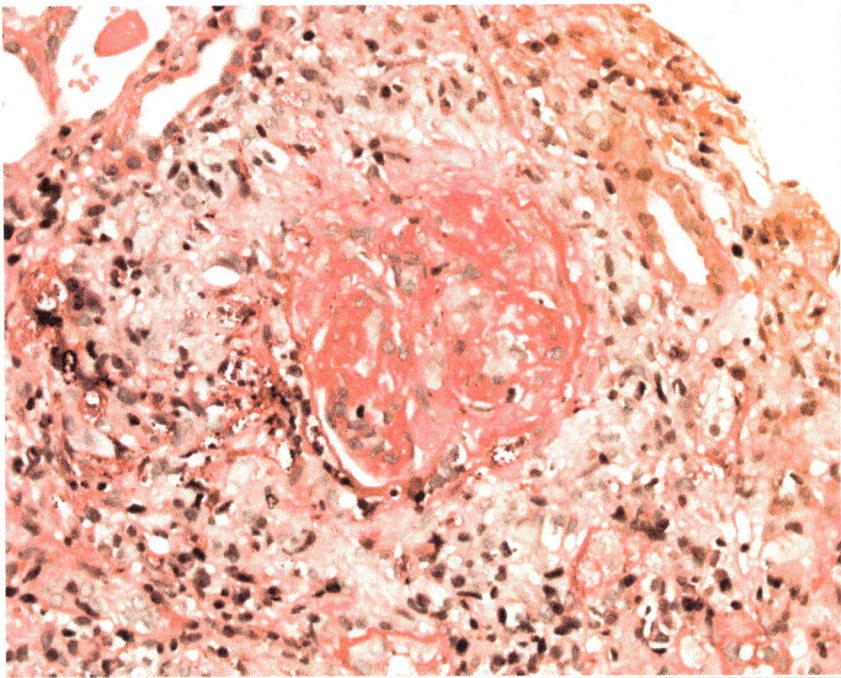

Figure 7.3: Focal segmental proliferative and necrotizing glomerulonephritis with periglomerular granuloma (PAS x 400)

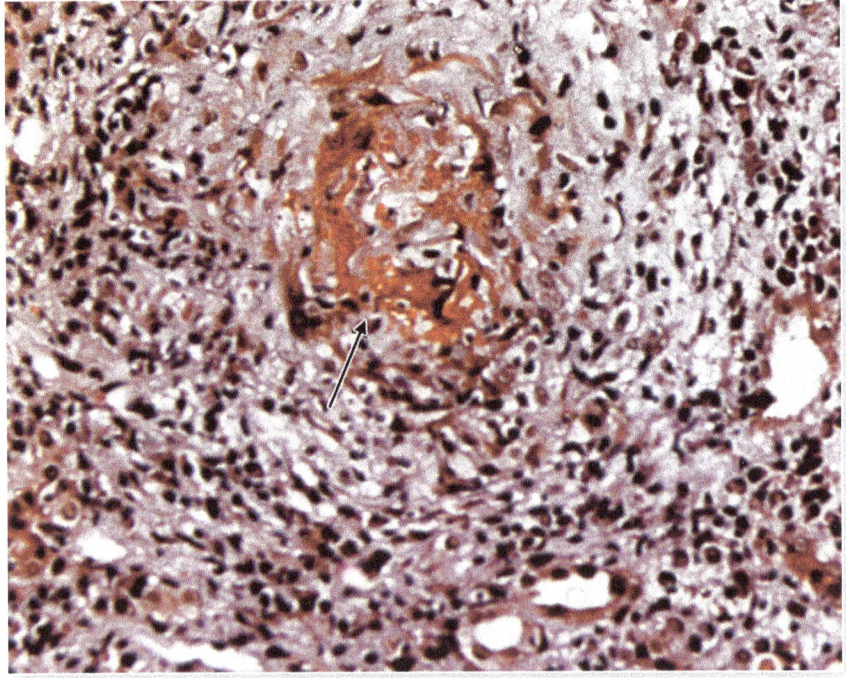

Figure 7.4: Fibrinoid glomerular tuft necrosis (Masson trichrome x 400)

Systemic and Renal Limited Vasculitides

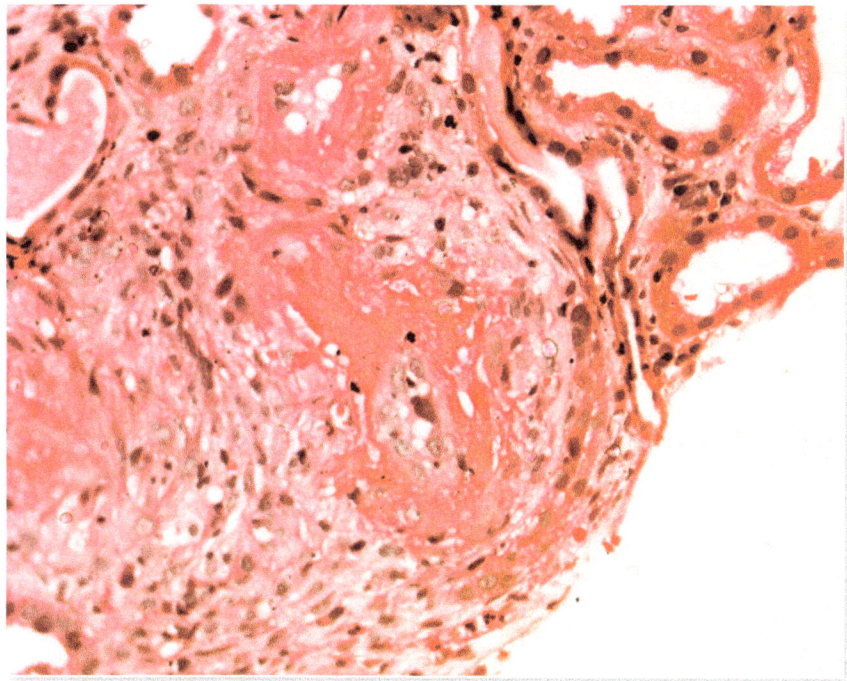

Figure 7.5: Fibrinoid necrosis of interlobular artery (H & E x 400)

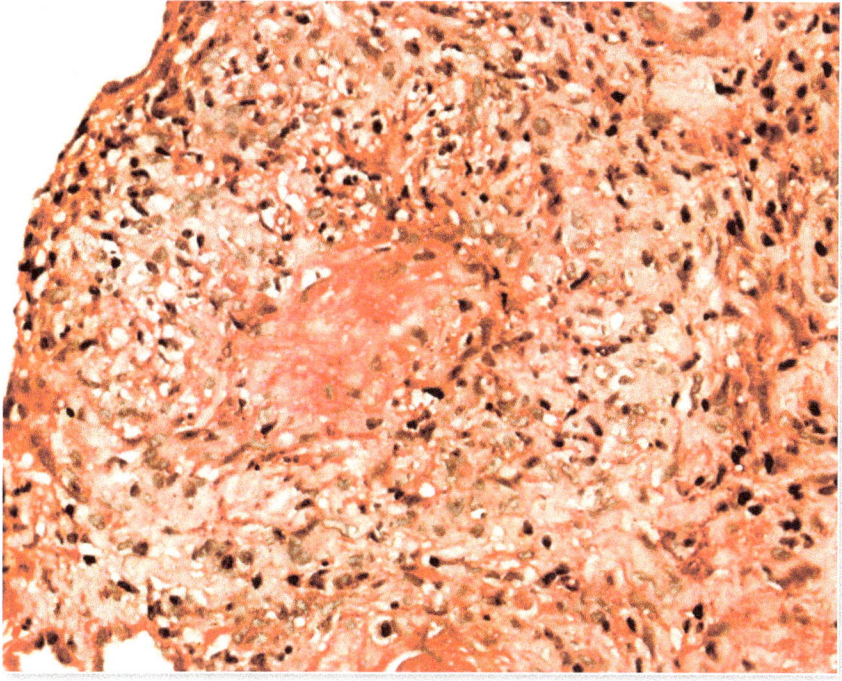

Figure 7.6: Perivascular granuloma (H & E x 400)

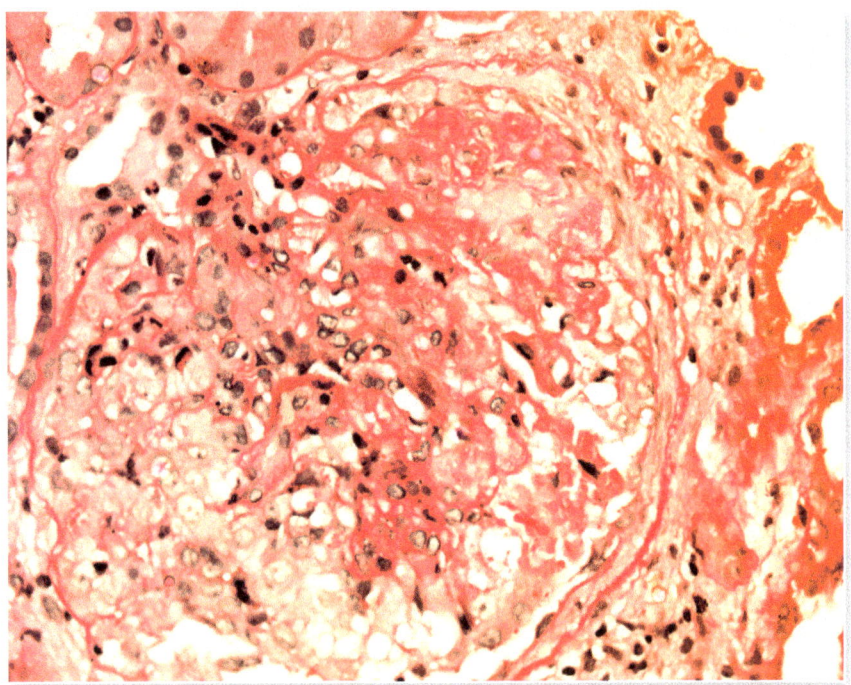

Figure 7.7: Focal segmental proliferative and sclerosing glomerulonephritis (PAS x 400)

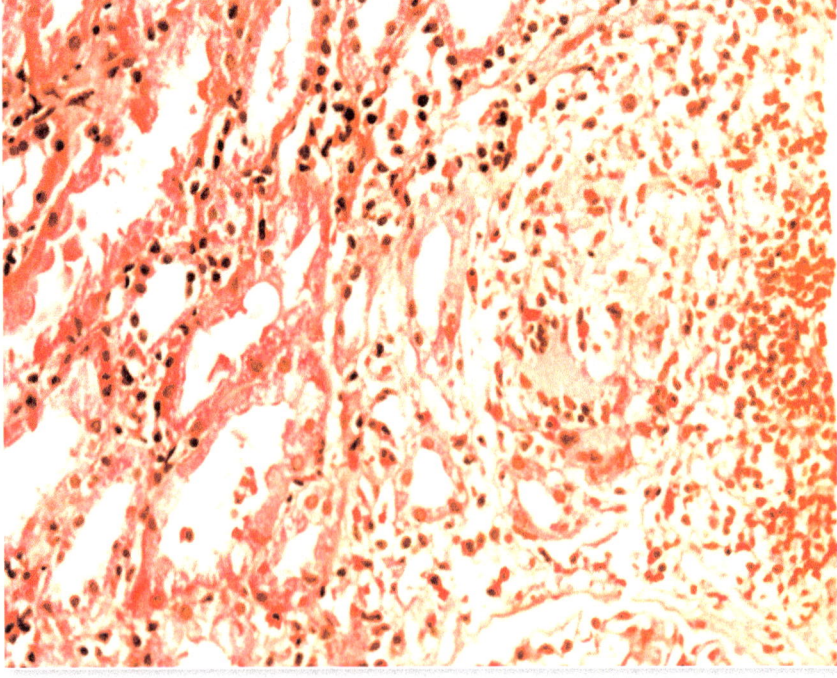

Figure 7.8: Interstitial granulomas with eosinophilia in Churg-Strauss disease (H & E x 400)

Systemic and Renal Limited Vasculitides

- Accentuated with trichrome stains on serial sections and Jones stains
- Neutrophilic infiltrates with leukocytoclasia and karyorrhectic nuclear fragments
- Cellular crescents found in 90% of cases in the acute phase
- Disruption of Bowman's capsule with periglomerular granulomata
- Interstitial granulomata centered around necrotic arterioles, specific for GPA
- Advanced fibrocellular crescents display alignment of epithelial cells: "tubularization"
- Segmental and global sclerosis with capsular synechiae and fibrosis in chronic phase
- Arteriolitis, arteritis (of interlobular arteries) and leukocytoclastic medullary angiitis in 10-20% cases
- Acute fibrinoid necrosis of these extraglomerular blood vessels with mural infiltrates of neutrophils, karyorrhectic nuclear fragments and occasional eosinophils and mononuclear cells
- Mural fibrosis and perivascular scarring are seen as chronic sequelae
- Associated tubulitis with leukocytes in tubular lumina in cortex and medulla.

Immunofluorescence

Focal deposits of C3 (1) to (2+) or negative staining in intact segments of glomerular tufts.

Electron Microscopy

- Focal endothelial necrosis with subendothelial fibrin deposits in early lesions
- Rupture of GBM and Bowman's capsule and associated electron dense fibrin tactoids with angular edges.

Microscopic polyangiitis (MPA): Displays similar microscopic features to GPA except for interstitial granulomas that are usually absent. Necrotizing glomerulonephritis (in 75-95%), pulmonary hemorrhage (10-15%) and mononeuritis multiplex (60-70%) are concomitant features. The majority are associated with perinuclear anti-myeloperoxidase ANCA (pANCA) on indirect immunofluorescence.[13]

Churg-Strauss disease (Eosinophilic granulomatosis with polyangiitis—EGPA): Differs from GPA and MPA by the association with severe allergic rhinitis and bronchial asthma and eosinophilia. There is a prodromal phase followed by eosinophilic pneumonia and vasculitic phase associated with a milder form of glomerulonephritis including crescents and eosinophilic interstitial infiltrates and granulomas. Pulmonary, neural and cutaneous involvement are more common with perinuclear pANCA positivity in the majority of cases.[14]

The new histopathologic classification of pauci-immune ANCA-mediated renal vasculitis,[15] proposed by AE Berden and Ingeborg Bajema of the International Working Group of Renal Pathologists (IWGRP) comprises four morphologic categories in a renal biopsy that is of prognostic value correlating with the outcome at 1year and 5 years follow-up. The baseline GFR and diagnostic category were independent predictors of outcome, utilizing this morphological classification.

IWGRP Classification of Renal ANCA-mediated Vasculitis

- Focal: ≥50% normal glomeruli (glomeruli without evidence of necrotizing vasculitic lesions)
- Crescentic: ≥50% glomeruli with cellular crescents

- Sclerotic: ≥50% globally sclerotic glomeruli
- Mixed: <50% normal glomeruli, <50% crescentic, <50% globally sclerotic glomeruli.

In this classification, the "focal" category contains predominantly normal glomeruli, while the "crescentic" type predominantly has cellular crescents, the "sclerotic" comprises advanced sclerotic lesions and the "mixed type" contains an admixture of the above in a renal biopsy.

Course and Prognosis

The focal lesions showed mild impairment of renal function when compared to the crescentic form that had markedly reduced renal function at onset with recovery on follow up and mixed lesions had an intermediate outcome whereas sclerotic lesions had the highest risk and poor survival. Validation studies of this classification from Chinese, US and Japanese cohorts showed similar results.[16-18]

In our recent study of 135 cases of biopsy proven cases of renal vasculitis, there were 107 cases of ANCA mediated vasculitis from CMC, Vellore (retrieved from March 2001 to March 2010) with a preponderance of the mixed category (55%) followed by crescentic (30%), focal (9%) and sclerotic (6%) respectively. Multiple linear regression analysis confirmed that interstitial fibrosis and the new classification (IWGRP) correlated with eGFR at presentation and the independent predictors of outcome were eGFR at entry and morphological subtype with statistical significance on 1 year follow up. The crescentic category showed active lesions and severely reduced renal function at entry but the highest increment of eGFR from the baseline at 1 year of follow up and the mixed subtype attained the highest GFR within a year. The focal and crescentic forms had a similar rate of recovery of renal function while the sclerotic category showed a progressive decrement of eGFR in 1 year.

LARGE VESSEL VASCULITIS[19-22]

Giant cell arteritis involves the temporal artery and major branches of the aorta in patients older than 50 years with polymyalgia rheumatica. The renal artery is rarely involved with stenotic lesions with ischemic cortical atrophy. Arcuate artery involvement is associated with intimal fibrosis with fragmentation of internal elastic lamina and infiltration by macrophages and occasional giant cells.

Takayasu arteritis mainly involves the aorta and major branches with granulomatous infiltrates with fragmentation of the medial elastica and segmental stenosis in females less than 50 years of age and renal hypertensive nephrosclerosis or ischemic cortical atrophy may occur.

MEDIUM-SIZED VESSEL VASCULITIS[22-24]

Polyarteritis Nodosa

It is a necrotizing arteritis of medium size arteries and small arteries without glomerulonephritis or involvement of arterioles, capillaries or venules. Arcuate and interlobar arteries are frequently involved by pseudoaneurysms with thrombosis, and associated infarction and hemorrhage.

Kawasaki disease

It involves medium size and small arteries and chiefly the coronary arteries with pseudoaneurysms and thrombosis. The mucocutaneous lymph node syndrome is the pathognomonic feature with a polymorphous erythematous rash, including the oropharyngeal mucosa and a concomitant non-suppurative lymphadenopathy. Renal interlobar and arcuate arterial involvement is less common with segmental inflammation, edema and infrequent fibrinoid necrosis.

REFERENCES

1. Jennette JC, Falk RJ. Small-vessel vasculitis. N Engl J Med.1997;337(21):1512-23.
2. Jennette JC, Falk RJ, Andrassy K, Bacon PA, Churg J, Gross WL, et al. Nomenclature of systemic vasculitides. Proposal of an international consensus conference. Arthritis Rheum.1994;37(2):187-92.
3. John R, Herzenberg AM. Vasculitis affecting the kidney. Semin Diagn Pathol. 2009;26(2):89-102.
4. Cohen BA, Clark WF. Pauci-immune renal vasculitis: natural history, prognostic factors, and impact of therapy. Am J Kidney Dis. 2000;36(5):914-24.
5. Jennette JC, Falk RJ. Pathogenesis of the vascular and glomerular damage in ANCA-positive vasculitis. Nephrol. Dial. Transplant. 1998;13 Suppl 1:16-20.
6. Jennette JC, Xiao H, Falk RJ. Pathogenesis of vascular inflammation by anti-neutrophil cytoplasmic antibodies. J Am Soc Nephrol. 2006;17(5):1235-42.
7. Hrusková Z, Marecková H, Ríhová Z, Rysavá R, Jancová E, Merta M, et al. T cells in the pathogenesis of ANCA-associated vasculitis: current knowledge. Folia Biol. (Praha). 2008;54(3):81-7.
8. Hua F, Wilde B, Dolff S, Witzke O. T-lymphocytes and disease mechanisms in Wegener's granulomatosis. Kidney Blood Press. Res. 2009;32(6):389-98.
9. Woywodt A, Haubitz M, Haller H, Matteson EL. Wegener's granulomatosis. Lancet. 2006;367(9519):1362-6.
10. Khasnis A, Langford CA. Update on vasculitis. J. Allergy Clin Immunol. 2009;123(6):1226-36.
11. Hauer HA, Bajema IM, de Heer E, Hermans J, Hagen EC, Bruijn JA. Distribution of renal lesions in idiopathic systemic vasculitis: a three-dimensional analysis of 87 glomeruli. Am J Kidney Dis. 2000;36(2):257-65.
12. D'Amico G, Sinico RA, Ferrario F. Renal vasculitis. Nephrol Dial Transplant.1996;11 (Suppl):9:69-74.
13. Guillevin L, Durand-Gasselin B, Cevallos R, Gayraud M, Lhote F, Callard P, et al. Microscopic polyangiitis: clinical and laboratory findings in eighty-five patients. Arthritis Rheum. 1999;42(3):421-30.
14. Noth I, Strek ME, Leff AR. Churg-Strauss syndrome. Lancet. 2003;361(9357):587-94.
15. Berden AE, Ferrario F, Hagen EC, Jayne DR, Jennette JC, Joh K, et al. Bajema IM. Histopathologic Classification of ANCA-Associated Glomerulonephritis. J Am Soc Nephrol. 2010:1-9.
16. Chang DY, Wu LH, Liu G, Chen M, Kallenberg CG, Zhao MH. Re-evaluation of the histopathologic classification of ANCA-associated glomerulonephritis: a study of 121 patients in a single center.Nephrol Dial Transplant. 2012;27(6):2343-9.
17. Ellis CL, Manno RL, Havill JP, Racusen LC, Geetha D. Validation of the new classification of pauci-immune glomerulonephritis in a United States cohort and its correlation with renal outcome. BMC Nephrology. 2013;14:210-6.
18. Iwakiri T, Fujimoto S, Kitagawa K, Furuichi K, Yamahana J, Matsuura Y, et al. Validation of a newly proposed histopathological classification in Japanese patients with anti-neutrophil cytoplasmic antibody-associated glomerulonephritis. BMC Nephrology. 2013;14:125-33.
19. Jennette JC, Falk RJ, Andrassy K, Bacon PA, Churg J, Gross WL, et al. Nomenclature of systemic vasculitides. Proposal of an international consensus conference. Arthritis Rheum.1994;37(2):187-92.
20. Gravanis MB. Giant cell arteritis and Takayasu aortitis: morphologic, pathogenetic and etiologic factors. Int J Cardiol. 2000;75:Suppl 1:S21-S33.
21. Johnston SL, Lock RJ, Gompels MM. Takayasu arteritis: a review. J Clin Pathol. 2002;55:481-6.
22. Weyand CM, Goronzy JJ. Medium and large–vessel vasculitis. N Engl J Med. 2003;349:160-9.
23. Ozen S, Ruperto N, Dillon MJ, Bagga A, Barron K, Davin JC, et al. EULAR/PReS endorsed consensus criteria for the classification of childhood vasculitides. Ann Rheum Dis. 2006;65:93-941.
24. Dillon MJ, Eleftherio D, Brogan PA. Medium vessel vasculitis. Pediatr Nephrol. 2010;25(9):1641-52.

HENOCH-SCHONLEIN PURPURA NEPHRITIS

It is an immune complex form of renal vasculitis presenting in children and adults in our recent study at CMC with an incidence of 12.6%. The classical tetrad of palpable purpura with polyarthralgia, abdominal pain and renal disease are usually present.

Microscopic Features[1-4]

- Focal proliferative GN as the most common type (in 52.9%)
- Mesangial proliferative GN (in 35.3%) (Fig. 7.9)
- Diffuse proliferative glomerulonephritis (in 5.9%)
- Focal segmental proliferative with segmental sclerosis and necrotizing crescentic glomerulonephritis (rarely).

Immunofluorescence

Dominant mesangial IgA deposits with less intense C3 deposits.

Course and Prognosis

Correlates with age, presenting clinical features and microscopic subtype. Adverse factors include older age, nephritic syndrome with gross hematuria and percentage of crescents of >50%, chronic lesions including glomerulosclerosis, tubulointerstitial scarring and extension of mesangial to dense subepithelial capillary wall deposits, with the risk of renal failure.[1-3,5]

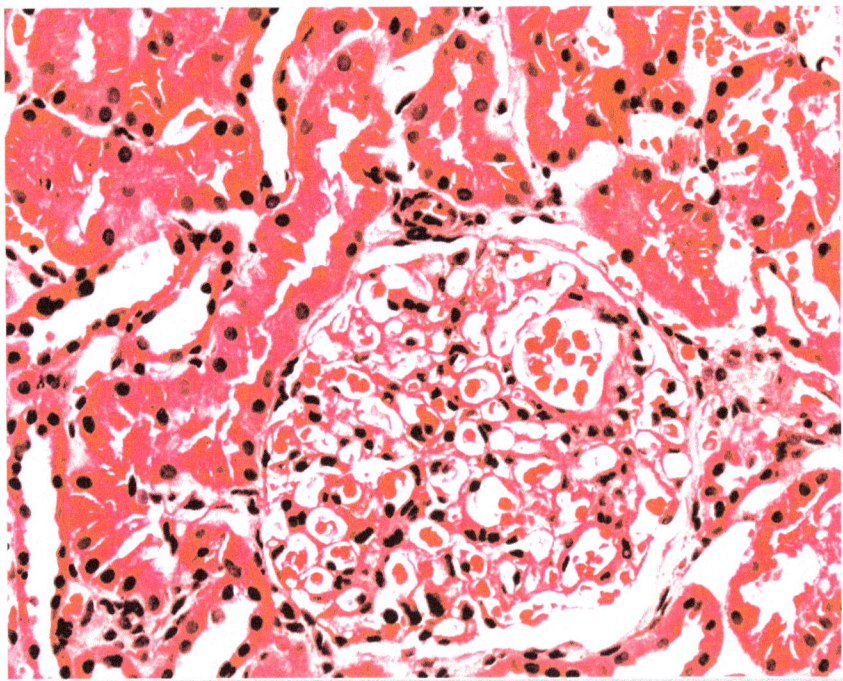

Figure 7.9: Mesangial proliferative glomerulonephritis in Henoch-Schonlein purpura nephritis (H & E x 400)

REFERENCES

1. Roberts PF, Waller TA, Brinker TM, Riffe IZ, Sayre JW, Bratton RL. Henoch-Schönlein purpura: a review article. South Med J. 2007;100(8):821-4.
2. Rai A, Nast C, Adler S. Henoch-Schönlein purpura nephritis. J Am Soc Nephrol. 1999;10(12):2637-44.
3. Szeto CC, Choi PC, To KF, et al. Grading of acute and chronic renal lesions in Henoch-Schönlein purpura. Mod Pathol. 2001;14(7):635-40.
4. Jauhola O, Ronkainen J, Koskimies O, Ala-Houhala M, Arikoski P, Holtta T, et al. Renal manifestations of Henoch-Schonlein purpura in a 6-month prospective study of 223 children. Arch Dis Child. 2010;95(11):877-82.
5. Pillebout E, Thervet E, Hill G, Alberti C, Vanhille P, Nochy D. Henoch-Schönlein purpura in adults: outcome and prognostic factors. J Am Soc Nephrol. 2002;13(5):1271-8.

CHAPTER 8

Anti-glomerular Basement Membrane Disease

> **ABSTRACT**
>
> The incidence of anti-glomerular basement membrane (GBM) in our medical center and the microscopic details of the typical glomerular lesions are concisely featured in this chapter. The pertinent differential diagnosis including other forms of crescentic glomerulonephritis, such as immune complex and pauci-immune vasculitic subtypes are mentioned together with collagen vascular diseases that can present with pulmonary–renal syndromes. The distinguishing aspects from necrotizing lesions of thrombotic microangiopathies, on immunofluorescence and electron microscopy are also highlighted. The coexisting ANCA-vasculitis that can occur concurrently is noted. The course and prognosis of the lesions and medical intervention required as well as the importance of serological testing for anti-GBM antibodies are alluded to for the benefit of clinical trainees in nephrology. Selected relevant references are included in their interests and for further information.

INTRODUCTION

Anti–glomerular basement membrane disease (anti-GBM) is a rare autoimmune disease comprising 6.7% of systemic vasculitis in our recent experience and includes renal limited anti-GBM glomerulonephritis, Goodpasture syndrome (with pulmonary and renal involvement) and anti-GBM pulmonary capillaritis, presenting with rapidly progressive renal failure and pulmonary hemorrhage. The most common target autoantigen is the non-collagenous domain 1 of α3 chain of type IV collagen with cross reactive autoantibodies to pulmonary capillary basement membrane in Goodpasture syndrome.[1-3]

ANTI-GBM GLOMERULONEPHRITIS

Microscopic Features[4,5]

- Focal segmental endocapillary proliferation with necrotizing lesions are seen
- Neutrophilic infiltrates in and around necrotic tufts and dissolution of capillary walls
- Disordered cellular crescents in >50% of glomeruli consisting of numerous macrophages and epithelial cells with occasional multinucleate giant cells
- Segmental to global scarring with fibrocellular to fibrous crescents (Fig. 8.1)
- Disruption of glomerular capillary walls and Bowman's capsule
- Periglomerular granulomas
- Interstitial edema with tubular necrosis and acute inflammatory cell infiltrates admixed with lymphocytes in acute phase
- Tubulointerstitial fibrosis and arteriosclerosis in chronic lesions.

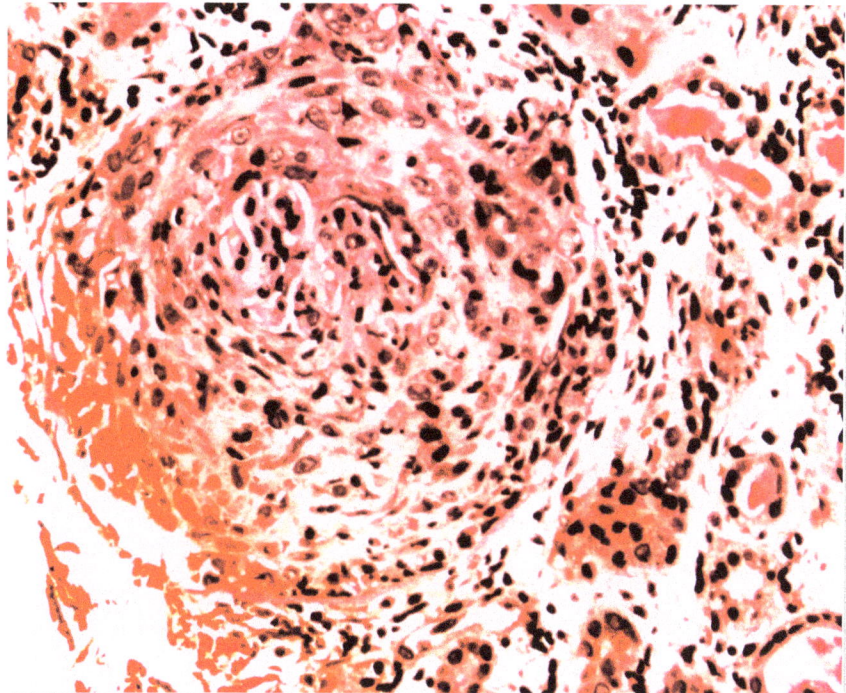

Figure 8.1: Circumferential fibrocellular crescent in anti-GBM disease (PAS × 400)

Immunofluorescence

Linear IgG deposits (3+) on glomerular capillary walls (Fig. 8.2).

Electron Microscopy

- Breaks in GBM and subendothelial lucent zones
- Absent immune complexes.

Differential Diagnosis[6]

1. *Immune complex crescentic GN* is distinguished from anti-GBM GN by glomerular hypercellularity and absence of fibrinoid tuft necrosis with orderly crescents and intact Bowman's capsule by light microscopy and distinct linear IgG deposits in the latter.
2. *Pauci-immune necrotizing and crescentic GN*: It can have similar features by light microscopy as anti-GBM crescentic GN and is differentiated by the IF features of the latter.
3. *Pulmonary-renal syndromes:* Including collagen vascular diseases, ANCA positive drug-induced vasculitis and thrombotic microangiopathies with similar microscopic features and require appropriate clinical correlation and laboratory investigation.[6]

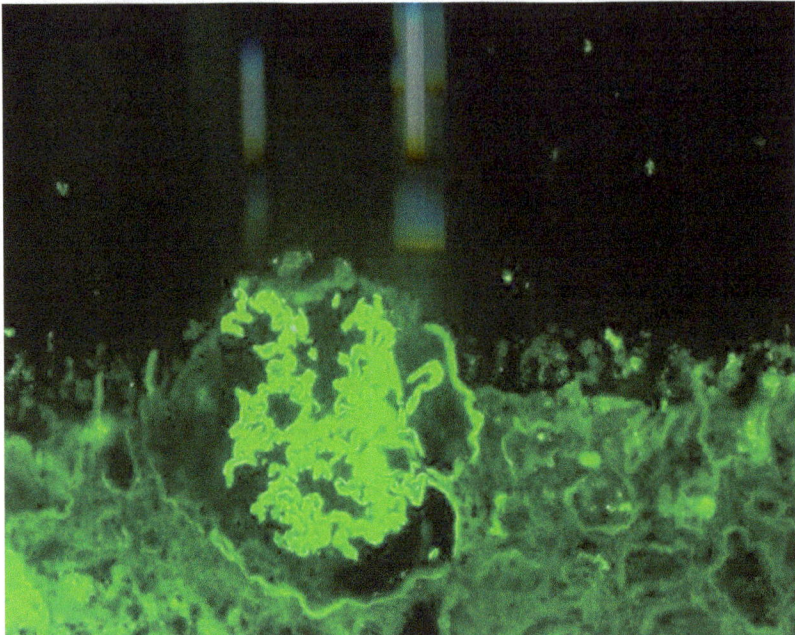

Figure 8.2: Linear IgG glomerular capillary wall deposits (IF × 400) in anti-GBM disease

Course and Prognosis

It is directly proportional to severity of renal failure, percentage of crescents and high titers of anti-glomerular basement membrane antibodies, requiring immediate intervention with high dose steroids, cytotoxic therapy, dialysis and plasmapheresis. **Concurrrent ANCA positive necrotizing small vessel vasculitis** of extraglomerular blood vessels can occur **in one-third of cases with a worse prognosis.**[7,8]

REFERENCES

1. Yang R, Hellmark T, Zhao J, Cui Z, Segelmark M, Zhao M, et al. Antigen and epitope specificity of anti-glomerular basement membrane antibodies in patients with Goodpasture disease with or without anti-neutrophil cytoplasmic antibodies. J Am Soc Nephrol. 2007;18(4):1338-43.
2. Cui Z, Zhao M-H. Advances in human anti-glomerular basement membrane disease. Nature Reviews Nephrology. 2011; 7: 697-705 doi:10.1038/nrneph.201.
3. OOI JD, Holdsworth SR, Kitching AR. Advances in the pathogenesis of Goodpasture's disease: From epitopes to autoantibodies to effector T cells. J Autoimm. 2008;31:295-301.
4. Jennette JC. Rapidly progressive crescentic glomerulonephritis. Kidney Int. 2003;63(3):1164-77.
5. Pusey CD. Anti-glomerular basement membrane disease. Kidney Int. 2003;64:1535-50 doi:10.1046/j.1523-1755.2003.00241.x.
6. Jara LJ, Vera-Lastra O, Calleja MC. Pulmonary-renal vasculitic disorders: differential diagnosis and management. Curr Rheumatol Rep. 2003;5(2):107-15.
7. Rutgers A, Slot M, van Paassen P, van Breda Vriesman P, Heeringa P, Tervaert JWC. Coexistence of anti-glomerular basement membrane antibodies and myeloperoxidase-ANCAs in crescentic glomerulonephritis. Am J Kidney Dis. 2005;46(2):253-62.
8. Kambham N. Crescentic glomerulonephritis: An update on Pauci-immune and anti-GBM diseases. Advances in Anatomic Pathology. 2012;19:111-24.

CHAPTER 9

Paraproteinemias/Dysproteinemias-associated Renal Disease

> **ABSTRACT**
>
> Monoclonal gammopathies of unknown significance (MGUS), multiple myeloma and Waldenstrom's macroglobulinemia are associated with heterogeneous renal lesions that are systematically elucidated in this chapter.
>
> Primary amyloidosis with deposition of monotypic light or rarely heavy chains have characteristic microscopic features that can be distinguished from secondary or uncommon hereditary forms of amyloid by immunohistochemical stains and by more advanced spectroscopic proteomic analysis of formalin fixed paraffin embedded material.
>
> Monoclonal immunoglobulin deposition disease consists of non-amyloidogenic congored negative deposits devoid of fibrillar or microtubular organized structure on electron microscopy.[1,2] Nodular glomerulosclerosis is the major feature that can be differentiated from similar lesions found in diabetic glomerulosclerosis and other glomerulopathies.
>
> Light chain cast nephropathy is also dealt with as a manifestation of myeloma and the pathognomonic features are clearly highlighted with illustrations. Light chain associated Fanconi syndrome is also mentioned together with course and prognosis of myeloma associated nephropathy.

INTRODUCTION

Plasma cell dyscrasias associated with paraproteinemias, such as monoclonal gammopathies of unknown significance (MGUS), multiple myeloma and Waldenstrom's macroglobulinemia can be associated with deposits of nephrotoxic light or heavy chain immunoglobulin deposits, with heterogeneous renal lesions as follows:
- Amyloidosis (Primary-AL or AH)
- Monoclonal immunoglobulin deposition disease (LCDD) light or heavy chain (HCDD)
- Light chain cast nephropathy (with acute tubulopathy and/or inflammatory tubulointerstitial nephritis).

AMYLOIDOSIS

Amyloidosis comprises disorders caused by misfolding of an amyloidogenic precursor protein and self-aggregation to generate protofilaments and form fibrils.[1,2] Amyloid fibrils have distinctive features on electron microscopy. Amyloid has a beta-pleated sheet configuration and ordered intercalation of Congo red dye into the fibrils produces the characteristic apple green birefringence under polarized light.[1] The incidence of amyloidosis in our case series was 1%.[3]

Primary amyloidosis (AL) is usually systemic and rarely localized, with extracellular deposition of fibrils, derived from immunoglobulin light chains, produced by clonal plasma cells. This category constitutes the major form (70–75%) of the disease in western countries, associated with multiple myeloma or B cell lymphoma or chronic lymphatic leukemia in 20% cases at presentation. In some cases, the plasma cell dyscrasia is detected 15 years after the diagnosis of amyloidosis is confirmed on a renal biopsy. In developing countries, the secondary form (Amyloid A), has to be excluded, which is composed of fragments derived from the acute phase reactant, serum amyloid A protein and commonly associated with chronic infections, granulomatous or autoimmune diseases. Hereditary forms of amyloidosis rarely involve the kidneys, and are derived from transthyretin (ATTR), apolipoprotein A-I and A-II (AApoAI and II) and other preamyloid fibrils such as lysozyme (ALys) and fibrinogen A (AFib), cystatin and gelsolin.[1,4] A rare and recently identified systemic form, known as as leukocyte cell-derived chemotaxin-2 (ALECT2) amyloidosis has been reported in Hispanics, Arabs and Punjabis.[5-9] The various forms of amyloid fibrils have been categorized and subtyped by laser microdissection and mass spectroscopic proteomic analysis as a recent and advanced technique on formalin fixed paraffin embedded tissue.[4] Beta-2 amyloidosis known as dialysis-related amyloidosis occurs in end-stage renal disease and involves mainly osteoarticular tissue. Senile systemic amyloidosis and localized amyloidosis do not involve the kidneys.[1]

Microscopic Features[1]

Light Microscopy

- Glomerular mesangial deposits of pale eosinophilic acellular deposits extending along capillary walls from the vascular pole (Fig. 9.1)

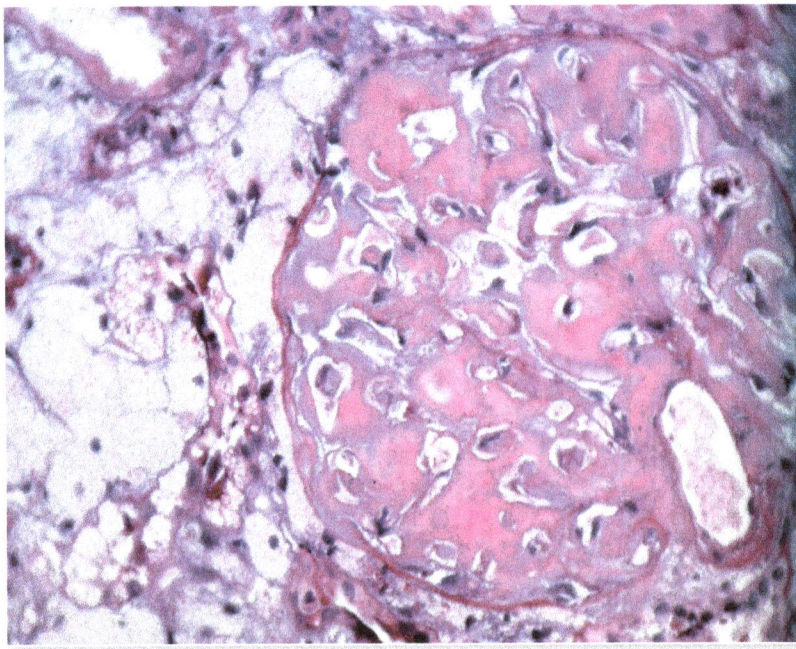

Figure 9.1: Renal amyloidosis (H & E 400X)

- Deposits are less eosinophilic than mesangial matrix or capillary basement membrane or Bowman's capsule
- Weakly periodic acid-Schiff (PAS) positive, pale blue on Masson trichrome and negative for Jones methenamine silver stain
- Segmental or diffuse mesangiocapillary to nodular or rarely predominantly perimembranous capillary wall deposits can occur
- Deposits are associated in foci with delicate spikes (cock's combs), on outer aspect
- Glomerular capillary luminal obliteration is seen in advanced global lesions
- Extraglomerular deposits are noted in walls of arterioles or interlobular arteries and interstitium.

Special Stains

- Congophilia in thick paraffin sections (8–10 microns thick) with apple green birefringence on polarized light is specific for amyloid (Fig. 9.2)
- Yellow fluorescence on the Thioflavin T stains is more sensitive and detects early deposits with UV light
- Red fluorescence with congo-red stain on UV light and a green filter.

Immunofluorescence

- Monoclonal light chain deposits in mesangium and capillary walls (kappa or lambda) is diagnostic of primary amyloidosis (AL) (Fig. 9.3)
- Heavy chain deposits are present in the uncommon AH type of primary amyloidosis.

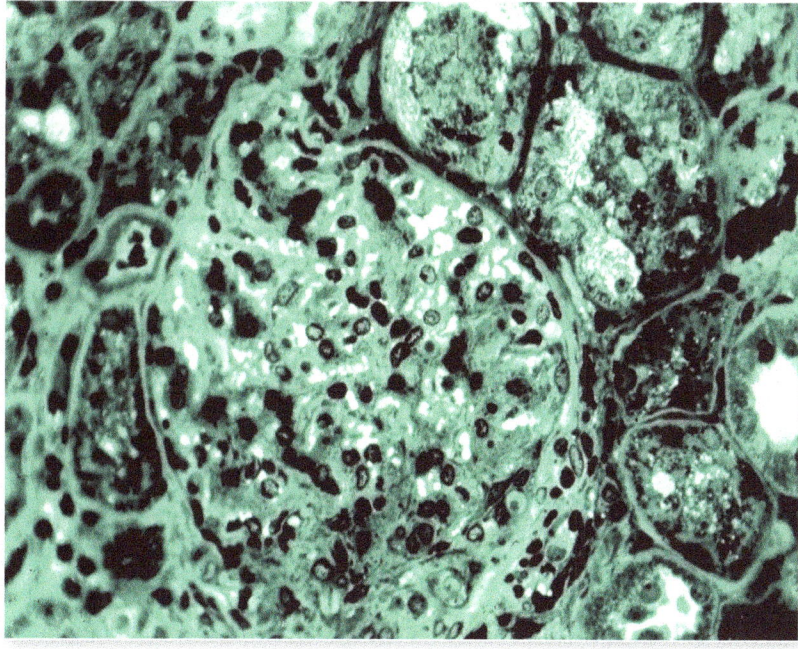

Figure 9.2: Glomerular amyloidosis (Congo red with polarizer X 250)

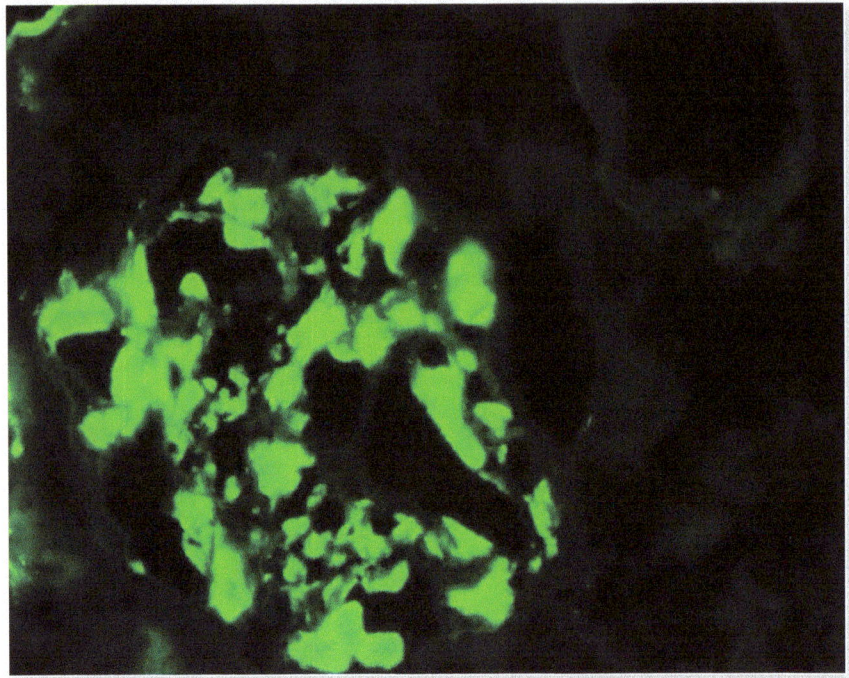

Figure 9.3: Mesangial lambda deposits in primary amyloidosis (IF x 400)

Electron Microscopy

Rigid, non-branching—fibrils 8–10 nm diameter (Fig. 9.4), randomly oriented, are found in the mesangium and focally in transmembranous location with parallel alignment extending into subepithelial region forming spikes and replacing lamina densa.

Differential Diagnosis[1]

1. *Diabetic glomerulosclerosis*: Intercapillary sclerotic material is intensely PAS and JMS positive and usually spares the peripheral capillary walls. The latter are dilated and are patent until the advanced stage when they are obliterated by the sclerotic matrix.
2. *Light chain deposition disease*: It can simulate nodular diabetic glomerulosclerosis by light microscopy and the deposits are negative for the Congo red stain. Linear deposits of monoclonal kappa and less often lambda light chains on glomerular capillary walls and tubular basement membranes are seen on immunofluorescence.
3. *Fibrillary glomerulopathy*: It has distinctive light microscopic, immunofluorescent and electron microscopic features with fibrils ranging in size from 15–20 nm and the deposits are negative for thioflavin T and Congo red stains.

Course and Prognosis

Primary amyloidosis has a worse prognosis than secondary amyloidosis and requires eradication of the underlying plasma cell dyscrasia with hemopoietic stem cell transplantation and melphalan associated with 25–50% response rate.[1,10] Suppression of SAA production has resulted

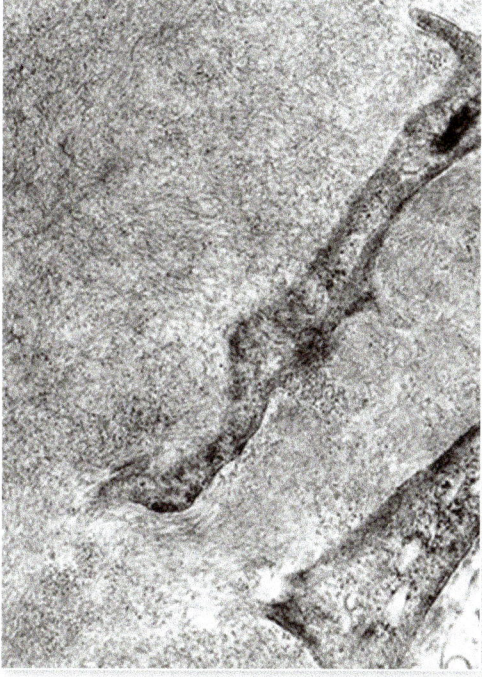

Figure 9.4: Renal amyloidosis (EM)

in functional improvement in secondary reactive amyloidosis.[1] A renal amyloid prognostic score has been proposed, based on extent of glomerular deposition with tubulointerstitial and vascular involvement with summated grades of severity, but has not been validated to date.[11]

REFERENCES

1. Dember LM. Amyloidosis-associated kidney disease. J Am Soc Nephrol. 2006;17: 3458-71.
2. Merlini G, Bellotti V. Molecular mechanisms of amyloidosis. N Engl J Med. 2003;349:583-96.
3. Narasimhan B, Chacko B, John GT, Korula A, Kirubakaran MG, Jacob CK. Characterization of kidney lesions in Indian adults: towards a renal biopsy registry. J Nephrol. 2006;19: 205-10.
4. Sethi S, Vrana JA, et al. Laser microdissection and mass spectrometry–based proteomics aids the diagnosis and typing of renal amyloidosis. Kidney International. 2012;82:226-34.
5. Benson MD, James S, Scott K, Liepnieks JJ, Kluve-Beckerman B. Leukocyte chemotactic factor 2: A novel renal amyloid protein. Kidney Int. 2008;74(2):218-22. PubMed PMID: 18449172.
6. Murphy CL, Wang S, Kestler D, Larsen C, Benson D, Weiss DT, et al. Leukocyte chemotactic factor 2 (LECT 2)-associated renal amyloidosis: a case series. Am J Kidney Dis. 2010;56(6):1100-7.
7. Larsen CP, Kossmann RJ, Beggs ML, Solomon A, Walker PD. Clinical, morphologic, and genetic features of renal leukocyte chemotactic factor 2 amyloidosis. Kidney Int. 2014;86(2):378-82. Pub Med PMID: 24522497.
8. Nasr SH, Dogan A, Larsen CP. Leukocyte cell-derived chemotaxin 2-associated amyloidosis: A recently recognized disease with distinct clinicopathologic characteristics. Clin J Am Soc Nephrol. 2015.pii: CJN.12551214. Review. PubMed PMID: 25873265.
9. Kulkarni U, Valson A, Korula A, Mathews V. Leukocyte derived chemotaxin 2 (ALECT2) amyloidosis. Mediterr J HematolInfect Dis. 2015,7(1):e2015043,DOI:http://dx.doi.org/10.4084/MJHID.2015.043.
10. Merlini G, Seldin DC, Gertz MA. Amyloidosis: pathogenesis and new therapeutic options. J Clin Oncol. 2011;29:1924-33.
11. Sait S, Banu S. A proposed histopathologic classification, scoring, and grading system for renal amyloidosis standardization of renal amyloid biopsy report. Arch Pathol Lab Med. 2010;134:532-44.

MONOCLONAL IMMUNOGLOBULIN DEPOSITION DISEASE

Renal diseases induced by monoclonal immunoglobulin molecule:
- Glomerular/Vascular diseases (Tubules and interstitium may be involved)
- AL amyloidosis
- AH amyloidosis
- Light chain deposition disease
- Heavy chain deposition disease
- Light and heavy chain deposition disease
- Monoclonal immunotactoid glomerulopathy
- Cryoglobulinemia-Types I and II.

Monoclonal immunoglobulin deposition disease is characterized by the deposition of non-amyloidogenic abnormally truncated immunoglobulin molecules in glomerular and tubular basement membranes, that are Congo red negative and devoid of fibrillar or microtubular organized structure on electron microscopy.[1,2]

Subtypes

- Light chain deposition disease (LCDD)
- Heavy chain deposition disease (HCDD)
- Light and heavy chain deposition disease (LHCDD).

LCDD is the most common, occurring in 19% of biopsy series, while HCDD and LHCDD are rarely reported.

Associated Features

Associated features include proteinuria with nephrotic syndrome and renal failure and detectable monoclonal immunoglobulins in serum or urine. Overt multiple myeloma is seen in 50% of cases and B cell lymphomas in a few cases. MGUS is found in about 17% of cases. In about 30% cases, there is no detectable paraproteinemia in serum or urine at the time of renal biopsy diagnosis. LCDD can occur concurrently with light chain cast nephropathy and renal amyloidosis.[3]

Light Microscopy[1,3]

- Diffuse symmetrical nodular expansion of glomerular mesangium (Fig. 9.5)
- Intensely PAS positive with lamellations
- Congo red negative, non-argyrophilic
- Variable mesangial hypercellularity
- Variable thickening of glomerular capillary walls with duplication
- Extraglomerular lesions: PAS positive thickening of tubular basement membranes
- Coarse PAS positive deposits around myocytes in blood vessel walls can also occur.
- LCDD when combined with light chain casts is usually dominated by the latter.
- Identical features are noted in HCDD and LHCDD.

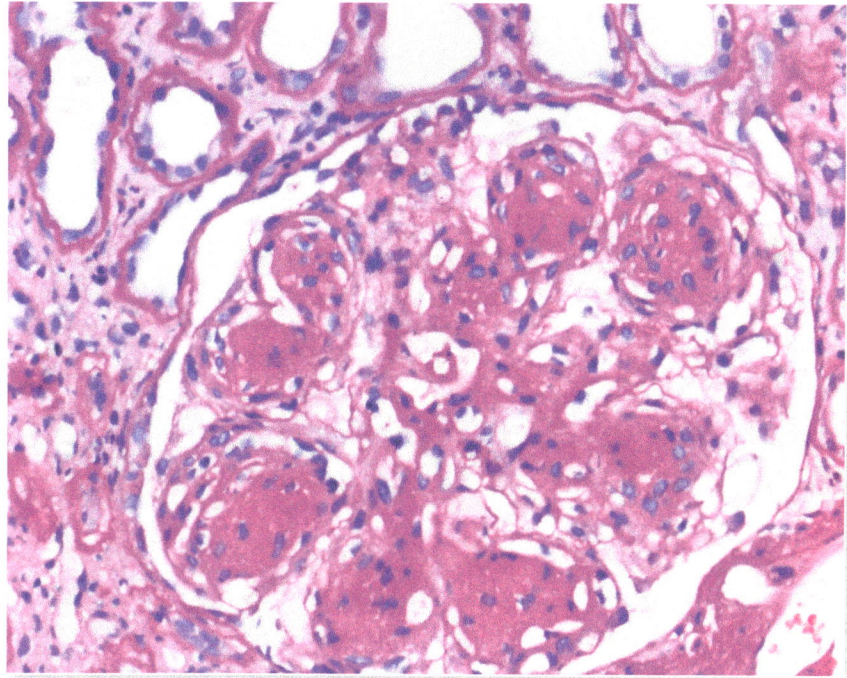

Figure 9.5: Light chain deposition disease with nodular glomerulosclerosis (PAS x 200)

Immunofluorescence

Linear deposits of monotypic light chains (usually kappa) on the peripheral capillary walls with concomitant staining of mesangial nodules in advanced lesions and linear staining of tubular basement membranes.

On direct IF with FITC labeled IgG1, IgG2, IgG3 and IgG4 monoclonal antibodies: Gamma heavy chain deposits are present in HCDD/LHCDD in the same distribution.

Electron Microscopy

Granular punctate electron dense subendothelial deposits on glomerular capillary walls replacing lamina densa in foci and on the inner aspect of paramesangial GBM and in the mesangium (Fig. 9.6).

Differential Diagnosis

Nodular diabetic glomerulosclerosis has similar but asymmetrical nodular lesions by light microscopy and can be distinguished by immunofluorescent features and electron microscopy from light chain nephropathy.

Primary (AL) amyloidosis with nodular deposits contain predominantly lambda light chains, by IF and characteristic fibrils on EM.

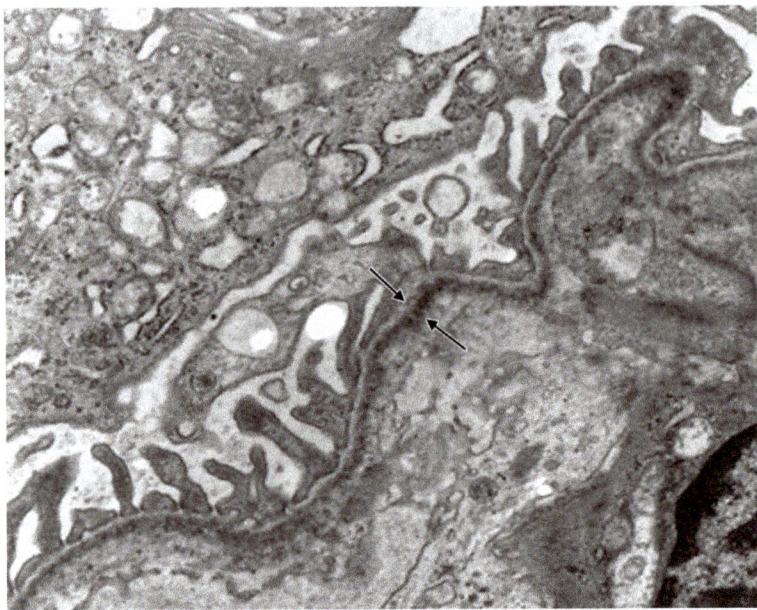

Figure 9.6: Light chain deposition disease (arrows) (EM) (Internet Resource)

Idiopathic nodular glomerulosclerosis do not contain monoclonal light chain deposits on immunofluorescence or immune deposits on electron microscopy.

Advanced membranoproliferative glomerulonephritis with nodular sclerosis displays perilobular capillary wall C3 deposits on immunofluorescence.

Course and Prognosis

It is dependent on early and aggressive treatment with high intensity chemotherapy and stem cell and bone marrow transplant for improved survival rates and renal function. Recurrence of disease occurs in renal allografts in >50% of patients, associated with incomplete remission of the underlying plasma cell dyscrasia. Extrarenal deposits can be present in the liver, heart, bone marrow, spleen, lymph nodes, pancreas, peripheral nerves and other rare sites.[1,4-6]

REFERENCES

1. Ronco P, Plaisier E, Mougenot B, Aucouturier P. Immunoglobulin light (heavy)-chain deposition disease: from molecular medicine to pathophysiology-driven therapy. Clin J Am Soc Nephrol. 2006;1(6):1342-50.
2. Buxbaum JN, Chuba JV, Hellman GC, Solomon A, Gallo GR. Monoclonal immunoglobulin deposition disease: light chain and light and heavy chain deposition diseases and their relation to light chain amyloidosis. Clinical features, immunopathology, and molecular analysis. Ann Intern Med. 1990;112(6):455-64.
3. Lin J, Markowitz GS, Kambham N, Sherman WH, Gerald G, Appel GG, et al. Renal monoclonal immunoglobulin deposition disease: The disease spectrum. J Am Soc Nephrol. 2001;12:1482-92.
4. Montseny J, Kleinknecht D, Meyrier A, Vanhille P, Simon P, Pruna A, et al. Long-term outcome according to renal histological lesions in 118 patients with monoclonal gammopathies. Nephrol Dial Transplant. 1998;13:1438-45.
5. Gertz AM, Lacy MQ, Dispenzieri A. Immunoglobulin light chain amyloidosis and the kidney. Kidney Int. 2002;61:1-9; doi:10.1046/j.1523-1755.2002.00085.x.
6. Buxbaum J, Gallo G. Non amyloidotic immunoglobulin deposition disease: Light-chain, heavy-chain, and light- and heavy-chain deposition diseases. Hematology/Oncology Clinics of North America.1999;13:1235-48.

LIGHT CHAIN CAST NEPHROPATHY

Light chain cast nephropathy (LCN) is caused by excessive production and excretion of monoclonal free immunoglobulin light chains presenting with acute renal failure in multiple myeloma, with an incidence of 40–60% in renal biopsies. There are identifiable precipitating factors such as dehydration, hypercalcemia, hyperuricemia, infections, nephrotoxins, non-steroidal inflammatory drugs and diuretics. LCN often occurs as the first manifestation of a myeloma, requiring laboratory work-up including bone marrow biopsy, serum/urine electrophoresis and immunofixation and serum free light chains assay with abnormal free kappa to lambda ratio (normal ratio = 0.26:1.65). Light chain casts are formed in the distal and collecting tubules bound and admixed with Tamm-Horsfall glycoprotein with luminal obstruction, giant cell reaction and interstitial fibrosis.[1-3]

Microscopic Features

- Marked dilatation of distal tubules and collecting ducts
- Angulated, brittle, eosinophilic, laminated/fractured casts with a rim of macrophages and multinucleate giant cells (Fig. 9.7)
- Necrotic cell debris admixed with casts
- Casts are Thioflavin T positive and can be congophilic
- Weakly PAS positive and contains focal crystalline structures
- Interstitial infiltrates of mononuclear cells and eosinophils
- Tubulointerstitial fibrosis and atrophy in chronic stages.

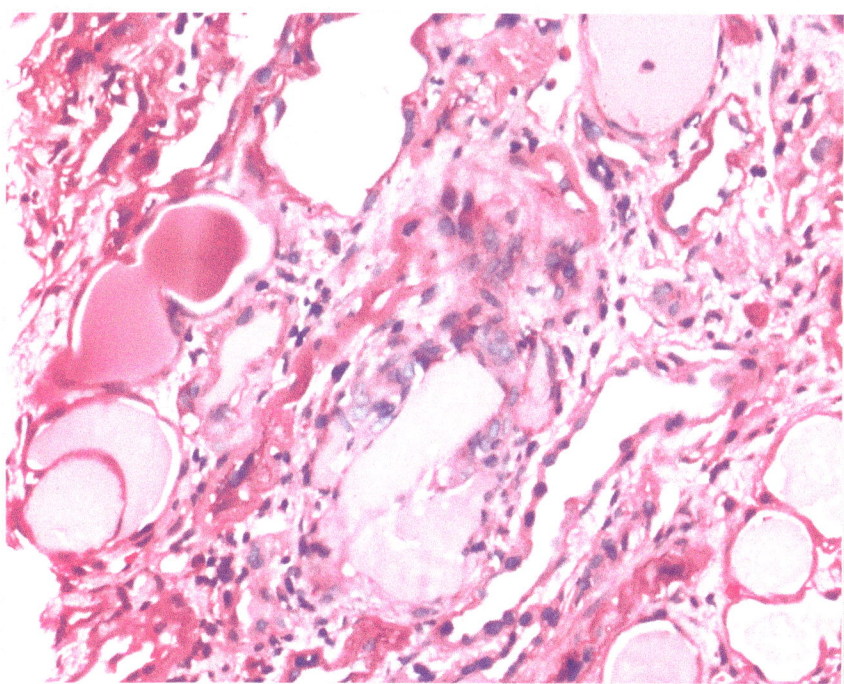

Figure 9.7: Light chain cast nephropathy (H & E 200X)

Immunofluorescence

Casts show monotypic light chain restriction or a predominance of one with trapping of the other in chronic cases. Concomitant light chain deposits in glomeruli can also be present less commonly in concurrent LCDD or amyloidosis.

Electron Microscopy

- Casts contain fibrillary material admixed with cellular debris and crystalline structures
- Concomitant glomerular amorphous or fibrillar amyloid/rarely non-amyloid organized deposits are reported.[4]

Light Chain-related Acquired Fanconi Syndrome

Proximal tubular dysfunction with impeded transport of amino acid, glucose and phosphate, is caused by crystalline cytoplasmic inclusions formed by endocytosis and localization of light chains in lysosomes. The variable regions of kappa or lambda light chains, resist protease degradation with unusual self-reactivity to form crystals, that accumulate within proximal tubular cells. Lysosomal overload causes release of proteolytic enzymes and cytoplasmic vacuolization, necrosis, apical blebs and loss of brush border. On electron microscopy, needle/rod-shaped and rhomboid electron dense crystalline intracytoplasmic structures are present.[5-9]

Course and Prognosis

Light chain cast nephropathy and the tubulointerstitial complications require dialysis, plasmapheresis and chemotherapy for the underlying multiple myeloma. LCN with concurrent LCDD or amyloidosis is rare and has a worse prognosis than MIDD alone.[1,3] Progressive loss of renal function occurs in the majority of cases of myeloma-associated nephropathy.

PROLIFERATIVE GLOMERULONEPHRITIS WITH MONOCLONAL IMMUNOGLOBULIN DEPOSITS

Proliferative glomerulonephritis, has rarely been reported with monoclonal gammopathy of undetermined significance (MGUS), that mimics immune complex glomerulonephritis. There is associated positive serum and/or urine electrophoresis and immunofixation electrophoresis and abnormal serum lambda/kappa free light chain ratio in about 30-50% of these cases.[10,11] Patients present with nephrotic syndrome, renal dysfunction and microhematuria.[11-13]

Microscopic Features[10,11]

Light Microscopy

- Predominantly membranoproliferative features in the majority[13]
- Endocapillary proliferative features are less common
- Mesangial or membranous features are seen rarely
- Focal cellular to fibrocellular crescents are infrequent

Immunofluorescence

- Granular to semilinear deposits of IgG (2+) on glomerular capillary walls and/or mesangium
- Monoclonal restriction of single kappa or lambda light chains
- IgG3 subclass is frequently present with C3 deposits.

Electron Microscopy

Subendothelial and mesangial or intramembranous and rare subepithelial deposits with double contours and neo-basement membrane formation.

Differential Diagnosis[11]

- Cryoglobulinemic glomerulonephritis-Type I with membranoproliferative/proliferative features is differentiated by intracapillary hyaline thrombi, monocyte infiltration and focal annular-tubular or fibrillar deposits on EM.
- Immunotactoid glomerulopathy is distinguished by presence of microtubular deposits, 30–50 nm in diameter with focal parallel alignment on EM.

Course and Prognosis

It is variable with partial to complete remission or persistent renal dysfunction and a quarter of cases progressing to end-stage renal disease in 2.5 years.[11]

REFERENCES

1. Korbet SM, Schwartz MM. Multiple myeloma. J Am Soc Nephrol. 2006;17:2533-45.
2. Masai R, Wakui H, Togashi M, Maki N, Ohtani H, Komatsuda A, Sawada K. Clinicopathological features and prognosis in immunoglobulin light and heavy chain deposition disease. Clin Nephrol. 2009;71(1):9-20.
3. Davenport A, Merlini G. Myeloma kidney: advances in molecular mechanisms of acute kidney injury open novel therapeutic opportunities. Nephrol Dial Transplant. 2012;27:3713-8.
4. Qian Q, Leung N, Theis JD, Dogan A, Sethi S. Coexistence of myeloma cast nephropathy, light chain deposition disease, and nonamyloid fibrils in a patient with multiple myeloma. Am J Kidney Dis. 2010;56(5):971-6.doi: 10.1053/j.ajkd.2010.06.018.Epub 2010 Sep 25.
5. Larsen CP, Bell JM, Harris AA, Messias NC, WangYH, Walker PD. The morphologic spectrum and clinical significance of light chain proximal tubulopathy with and without crystal formation. Modern Pathology. 2011;24:1462-9.
6. Lacy MQ, Gertz MA. Acquired Fanconi's syndrome associated with monoclonal gammopathies. Hematol Oncol Clin North Am. 1999;13:1273-80.
7. Ma CX, Lacy MQ, Rompala JF, Dispenzieri A, Rajkumar SV, Greipp PR, et al. Acquired Fanconi syndrome is an indolent disorder in the absence of overt multiple myeloma. Blood. 2004;104: 40-2.
8. Messiaen T, Deret S, Mougenot B, Bridoux F, Dequiedt P, Dion JJ, et al. Adult Fanconi syndrome secondary to light chain gammapathy. Clinicopathologic heterogeneity and unusual features in 11 patients. Medicine. 2000;79:135-54,
9. Orfila C, Lepert JC, Modesto A, Bernadet P, Suc JM. Fanconi's syndrome, kappa light-chain myeloma, non-amyloid fibrils and cytoplasmic crystals in renal tubular epithelium. AmJ Nephrol. 1991;11:345-9.
10. Nasr SH, Markowitz GS, Stokes MB, Seshan SV, Valderrama E, Appel GB, et al. Proliferative glomerulonephritis with monoclonal IgG deposits: A distinct entity mimicking immune-complex glomerulonephritis. Kidney Int. 2004;65: 85-96.
11. Nasr SH, Satoskar A, Markowitz GS, Valeri AM, Appel GB, Stokes MB, et al. Proliferative glomerulonephritis with monoclonal IgG deposits. J Am Soc Nephrol. 2009;20:2055-64.
12. Geldenhuys L, Jones B. Glomerulonephritis with monoclonal immunoglobulin deposits. J Am Soc Nephrol. 2008;19:671A.
13. Sethi SZ, Leung L, Smith N, Jevremonic RJH, Hermann D, Fervenza SSF. Membranoproliferative glomerulonephritis secondary to monoclonal gammopathy. Clin JAm Soc Nephrol. 2010;5:770-82.

CHAPTER 10

Glomerulonephritis with Organized Immune Deposits

ABSTRACT

Glomerulonephritis with organized immune deposits encompasses the major entities of fibrillary, immunotactoid glomerulopathy and cryoglobulinemic glomerulonephritis. Their incidence, common disease associations and microscopic features are comprehensively elucidated with appropriate photographic illustrations. The differential diagnosis from other hereditary nephropathies with non-immune derived organized deposits such as collagenofibrotic glomerulopathy and fibronectin glomerulopathy are highlighted.

Cryoglobulinemic glomerulonephritis has distinctive features by light and immunofluorescence microscopy with organized immune deposits that display a substructure that can be resolved and differentiated from immunotactoid glomerulopathy by electron microscopy. The associated features of monoclonal gammopathies, infections and autoimmune diseases in the subtypes of cryoglobulinemic glomerulonephritis are also noted.

Selected references for an algorithmic approach to the diagnosis are included to facilitate further interests of postgraduates in this specialty.

This entity includes two major categories known as fibrillary and immunotactoid glomerulopathy that are associated with Congo red negative, non-amyloid glomerular deposits derived from homogeneous fragments of immunoglobulins with distinctive electron microscopic features.[1-5] Cryoglobulinemic glomerulonephritis can also be associated with immunoglobulin-derived organized deposits and hence is detailed in this chapter.

Fibrillary Glomerulopathy

Fibrillary glomerulopathy has an incidence of about 1% presenting with hematuria, proteinuria with nephrotic syndrome and renal failure with hypertension, occurring in the age group, 10 to 81 years, associated with monoclonal gammopathy, malignancy (multiple myeloma or leukemia), autoimmune diseases (SLE, Crohn's disease, Graves' disease and immune thrombocytopenia) and Hepatitis C viral infection.[6,7]

MICROSCOPIC FEATURES[7-10]

Light Microscopy

- Mesangial matrix expansion with amorphous acellular eosinophilic deposits (Figs 10.1 and 10.2) (PAS positive and JMS/Congo red negative)

Glomerulonephritis with Organized Immune Deposits

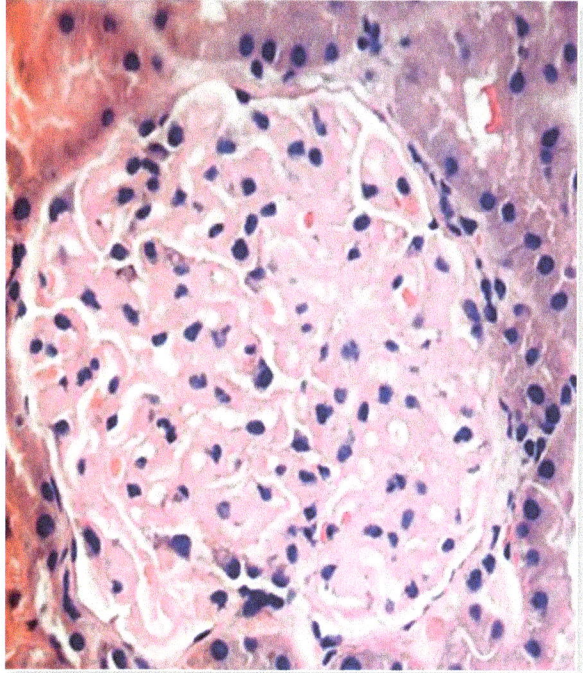

Figure 10.1: Fibrillary glomerulopathy (H & E × 400)

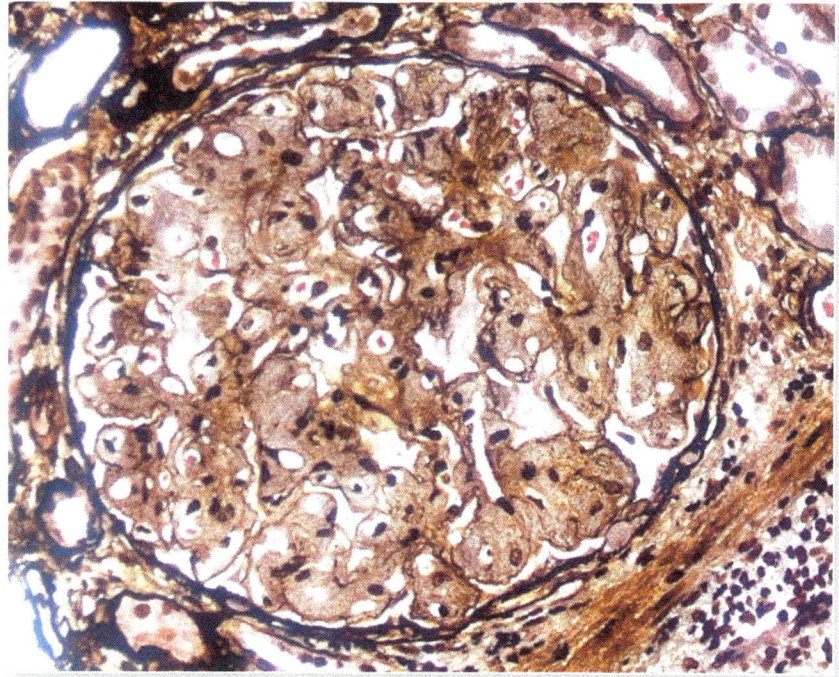

Figure 10.2: Fibrillary glomerulopathy (JMS × 400)

- Thickening of paramesangial capillary walls with focal mesangial hypercellularity and mesangial sclerosis
- Membranous or membranoproliferative features can be present in some cases.

Immunofluorescence

- Granular to linear deposits of IgG (3+) and less intense C3 deposits in mesangium and glomerular capillary walls (Fig. 10.3)
- Polyclonal kappa and lambda light chain deposits are usually present.

Electron Microscopy

- Subendothelial and intramembranous, fibrillar deposits 16 to 24 nm in diameter
- Randomly arranged with replacement and disruption of GBM (Fig. 10.4).

Differential Diagnosis[8,10]

1. *Immunotactoid glomerulopathy* has different ultrastructural features and can rarely overlap or concomitantly occur with a predominantly fibrillary substructure.[10]
2. *Amyloidosis* is differentiated by special histochemical stains and is Congo red positive with randomly arranged 8–10 nm fibrils on EM.
3. *Non-immune derived fibrillary glomerulopathies including* fibronectin glomerulopathy and Collagenofibrotic glomerulopathy as detailed under heredofamilial nephropathies.

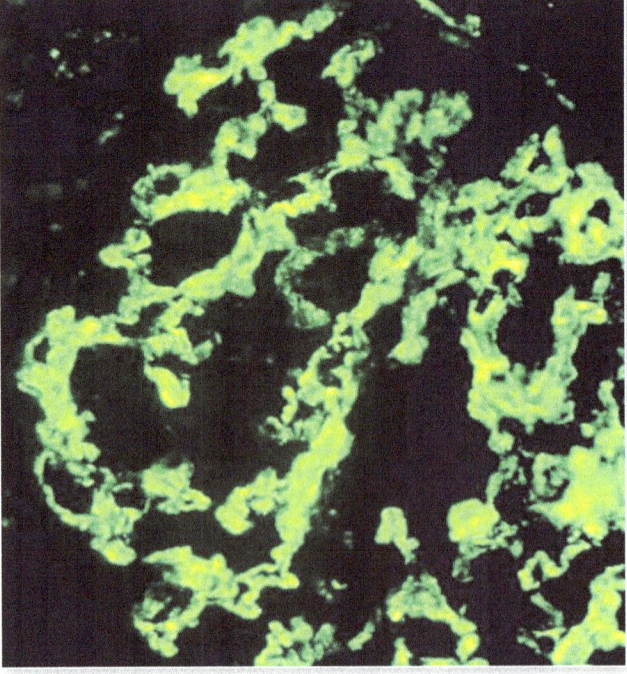

Figure 10.3: Mesangial and capillary wall deposits of IgG 3+ (IF × 400)

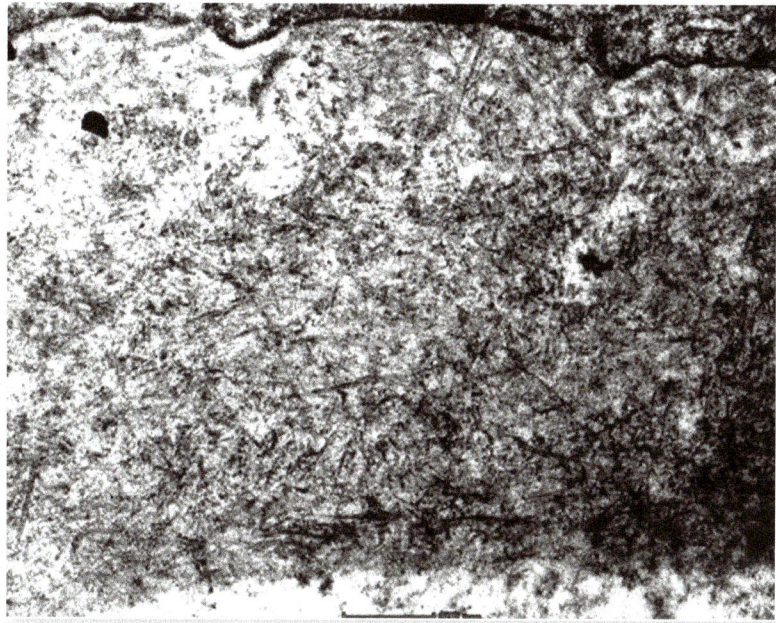

Figure 10.4: Fibrillar deposits (15 nm) replacing GBM (EM)

Course and Prognosis[6]

Persistent and progressive renal disease occurs with end-stage renal failure. Recurrence of fibrillary glomerulopathy in renal transplants can occur.

IMMUNOTACTOID GLOMERULOPATHY

Defined by the immune-derived component and polymeric substructure has a similar clinical presentation associated mainly with lymphoproliferative disorders including chronic lymphatic leukemia and B cell lymphoma and paraproteinemia with an age predilection of 12 to 68 years.

Light Microscopic Features[7,9-12]

- Marked enlargement of glomerular with lobular accentuation and endocapillary hypercellularity (Fig. 10.4)
- Thickening of peripheral capillary walls with reduplication and obliteration of capillary walls
- Focal parietal cell proliferation forming crescents
- Segmental hyalinosis and occasional hyaline thrombi with massive immunotactoid deposits
- Jones methenamine stain (JMS) and Masson trichrome stain shows mesangial expansion by mottled material
- Negative for silver stains admixed with residual silver positive collagenous material.

Immunofluorescence

- Confluent flocculent mesangial and capillary wall deposits of IgG (3+)
- Monoclonal kappa or lambda light chain deposits are present.

Electron Microscopy

- Microtubular deposits, 30–50 nm in diameter with electrolucent core (at 5000 to 10,000 magnification) (Fig. 10.5)
- Focal parallel alignment and located subjacent to GBM.

Differential Diagnosis[7,10,13-14]

1. *Cryoglobulinemic glomerulonephritis* can be differentiated with immunofluorescence by the presence of predominant monoclonal IgM deposits and curved shorter microtubular deposits in subendothelial region and capillary lumen within the massive hyaline thrombi in a background of amorphous, more electron dense material on EM.
2. *Lupus nephritis* with wire loop lesions and hyaline thrombi have "full house" deposits of immunoglobulins and C1q and C4 on glomerular capillary walls on IF and organized finger print type of whorled deposits and tubuloreticular inclusions in endothelial cells on EM.

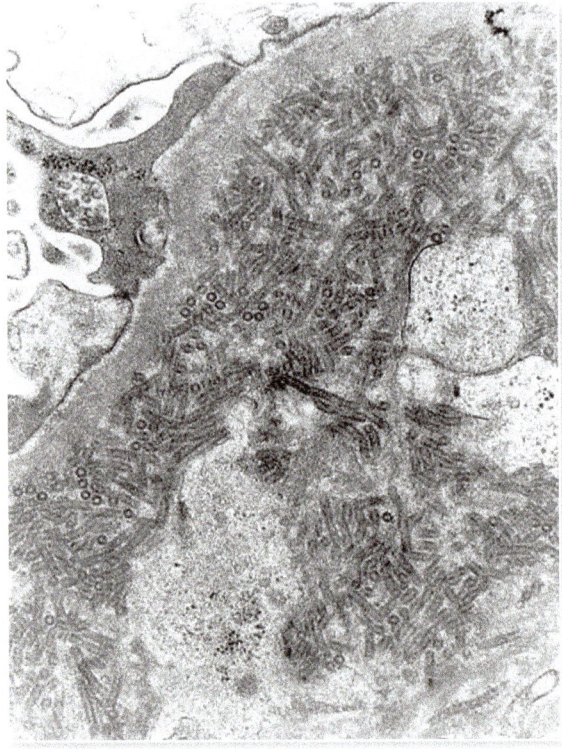

Figure 10.5: Immunotactoid glomerulopathy (EM × 20,000)

Course and Prognosis

Depends on treatment of underlying B cell lymphoma with appropriate chemotherapy and high dose steroids with cyclophosphamide for the glomerulopathy. The disease recurs in the transplant, with a slower rate of progression than in native kidneys.[7,14-16]

REFERENCES

1. Brady HR. Fibrillary glomerulopathy. Kidney Int. 1998;53:1421-9.
2. Iskandar SS, Herrera G. Glomerulopathies with organized deposits. Semin Diagn Pathol. 2002;19:116-32.
3. Alpers ChE. Fibrillary glomerulonephritis, and immunotactoid glomerulopathy: two entities, not one. Am J Kidney Dis. 1993;22:448-51.
4. Fogo A, Qureshi N, Horn RG. Morphologic and clinical features of fibrillary glomerulonephritis versus immunotactoid glomerulopathy. Am J Kidney Dis. 1993;22(3):367-77.
5. Rosenstock JL, Markowitz GS, Valeri AM, et al. Fibrillary and immunotactoid glomerulonephritis: distinct entities with different clinical and pathologic features. Kidney Int. 2003;63:1450-61.
6. Iskandar SS, Falk RJ, Jenette JC. Clinical and pathologic features of fibrillary glomerulonephritis. Kidney Int. 1992; 42:1401-7.
7. Pronovost PH, Brady HR, Gunning ME, Espinoza O, Rennke HG. Clinical features, predictors of disease progression and results of renal transplantation in fibrillary/immunotactoid glomerulopathy. Nephrol Dial Transplant. 1996;11: 837-42.
8. Herrera GA, Turbat-Herrera EA. Renal diseases with organized deposits: an algorithmic approach to classification and clinicopathologic diagnosis. Archives of Pathology and Laboratory Medicine. 2010;134(4):512-31.
9. Nasr SH, Valeri AM, Cornell LD, et al. Fibrillary glomerulonephritis: a report of 66 cases from a single institution. Clin J Am Soc Nephrol. 2011;6:775.
10. Schwartz MM, Korbet SM, Lewis EJ. Immunotactoid glomerulopathy. J Am Soc Nephrol. 2002;13:1390-7.
11. Korbet SM, Schwartz MM, Lewis EJ. Immuotactoid glomerulopathy (Fibrillary glomerulonephritis). Clin J Am Soc Nephrol. 2006:1351-6. doi: 10.2215/CJN.01140406.
12. Korbet SM, Schwartz Lewis EJ. The fibrillary glomerulopathies. Am J Kidney Dis. 1994;23:751-65.
13. Korbet SM, Schwartz MM, Lewis EJ. Immmunotactoid glomerulopathy. Am J Kidney Dis. 1991;17:247-57.
14. Bridoux F, Hugue V, Coldefy O, et al. Fibrillary glomerulonephritis and immunotactoid (microtubular) glomerulopathy are associated with distinct immunologic features. Kidney Int. 2002;62:1764-75.
15. D'Agati, Sacchi G, Truong L, et al. Fibrillary glomerulopathy: defining the disease spectrum. J Am Soc Nephrol. 1991;2:591.
16. Devaney K, Sabnis SG, Antonovych TT. Nonamyloidotic fibrillary glomerulopathy, immunotactoid glomerulopathy, and the differential diagnosis of filamentous glomerulopathies. Mod Pathol. 1991;4:36-45.

Cryoglobulinemic Glomerulonephritis

Cryoglobulinemic glomerulonephritis (CGn) is associated with circulating cryoglobulins that are soluble at 37°C, precipitate on refrigeration and redissolve when heated. The decreased solubility of component immunoglobulins occurs due to temperature-induced alterations in protein conformation. There are three types of cryoglobulinemias according to Brouet's classification, with reported frequencies of 25-50%.[1] Renal involvement presents with nephrotic range proteinuria with hypertension and acute renal failure.

Type I: With an isolated monoclonal component, usually IgM associated with monoclonal gammopathies such as Waldenstrom's macroglobulinemia, multiple myeloma, B cell lymphomas/chronic lymphatic leukemia[2-4] and associated hyperviscosity syndrome and/or thrombosis with cryoprecipitation.

Type II: With monoclonal IgM and rheumatoid factor activity against polyclonal IgG, associated with palpable purpura, myalgia and arthralgia caused by:
- Viral infections: Hepatitis C (40-65%), Hepatitis B, Epstein Barr and HIV[5] bacterial endocarditis and auto-immune diseases (15-25%) in SLE, rheumatoid arthritis and Sjogren's syndrome.

Type III: With mixed polyclonal immunoglobulins in autoimmune diseases and infections, and is less frequently implicated in the development of glomerulonephritis than type II CGn.

MICROSCOPIC FEATURES

Usually associated with type II CgN.

Light Microscopy[2,5-7]

- Markedly enlarged glomeruli with lobular accentuation and capillary wall thickening
- Variable mesangial hypercellularity and endocapillary cell proliferation
- Foci of reduplication of capillary walls with monocyte interposition and intracapillary hyaline thrombi
- Massive hyaline thrombi can be present in type I CGn (Fig. 10.6)
- Numerous intracapillary monocytes and focal neutrophils are noted
- Concomitant vasculitis is seen in 25-30% of cases.

Immunofluorescence

- Spotty granular to pseudolinear intensely positive capillary wall deposits of IgM (2 to 3+)
- Monoclonal (kappa or lambda) light chain capillary wall deposits
- Intracapillary thrombi stain for IgM.

Electron Microscopy

- Curved microtubular or annular structures (10 to 25 nm) are found in electron dense amorphous deposits in the subendothelial region and intraluminally within the thrombi (Figs 10.7 and 10.8)

Glomerulonephritis with Organized Immune Deposits

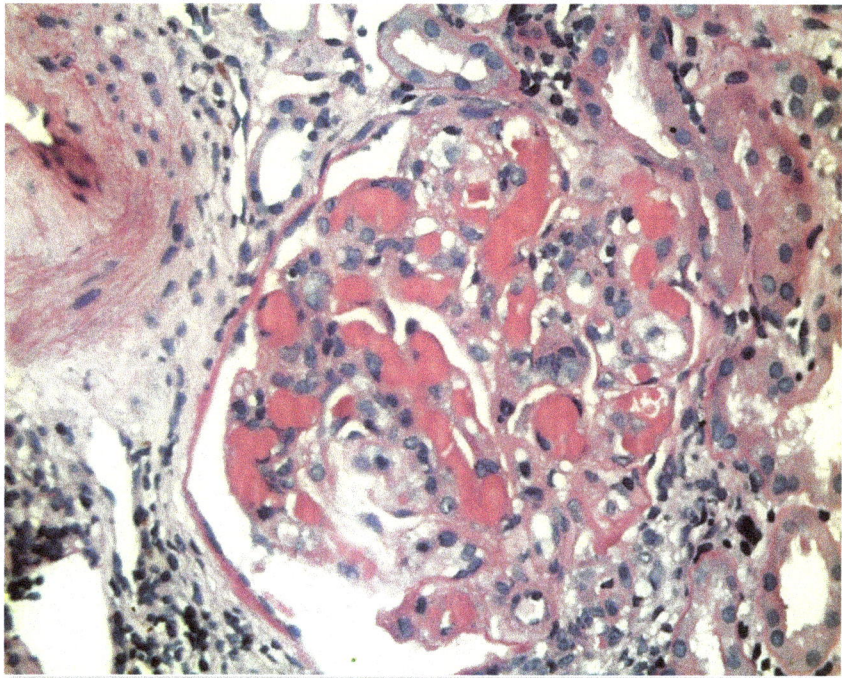

Figure 10.6: Cryoglobulinemic glomerulonephritis with massive hyaline thrombi (PAS x 400)

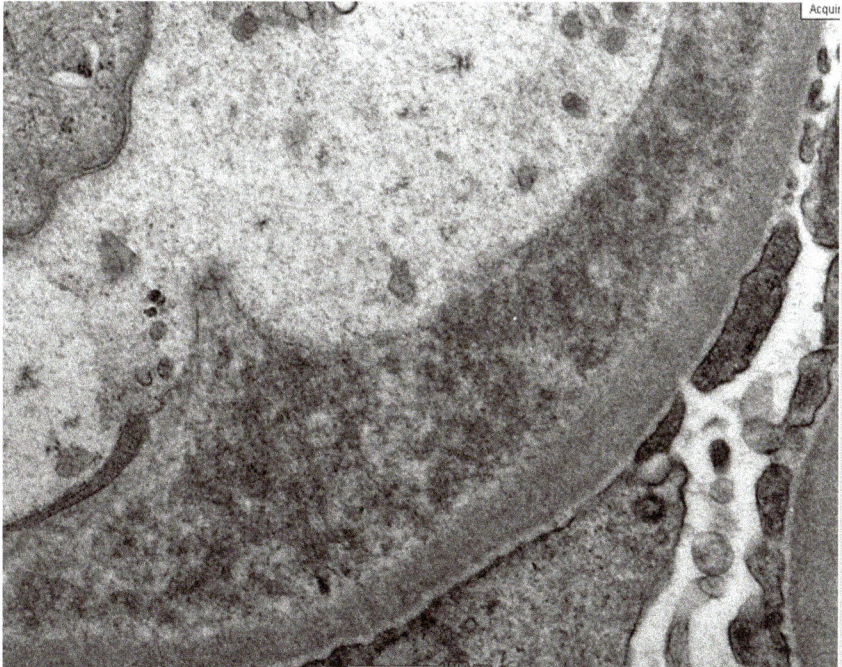

Figure 10.7: Subendothelial organized microtubular deposits in cryoglobulinemic GN type I (EM)

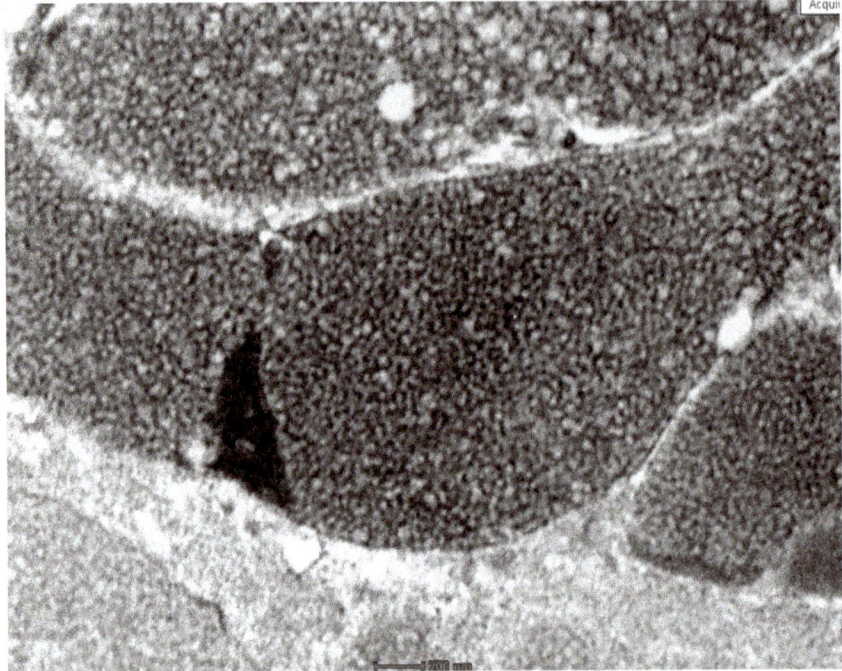

Figure 10.8: Short, curved microtubular deposits within hyaline thrombus (EM x 26,500)

- Monocyte interposition and capillary wall reduplication can be seen
- Intraluminal monocytes with ingested granular or amorphous material are present.

Differential Diagnosis[2]

1. Lupus nephritis class IV with typical IF and EM features can be distinguished from CGn.
2. Immunotactoid glomerulopathy- with distinctive ultrastructural features and size of organized microtubular immune deposits >30 nm in diameter.
3. Waldensrom's macroglobulinemia (WM): Displays massive intraglomerular capillary hyaline thrombi and can be associated with neoplastic lymphoplasmacytic infiltrates in the parenchyma (Fig. 10.9) and detectable circulating cryoglobulins with similar immune deposits on IF and EM.[4] Membranoproliferative glomerulonephritis has rarely been reported with WM.[8]

Course and Prognosis

It is usually associated with exacerbations and remissions and infrequently progressing to end stage renal failure requiring dialysis or plasmapheresis.[5]

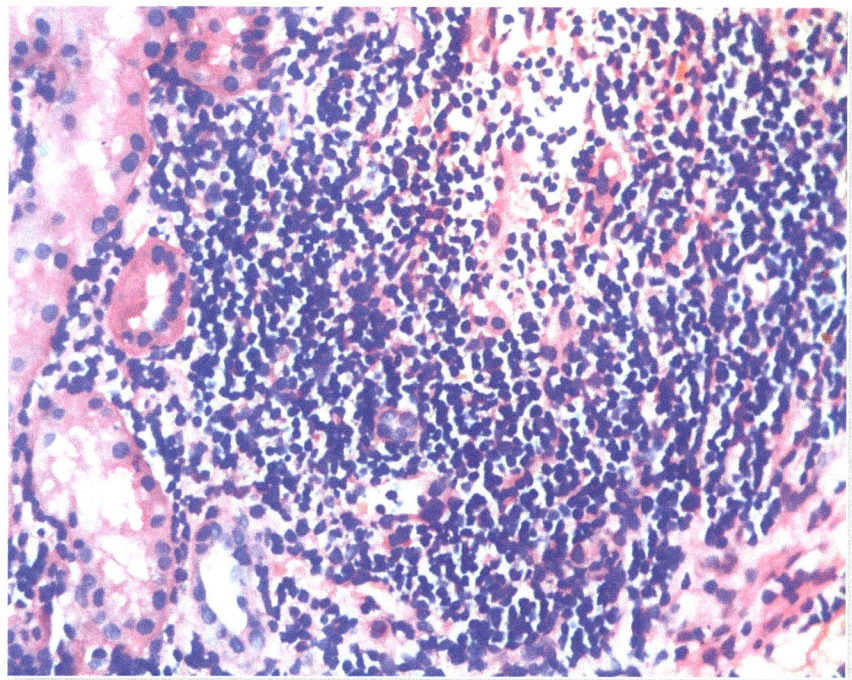

Figure 10.9: Neoplastic tubulointerstitial lymphoid infiltrate—in WM, associated with type I CGN (PAS x 400)

REFERENCES

1. Brouet JC, Clauvel JP, Danon F, Klein M, Seligmann M. Biologic and clinical significance of cryoglobulins: a report of 86 cases Am J Med. 1974;57:775-88.
2. Audard V, Georges B, Vanhille P, Toly C, Deroure B, Fakhouri F. Renal lesions associated with IgM Secreting monoclonal proliferations: revisiting the disease spectrum. Clin J Am Soc Nephrol. 2008;3:1339-49.
3. Veltman GAM, Veen SV, Kluin-Nelemans JC, Bruijn JA, Van EsLA. Renal disease in Waldenstrom's macroglobulinaemia. Nephrol Dial Transplant. 1997;12:1256-9.
4. Ghobrail IM, Gertz MA, Fonseca R. Waldenstrom macroglobulinemia. The Lancet Oncology. 2003;4(11):679-85.
5. D'Amico G. Renal involvement in hepatitis C infection: Cryoglobulinemic glomerulonephritis. Kidney Int. 1998; 54:650-71.
6. Roccatello D, Fornasieri A, Giachino O, Rossi D, Beltrame A, Banfi G, et al. Multicenter study on hepatitis C virus-related cryoglobulinemic glomerulonephritis. Am J Kidney Dis. 2007;49(1):69.
7. D'Amico G. Renal involvement in essential mixed cryoglobulinemia. Kidney Int. 1989;35:1004-4.
8. Kratochvil D, Amann K, Buttner BH. Membranoproliferative glomerulonephritis complicating Waldenstrom's macroglobulinemia. BMC Nephrology. 2012;13:172.

CHAPTER 11

HIV-associated Nephropathy

> **ABSTRACT**
>
> The pan-nephropathy of HIVAN is detailed in this chapter with an emphasis on the pathognomonic lesion of collapsing glomerulopathy with viral DNA leading to dysregulation and proliferation of the podocytes and cytokine production with glomerulosclerosis and tubulointerstitial scarring. The typical ultrastructural features are highlighted, including the tubuloreticular inclusions of endothelial cells and confronting cylindrical cisternae.
>
> The course and prognosis of the disease and concurrent glomerular lesions are noted, including the CMC, Vellore experience, particularly lupus-like glomerulonephritis, immune complex mediated PIGN and hepatitis B and C membranous and membranoproliferative glomerulonephritis.
>
> Pertinent and current references and photomicrographs are included for completion of this succinct chapter.

INTRODUCTION

HIV-associated nephropathy (HIVAN) is a pan-nephropathy with typical glomerular, tubular and interstitial lesions, associated with severe non-selective proteinuria and progressive renal failure. The HIV genome has been detected by molecular studies with viral DNA leading to dysregulation and proliferation of the podocytes and cytokine production with glomerulosclerosis and tubulointerstitial scarring.[1-4] In situ hybridization for HIV-1 mRNA has revealed HIV-RNA in podocytes and tubular epithelial cells during the infection and after treatment.[4] There is a racial and genetic predilection for black African-Americans[5] with few published case reports from Asia or India.[6] In HIV-associated nephropathy, a form of collapsing glomerulopathy occurs due to dedifferentiation of podocytes, with loss of maturation markers and expression of proliferation markers on immunohistochemistry.[7,8]

MICROSCOPIC FEATURES

Light Microscopy[1-4,9-11]

HIV-Glomerulopathy

- Wrinkling, collapse of capillary tufts and narrowing of glomerular capillary lumina (Fig. 11.1)
- Mesangial sclerosis, luminal obliteration and solidification of tufts
- Hyperplasia and hypertrophy of podocytes with coarse vacuolization and protein droplets
- Dilatation of Bowman's space and insudation of hyaline material.

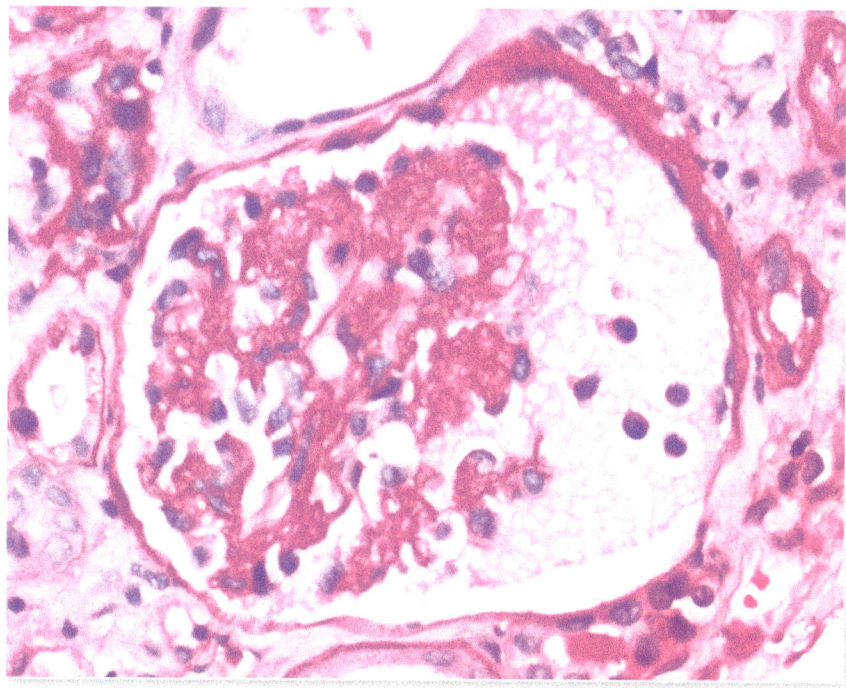

Figure 11.1: Collapsing glomerulopathy: HIVAN (PAS x 200)

Tubulointerstitial Features

- Tubular dilatation with flattening of lining epithelium and loss of brush border of proximal tubules with microcysts (Fig. 11.2)
- Desquamated cellular luminal debris admixed with plasma proteins and hyaline casts
- Interstitial edema with mononuclear cell infiltrate in initial phase
- Fibrosis with tubular atrophy in chronic phase.

Immunofluorescence

Focal and segmental trapping of IgM and C3 in sclerotic tufts.

Immunohistochemistry

Increased K1-67 (MIB-1) positivity in proliferated podocytes.

Electron Microscopy[1]

- Marked enlargement and detachment of podocytes with membrane bound vacuoles and secondary lysosomes
- Wrinkling of GBM and obliteration of lumina by matrix and collapse of capillary walls
- Intraluminal monocytes with foamy lipid material
- Swollen endothelial cells, degeneration and detachment from thin layers of neo-basement membrane material

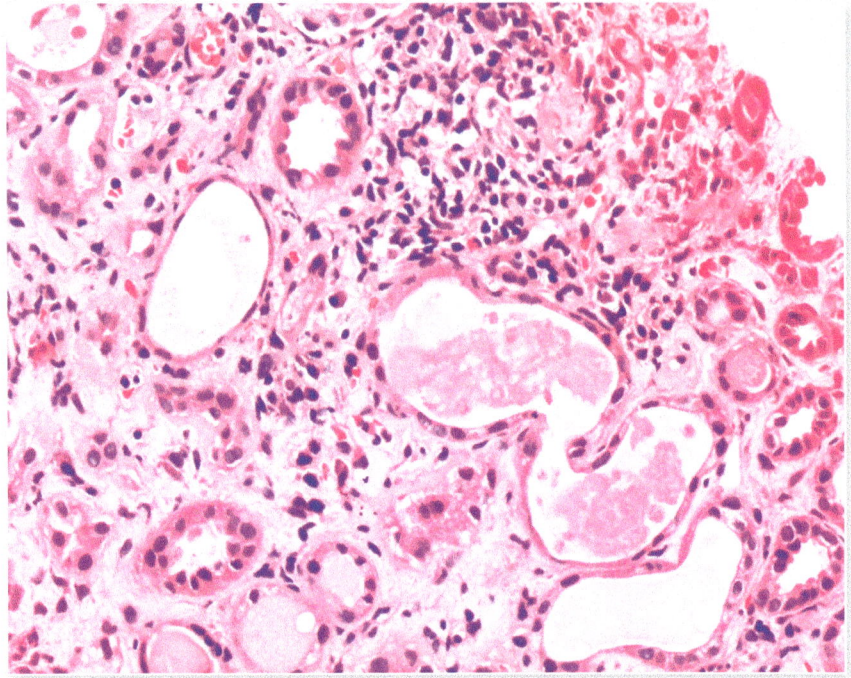

Figure 11.2: Microcystic tubular dilatation with tubular necrosis (H & E x 100)

- Tubuloreticular structures (25 nm) in endoplasmic reticulum of endothelial cells
- "Confronting cylindrical cisternae" (fused cell membranes) in interstitial cells
- Nuclear bodies and granular/granulofibrillar transformation of tubular epithelial cells (in HIV infection).

Course and Prognosis

It is modified by highly active antiretroviral therapy, ACE inhibitors and corticosteroids with reversibility of lesions[4] and less rapid progression to end-stage renal failure.[12]

Concurrent glomerular lesions include:
- IgA nephropathy
- Lupus-like glomerulonephritis
- Hepatitis B and C associated membranous or membranoproliferative glomerulonephritis
- Immune complex mediated, or postinfectious glomerulonephritis
- Immunotactoid/fibrillary glomerulonephritis
- Light chain nephropathy
- Cryoglobulinemia
- Amyloidosis
- Thrombotic microangiopathy.[2,9]

In the CMC experience, renal biopsies done in HIV positive patients comprised cases of collapsing glomerulopathy, PIGN, lupus-like glomerulonephritis and hepatitis B/C viral associated immune complex glomerulonephritis.

Transplantation after anti-retroviral therapy and stable CD4 counts with undetectable plasma HIV-RNA levels has a reported graft survival of 95.4%.[13,14]

REFERENCES

1. D'Agati V, Suh J-I, Carbone L, et al. Pathology of HIV-associated nephropathy: a detailed morphologic and comparative study. Kidney Int. 1989;35:1358-70.
2. D'Agati V, Appel GB. Renal pathology of human immunodeficiency virus infection. Semin Nephrol. 1998;18:406-21.
3. Rao TK. Human immunodeficiency virus (HIV) associated nephropathy. Annu Rev Med.1991;42:391-401.
4. Winston JA, Bruggeman LA, Ross MD, et al. Nephropathy and establishment of a renal reservoir of HIV type 1 during primary infection. N Engl J Med. 2001;344:1979-84.
5. Rao TK, Filippone EJ, Nicastri AD, et al. Associated focal and segmental glomerulosclerosis in the acquired immunodeficiency syndrome. N Engl J Med. 1984;310:669-73.
6. Gupta V, Gupta S, Sinha S, Sharma SK, Dinda AK, Agarwal SK, et al. HIV associated renal disease: a pilot study from north India. Indian J Med Res. 2013;137(5):950-6.
7. Barisoni L, Kriz W, Mundel P, D'Agati V. The dysregulated podocyte phenotype: a novel concept in the pathogenesis of collapsing idiopathic focal segmental glomerulosclerosis and HIV-associated nephropathy. J Am Soc Nephrol. 1999;10(1):51-61.
8. Schwartz EJ, Klotman PE. Pathogenesis of human immunodeficiency virus (HIV)-associated nephropathy. Semin Nephrol. 1998;18(4):436-45.
9. Wyatt CM, Morgello S, Katz-Malamed R, et al. The spectrum of kidney disease in patients with AIDS in the era of antiretroviral therapy. Kidney Int. 2009;75(4):428-34.
10. Kalim S, Szczech LA, Wyatt CM. Acute kidney injury in HIV-infected patients. Semin Nephrol. 2008;28(6):556-62.
11. Phair J, Palella F. Renal disease in HIV-infected individuals. Curr Opin HIV Aids. 2011;6(4):285-9.
12. Carbone L, D'Agati V, Cheng JT, et al. The course and prognosis of human immunodeficiency virus associated nephropathy. Am J Med. 1989;87:389-95.
13. Foy MC, Estrella MM, Lucas GM, Tahir F, Fine DM, Moore RD, et al. Comparison of risk factors and outcomes in HIV immune complex kidney disease and HIV-associated nephropathy. Clin J Am Soc Nephrol. 2013;8(9):1524-32.
14. Locke JE, Montgomery RA, Warren DS, et al. Renal transplant in HIV-positive patients: long-term outcomes and risk factors for graft loss. Arch Surg. 2009;144:83-6.

CHAPTER 12

Heredofamilial Glomerulopathies

ABSTRACT

This chapter deals with collagenopathies, fibronectin glomerulopathy, lipid storage diseases and congenital nephrotic syndrome. Among the Type IV collagenopathies, the major emphasis is on the pathogenesis and histopathology of Alport's syndrome, including the X-linked, autosomal recessive and autosomal dominant variants with their distinctive features on immunofluorescence and electron microscopy. Thin basement membrane disease is also considered in comparison to these entities.

Collagenofibrotic and Nail-patella syndrome comprise the Type III collagenopathies and have been detailed.

Fibronectin glomerulopathy is mentioned here as a rare autosomal dominant form of glomerular disease with organized non-immune deposits.

The lipid storage diseases included are Fabry's disease, familial lecithin cholesterol acyl transferase deficiency (LCAT) and lipoprotein glomerulopathy, categorized together with differential diagnosis, illustrations and selected references.

The congenital nephrotic syndrome with the inherited genetic mutations, include the finnish type and diffuse mesangial sclerosis, syndromic and non-syndromic variants of minimal change nephrotic syndrome and focal and segmental sclerosis.

Podocytopathies are classified based on histopathology, defined by podocyte number and four different morphological types and the etiology including idiopathic, genetic and reactive forms associated with podocyte injury. The four distinct pathways of podocyte injury caused by various intrinsic and extrinsic factors are detailed with appropriate illustrations.

Collagen Nephropathies

Collagen nephropathies include type IV and type III collagen abnormalities.

TYPE IV COLLAGEN NEPHROPATHIES

Type IV collagen molecule is a heterotrimer or protomer of subunits called alpha chains forming a triple helical structure. There are 6 isomers of the alpha chains encoded by COLA 1 to A6 genes located in pairs on three different chromosomes. The alpha peptide network-3, 4 and 5 is found in the mature glomerular capillary basement membranes and the 5,5 and 6 protomer in the Bowman's capsule, in contrast to that of early embryogenesis and the fetal kidneys where the alpha 1 and alpha 2 isoforms predominate.

Absence of any of the alpha chains due to genetic mutations limits incorporation of other chains and formation of the intricate collagen network. The primary aberration of glomerular basement membrane (GBM) is in the non-collagenous domain of the C terminal of alpha-5 (IV) chain in the X-linked type and that of alpha-3 (IV) and alpha-4 (IV) chains in autosomal recessive and autosomal dominant type of Alport's syndrome. The anomalous persistence of alpha1 and alpha 2 isoforms occurring with developmental maturation arrest in Alport's syndrome leads to increased susceptibility to proteolytic enzyme degradation, leading to splitting of the GBM. There is evidence to suggest that alterations in glomerular homeostasis from loss of normal alpha chains leads to thickening of GBM and impairment of macromolecular permselectivity, glomerulosclerosis, interstitial fibrosis and renal failure.[1-3]

Classification of Type IV Collagenopathies

Alport's Syndrome (AS)
- X-linked Alport's syndrome (XLAS)
- Autosomal recessive Alport's syndrome (ARAS)
- Autosomal dominant Alport's syndrome (ADAS).

Thin Basement Membrane Disease/Benign familial hematuria.

Alport's Syndrome

Alport's syndrome has an incidence of 3% in children and 0.2% in adults with an estimated gene frequency of 1 in 5000 comprising three major forms of mutations:

X-linked type: Accounts for 85% of Alport's syndrome and has juvenile and adult forms involving mutations of *Col4A5* gene on chromosome Xq 26-48 with loss of alpha 5 peptide chain of type IV collagen, affecting the basement membranes of the glomeruli, cochlea and lens capsule. Males are predominantly affected with renal manifestations such as persistent hematuria, progressive proteinuria and hypertension with renal failure. This is associated with sensorineural deafness and ocular lesions including anterior lenticonus and dot and fleck retinopathy.[1]

Microscopic Features

Light Microscopy[1,2,5-7]

- Mild mesangial expansion to focal mesangial hypercellularity
- Segmental to global mesangial expansion with hypercellularity
- Thickening of capillary walls with splitting on JMS stain
- Thickening of Bowman's capsule, progression to segmental and global sclerosis with hyalinosis (Fig. 12.1)
- Interstitial expansion with aggregates of foam cells is characteristic (Fig. 12.2)
- Interstitial fibrosis with tubular atrophy and arteriosclerosis in chronic phase.

Immunofluorescence

- Negative for alpha-5 peptide chain in GBM of glomeruli and Bowman's capsule/distal tubules
- Nonspecific trapping of IgM and C3 in segments of sclerosis.

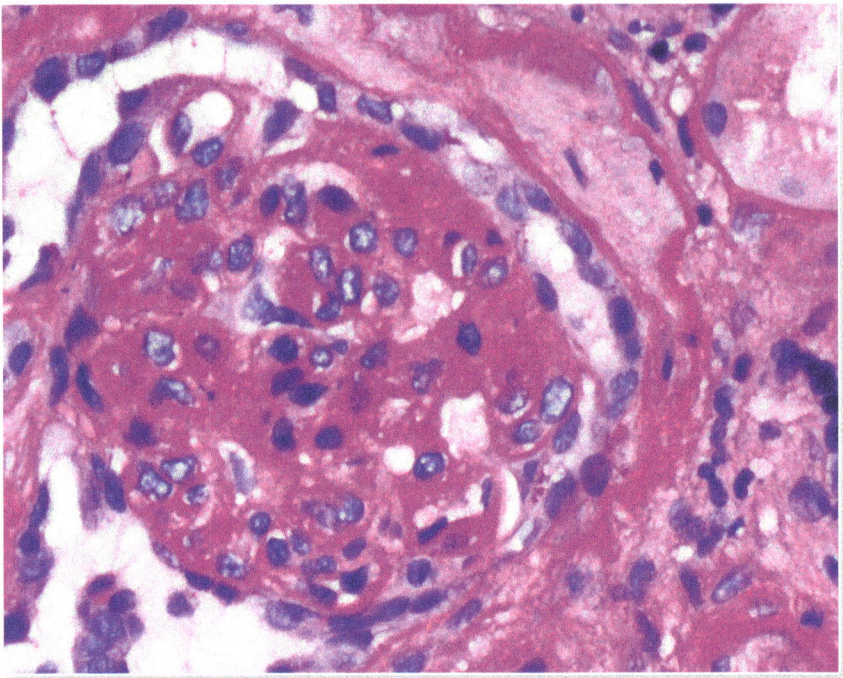
Figure 12.1: Global mesangial sclerosis with hypercellularity (PAS × 400)

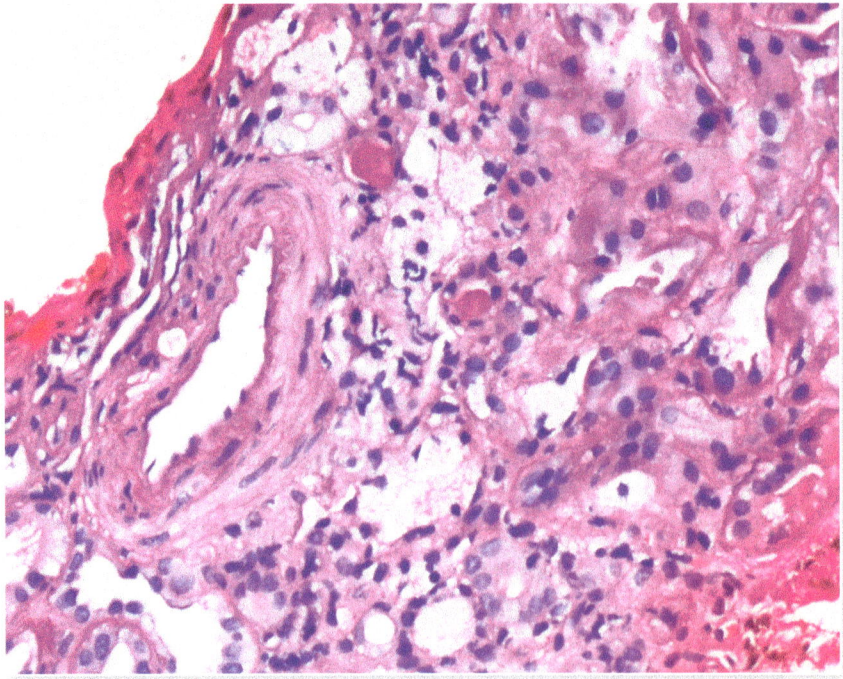
Figure 12.2: Interstitial foam cells in Alport's syndrome (PAS × 200)

Electron Microscopy (Fig. 12.3)

- Thickening of GBM, measuring 800 to 1200 nm, involving >50% of capillary loops
- Irregular outer and inner contours of the GBM
- Splitting with lamellation of lamina densa, forming "basket weave" pattern
- Small electron dense granules in lucent zones of lamina densa
- In children and younger adults, thickened and split foci of GBM are seen
- Alternating with thin, attenuated segments, measuring 100-200 nm
- Foci of mesangial expansion with hypercellularity and subendothelial mesangial expansion
- Focal effacement of foot processes is also noted.

Autosomal recessive Alport's syndrome (ARAS) accounts for 10-15% of cases with identical morphological features. Biallelic mutations are present in either *COL4 A3* or *A4* genes on chromosome 2. The manifestations are equally severe in male and female homozygotes and parents are symptomatic carriers of the disease.[1,2]

Immunofluorescent microscopy shows absence of alpha 3, 4 and 5 chain network of type IV collagen in the GBM and persistence of alpha 5 (IV) chains in the Bowman's capsule and collecting ducts, in contrast to XLAS.

Autosomal dominant Alport's syndrome accounts for <5% of cases of AS with a slower progression, heterozygous mutations of *COL4 A3* and *A4* genes on chromosome 2 and absence of ocular involvement with a milder and more variable clinical phenotype than the X-linked dominant form.

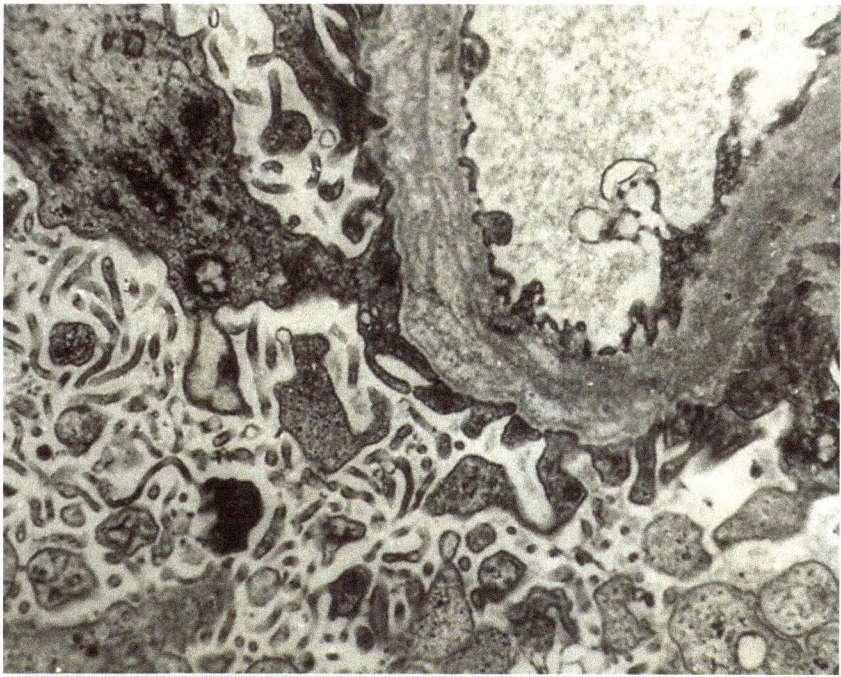

Figure 12.3: Lamellation of lamina densa with electrolucent zones and focal electron dense granules in Alport's syndrome (EM)

Immunofluorescent microscopy can show a normal distribution of alpha chains while EM shows thickening, splitting or diffuse thinning of GBM.

Course and Prognosis

The majority of hemizygous males with the X-linked form progress to end-stage renal disease by the age of 40 years, requiring renal transplantation and the disease does not recur in the transplant. Anti-GBM disease develops in the transplanted kidney in 3–5% of cases with formation of alloantibodies to alpha 5 chains of type IV collagen in XLAS and alpha 3 and 4 chains in ARAS, presenting with crescentic glomerulonephritis, linear immune deposits on GBM and renal failure. The prognosis of autosomal recessive Alport's syndrome is poor in both males and females.[1,8,9]

REFERENCES

1. Hudson BG, Tryggvason K, Sundaramoorthy M, Neilson EG. Alport's syndrome, Goodpasture's syndrome, and Type IV collagen. N Engl J Med. 2003;348:2543-56.
2. Haas M. Alport syndrome and thin glomerular basement membrane nephropathy: a practical approach to diagnosis. Arch Pathol Lab Med. 2009;133:224-32.
3. Hudson BG. The molecular basis of Goodpasture and Alport syndromes: beacons for the discovery of the collagen IV family. J Am Soc Nephrol. 2004;15:25.
4. Savige J, Gregory M, Gross O, Kashtan C, Ding J, Flinter F. Expert guidelines for the management of Alport syndrome and thin basement membrane nephropathy. Am Soc Nephrol. 2013;24:364-75.
5. Kashtan CE. Familial hematuria due to type IV collagen mutations: Alport syndrome and thin basement membrane nephropathy. Curr Opin Pediatr. 2004;16:177-81.
6. Gubler M, Levy M, Broyer M, et al. Alport's syndrome: a report of 58 cases and a review of the literature. Am J Med.1981;70:493-505.
7. Heidet L, Gubler MC. The renal lesions of Alport syndrome. J Am Soc Nephrol. 2009;20(6):1210-5.
8. Kashtan CE, Michael AF. Alport syndrome Kidney Int. 1996;50;1445-63.
9. Kashtan CE Alport syndrome and thin glomerular basement membrane disease. J Am Soc Nephrol. 1998;9(9):1736-50.

THIN BASEMENT MEMBRANE DISEASE/BENIGN FAMILIAL HEMATURIA

Thin basement membrane disease (TBMD)/Benign familial hematuria presents in 1% of cases with persistent microscopic hematuria, normal serum creatinine and negative serologies. There is no evidence of proteinuria or clinical, renal or extrarenal features of Alport's syndrome in benign familial hematuria. 40% of TBMD cases are heterozygous carriers for ARAS with genetic mutations of *COL A3* and *A4* for alpha 3 and alpha 4 chains respectively.[1-4]

Light Microscopy

Light microscopy shows no significant glomerular lesions. Erythrocytes can be present in the Bowman's space and tubular lumina.[5,6]

Electron Microscopy

Electron microscopy shows diffuse uniform thinning of GBM with smooth contours, and a width of <200 nm in children and <250 nm in adults depending on the cut-off values in each laboratory.[1,5,6]

Course and Prognosis

It is usually excellent although some patients develop proteinuria, hypertension and renal failure and require follow-up due to the different implications of the structural defects present.[1,4,7,8] Concomitant IgA nephropathy in 2–39% in different case series and focal and segmental sclerosis in about 5% of cases have been reported.[4,8]

REFERENCES

1. Kashtan CE. Alport syndrome and thin glomerular basement membrane disease. J Am Soc Nephrol. 1998;9:1736-50.
2. Buzza M, Wang YY, Dagher H, Babon JJ, Cotton RG, Powell H, et al. COL4A4 mutation in thin basement membrane disease previously described in Alport syndrome. KidneyInt. 2001;60:480-3.
3. Buzza M, Dagher H, Wang Y Y, Wilson D, Babon JJ, Cotton RG, et al. Mutations in the COL4A4 gene in thin basement membrane disease. Kidney Int. 2003;63:447-53.
4. Savige J, Rana K, Tonna S, Buzza M, Dagher H, Wang YY. Thin basement membrane nephropathy. Kidney Int. 2003;64: 1169-78.
5. Haas M. Thin glomerular basement membrane nephropathy: incidence in 3471 consecutive renal biopsies examined by electron microscopy. Arch Pathol Lab Med. 2006;130:699-706.
6. Haas M. Alport syndrome and thin glomerular basement membrane nephropathy: a practical approach to diagnosis. Arch Pathol Lab Med. 2009;133:224-32.
7. Longo I, Porcedda P, Mari F, et al. COL4A3/COL4A4 mutations: from familial hematuria to autosomal-dominant or recessive. Alport syndrome. Kidney Int. 2002;61:1947-56.
8. Voskarides K, Damianou L, Neocleous V, Christodoulidou S, et al. COL4A3/COLA4 mutations producing focal segmental glomerulosclerosis and renal failure in thin basement membrane nephropathy. JASN. 2007;18:3004-16.

Type III Collagen Nephropathy

This includes two major entities as follows:
- Collagenofibrotic glomerulopathy
- Nail-patella syndrome.

COLLAGENOFIBROTIC GLOMERULOPATHY

It is a rare autosomal recessive renal disease associated with deposition of **banded collagen fibrils (type III) and circulating procollagen type III polypeptides**, involving the glomerular mesangium and subendothelial region.[1-5] This occurs in children and adults, from 6 to 72 years with no gender predilection. These cases presenting with proteinuria, hematuria and hypertension have a reported higher prevalence among Asians, including Indians and were originally detected in the Japanese.[6,7] A phenotypic alteration of mesangial cells and myofibroblastic transformation with type III collagen production, is implicated in the pathogenesis.[7-9]

Microscopic Features[6,7,10,11]

Light Microscopy

- Global mesangial expansion and capillary wall thickening by amorphous eosinophilic material (Fig. 12.4)
- Stains weakly with PAS, Masson trichrome and JMS +/-

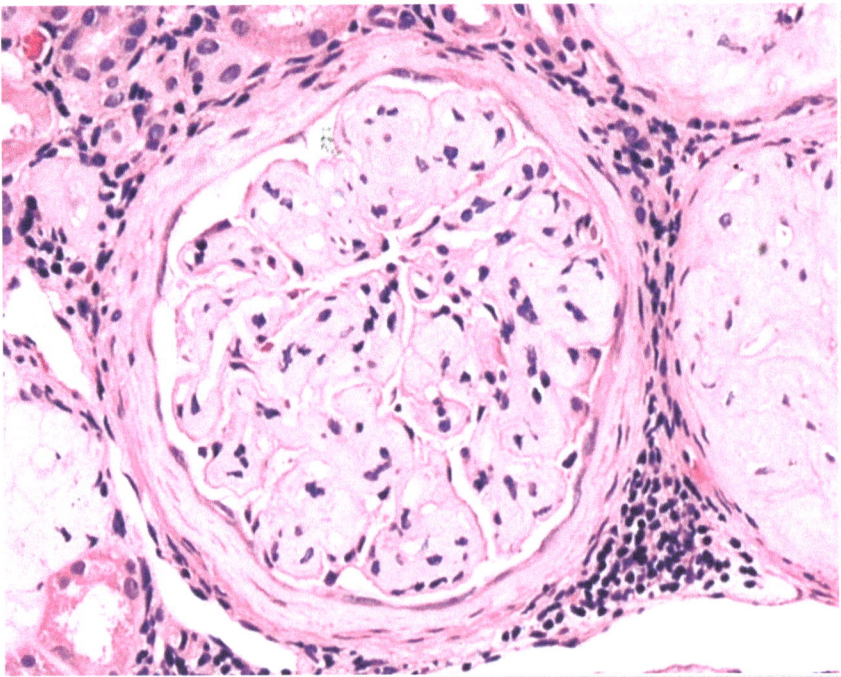

Figure 12.4: Collagenofibrotic glomerulopathy (H & E x 400)

Heredofamilial Glomerulopathies

- Thioflavin T and Congo red negative
- Inner subendothelial band of newly formed GBM or more organized abnormal collagen deposits
- Staining intensely with trichrome and silver stains, seen with high power magnification.

Immunofluorescence

- Negative for immunoglobulins and complement
- Mesangium and subendothelium stains positive with antisera to type III collagen.

Electron Microscopy

- Typical curved collagen fibrils with frayed ends in subendothelial region and mesangium (Fig. 12.5)
- Periodicity of banded collagen of 60 nm is seen (Fig. 12.6)
- Normal lamina densa in contrast to nail-patella syndrome
- Effacement of foot processes of podocytes.

Differential Diagnosis[6,7]

1. **Membranoproliferative glomerulonephritis** has distinctive diagnostic features on IF and EM, that can be excluded.
2. **Nail-patella syndrome**: An **autosomal dominant syndrome** with specific clinical dysmorphic features and electron lucencies in GBM, including lamina densa, containing fibrillar collagen on EM.

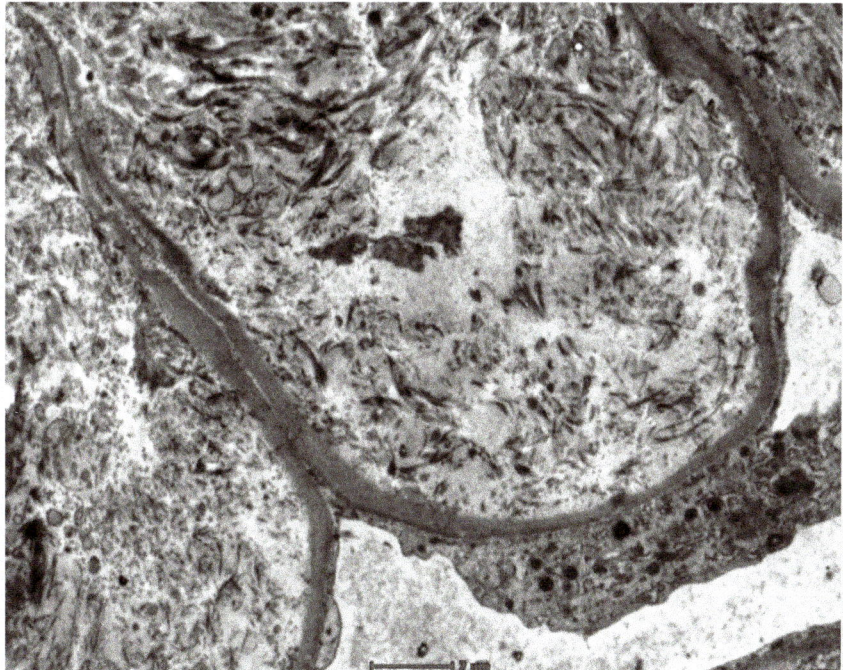

Figure 12.5: Electron micrograph with subendothelial and mesangial collagen fibrils

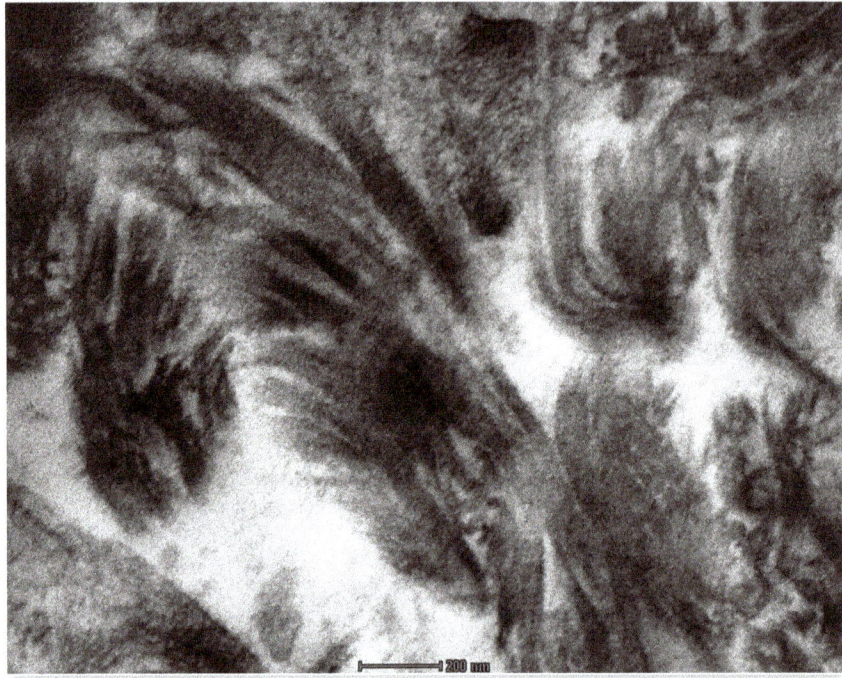

Figure 12.6: Collagenofibrotic glomerulopathy with banded collagen fibrils (EM x 43000)

3. **Fibrillary glomerulopathies**: are distinguished by Congo red negative mesangial and capillary wall deposits with different organized immune-derived deposits seen on IF and EM.
4. **Amyloidosis** has characteristic features on histochemical stains, immunochemistry and EM as detailed in the previous chapter.

Course and Prognosis

The disease has an unpredictable course with no specific treatment and a subset progresses to end-stage renal failure. Occasional cases have been associated with factor VIII deficiency, hemolytic uremic syndrome and hemolytic anemia.[6,7]

NAIL-PATELLA SYNDROME (HEREDITARY OSTEO-ONYCHODYSPLASIA)

Nail-patella syndrome is a rare autosomal dominant skeleletal disease caused by *LMX1B* gene mutation on chromosome 9q34.1, known as LIM-homeodomain transcription factor gene; involved in limb development, collagen expression and maturation of basement membranes of the glomeruli, anterior chamber of eye and inner ear; dopaminergic and serotonergic neurons.[13,14] LMX1B is primarily present in the podocytes and regulates the expression of podocyte slit diaphragm proteins and alpha 3 and alpha 4 chains of type IV collagen of the GBM.[13,15-17] There is associated classical clinical tetrad of dysplasia of the nails, patella, elbows,bilateral iliac horns.Other variable features include swan neck deformity of proximal and distal interphalangeal joints, foot deformities, scoliosis and joint contractures, open angle glaucoma and hearing impairment. Renal involvement occurs in about 35–40% of cases with proteinuria, microscopic hematuria and renal failure.[13]

Microscopic Features

Light Microscopy[18,19]

- Focal mild mesangial expansion with mild thickening of capillary walls
- Focal and segmental sclerosis
- Foci of interstitial fibrosis, tubular atrophy and arteriolar hyalinosis.

Immunofluorescence Microscopy

Negative or nonspecific trapping of IgM and C3 in sclerotic tufts.

Electron Microscopy

- Irregular thickening of GBM with mottled electron lucent areas
- Banded collagen fibrils, with periodicity of interstitial type collagen
- Located in lucent foci including mid-lamina densa
- Stained with phosphotungstic acid
- Focal effacement of foot processes, also present.

Differential Diagnosis

1. **Collagenofibrotic glomerulopathy:** Displays PAS-negative expansion of mesangium with capillary wall thickening and lacks "moth-eaten" lucencies of the GBM, on EM
2. **Banded collagen fibrils** are present in subendothelial region and mesangium.

Course and Prognosis

It is unpredictable and EM changes can occur in the absence of renal symptoms. Progression to renal failure occurs in about 30% of symptomatic cases.[13,14]

REFERENCES

1. Alchi B, Nishi S, Narital, Gejyo F. Collagenofibrotic glomerulopathy: clinicopathologic overview of a rare glomerular disease. Am J Kidney Dis. 2007;49:499-506.
2. Cohen AH. Collagen type III glomerulopathies. Advances In Chronic Kidney Diseases. 2012;19:101-6.
3. Gubler MC, Dommergues JP, Foulard M, et al. Collagen type III glomerulopathy: A new type of hereditary nephropathy. Pediatr Nephrol. 1993;7:354-60.
4. Ikeda K, Yokoyama H, Tomosugi N, et al. Primary glomerular fibrosis: a new nephropathy caused by diffuse intra-glomerular increase in atypical type III collagen fibres. Clin Nephrol. 1990;33:155-9.
5. Imbasciati E, Gherardi G, Morozumi K, et al. Collagen type III glomerulopathy: A new idiopathic glomerular disease. Am J Nephrol. 1991;11:422-9.
6. Herrera GA, Turbat-Herrera EA. Renal diseases with organized deposits: an algorithmic approach to classification and clinicopathologic diagnosis. Archives of Pathology and Laboratory Medicine. 2010;134(4):512-31.
7. Duggal R, Nada R, Rayat CS, Rane SU, Sakhuja V, Joshi K. Collagenofibrotic glomerulopathy—a review. Clin Kidney J. 2012;5:7-12.

8. Scheinman JI, Tanaka H, Haralson H, et al. Specialized collagen mRNA and secreted collagens in human glomerular epithelial, mesangial and tubular cells. J Am Soc Nephrol. 1992;2:1475-83.
9. Naruse K, Ito H, Moriki T, et al. Mesangial cell activation in the collagenofibrotic glomerulopathy. Case report and review of the literature. Virchow Arch. 1998;433:183-8.
10. Khubchandani SR, Chitale AR, Gowrishankar S. Banded collagen in the kidney with special reference to collagenofibrotic glomerulopathy. Ultrastruct Pathol. 2010;34:68-72.
11. Patro KC, Jha R, Sahay M, Swarnalatha G. Collagenofibrotic glomerulopathy - Case report with review of Literature. Indian J Nephrol. 2011;21:52-55.
12. Soni SS, Gowrishankar S, Nagarik AP, et al. Collagenofibrotic glomerulopathy in association with Hodgkin's lymphoma. Saudi J Kidney Dis Transpl. 2011;22:126-9.
13. Sweeney E, Fryer A, Mountford R, Green A, McIntosh I. Nail patella syndrome: a review of the phenotype aided by developmental biology. J Med Genet 2003;40:153-62.
14. Bennett WM, Musgrave JE, Campbell RA, Elliot D, Cox R, Brooks RE, et al. The nephropathy of the nail-patella syndrome.Clinicopathologic analysis of 11 kindred. Am J Med. 1973;54:304-19.
15. Morello R, Zhou G, Dreyer S, Harvey S, Ninomiya Y, Thorner P, et al. Regulation of glomerular basement membrane collagen expression by LMX1B contributes to renal disease in nail patella syndrome. Nat Genet. 2001;27:205-8.
16. Morello R, Lee B. Insight in to podocyte differentiation from the study of human genetic disease: nail-patella syndrome and transcriptional regulation in podocytes. Pediatr Res. 2002;51:551-8.
17. Miner J, Morello R, Andrews K, Li C, Antignac C, Shaw A, et al. Transcriptional induction of slit diaphragm genes by Lmx1b is required in podocyte differentiation. J Clin Invest. 2002;109:1065-72.
18. Lemley KV. Kidney disease in nail–patella syndrome. Pediatr Nephrol. 2009;24(12):2345-54.
19. Heidet L, Bongers EMHF, Sich M, Zhang S-Y, Loirat C, Meyrier A. In vivo expression of putative LMX1B Targets in Nail-Patella syndrome Kidneys. Am J Pathol. 2003;163(1):145-55.

Fibronectin Glomerulopathy

Fibronectin glomerulopathy is a rare autosomal dominant genetic disease, caused by the glomerular deposition of fibronectin, a large dimeric adhesive glycoprotein, derived from the soluble plasma isoform and involving chromosome, 1q32 and the regulation of complement activation gene. This is associated with proteinuria, varying degrees of hematuria and renal failure occurring in the third or fourth decade.[1-6]

MICROSCOPIC FEATURES

Light Microscopy[1]

- Marked lobular expansion by pale eosinophilic, acellular amorphous mesangial and capillary deposits (Fig. 12.7)
- Obliteration of capillary lumina is seen
- PAS positive, JMS negative and Congo red negative material is noted
- Focal fuschinophilia is seen on Masson trichrome.

Immunofluorescence

- Homogeneous staining of mesangium and capillary walls by antiserum specific for plasma fibronectin
- Negative for immunoglobulins and complement.

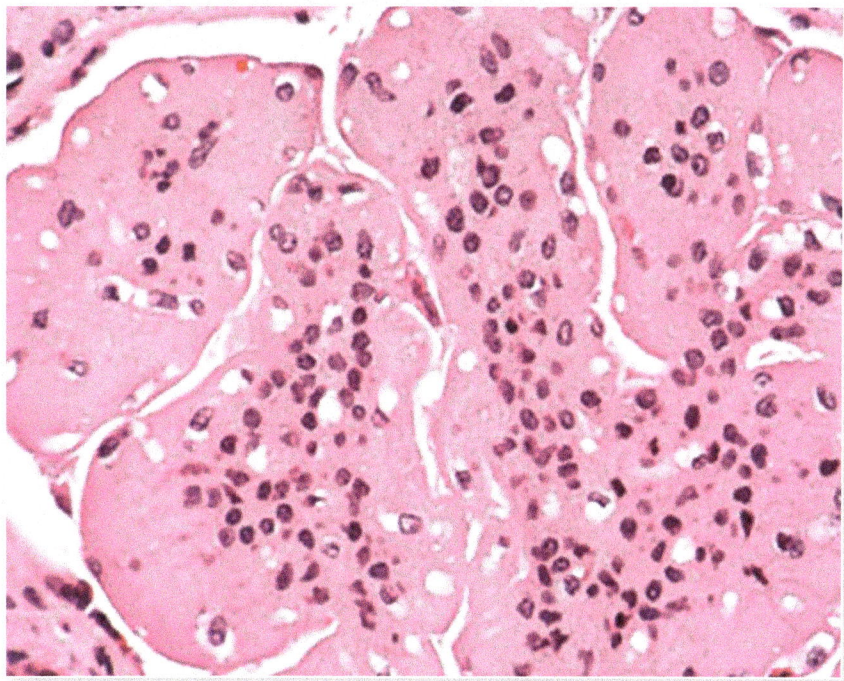

Figure 12.7: Fibronectin glomerulopathy (H & E x 400)

Electron Microscopy

- Homogeneous to finely granular electron dense deposits in mesangium and subendothelial region (Fig. 12.8)
- Fibrillar substructure, 12 nm in width, is noted in occasional cases.

Differential Diagnosis

This includes membranoproliferative glomerulonephritis, monoclonal immunoglobulin deposition disease (MIDD), cryoglobulinemic GN and fibrillary glomerulonephritis. The distinct IF/EM features and absence of immunoglobulin deposits and complement confirms the diagnosis and excludes these entities. Currently, molecular proteomics with laser capture microdissection on formalin fixed renal biopsies of fibronectin glomerulopathy, have proved the presence of fibronectin with fibulin-1 in glomeruli, associated with disrupted mesangial and podocyte function and proteinuria.[7]

Course and Prognosis

The disease progresses to end-stage renal failure in 15 to 20 years and recurs in renal transplants.[8,9]

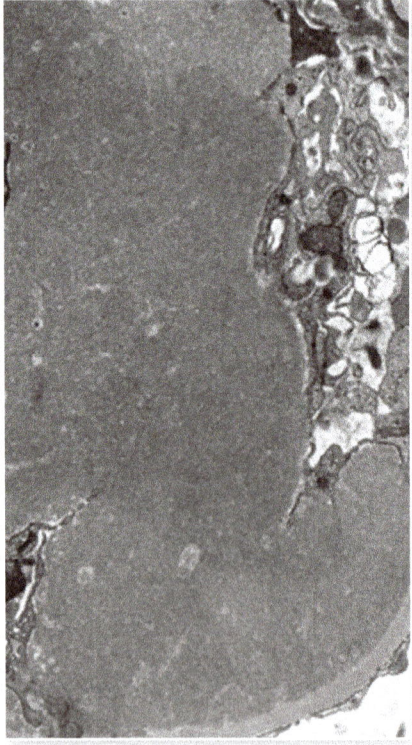

Figure 12.8: Homogeneous to finely granular subendothelial deposits (EM x 6000) (Internet Resource)

REFERENCES

1. Strom EH, Banfi G, Krapf R. Glomerulopathy associated with predominant fibronectin deposits: a newly recognized hereditary disease. Kidney Int. 1995;48;163-70.
2. Abt AB, Wasner SJ, Moran J. Familal lobular glomerulopathy. Hum Pathol. 1991;2:825-9.
3. Mazzucco G, Maran E, Rolino C, Monga G. Glomerulonephritis with organized deposits: a mesangiopathic, not immune complex-mediated disease? Hum Pathol. 1992;23:63-68.
4. Assmann KJ, Koene RA, Wetzels JF. Familial glomerulonephritis characterized by massive deposits of fibronectin. Am J Kidney Dis. 1995;25(5):781.
5. Sato H, Matsubara M, Marumo R, Soma J, Kurosawa K, Taguma Y, et al. Familial lobular glomerulopathy: first case report in Asia. Am J Kidney Dis. 1998;31(6):E3.
6. Jung M, Ruschendorf F, Rainer R, Weinker T. The gene for human fibronectin glomerulopathy maps to 1q32, in the region of the regulation of complement activation gene cluster. AJHG. 1998;63:1724-31.
7. Satoskar AA, Shapiro JP, Bott C. Characterization of glomerular diseases using proteomic analysis of laser capture microdissected glomeruli. Mod Pathol. 2012;25(5):709-21.
8. Tuttle SE, Sharma HM, Bay W, Heber L. A unique familial lobular glomerulopathy. Arch Pathol Lab Med.1987;111:726-31.
9. Gemperle O, Neuweiler J, Reutter FW, Hildebrandt F, Krapf R. Familial glomerulopathy with giant fibrillar (fibronectin-positive) deposits: 15-year follow-up in a large kindred. Am J Kidney Dis. 1996;28(5):668-75.

Lipid Storage Diseases

Lysosomal storage diseases are caused by deficiency of lysosomal enzymes with excessive accumulation of substrates such as glycosphingolipids, glycogen, glycoproteins, lipoproteins and mucolipids. **The major primary lipid storage diseases involving the renal parenchyma are:**
- Fabry's disease
- Familial lecithin cholesterol acyltransferase, (LCAT) deficiency
- Lipoprotein glomerulopathy.

FABRY'S DISEASE

Fabry's disease (Angiokeratoma corporis diffusum) is an X-linked recessive disorder due to deficient activity of the lysosomal hydrolase alpha galactosidase A, resulting in the deposition of the neutral glycosphingolipid, globotriaosylceramide (ceramide trihexoside) in vascular endothelium and smooth muscle, dorsal root and autonomic ganglia.[1,2] The manifestations of cutaneous angiokeratomas in the lower trunk and thighs, corneal opacities, acroparaesthesias, hypohidrosis, renal and cardiac involvement affect hemizygous males with a variable expression in heterozygous female carriers. The disease occurs in all racial and ethnic populations with a prevalence of 0.16–1.2%.[3,4] Renal involvement with proteinuria, renal failure, reduced glomerular filtration rate and hypertension are presenting features in young adults and in children.[1]

Microscopic Features

Light Microscopy[5-9]

- Glomeruli display enlarged podocytes with foamy vacuolization as the classical lesion (Fig. 12.9)
- Variable vacuolation of endothelial, mesangial cells and parietal epithelial cells of Bowman's capsule
- In frozen sections, the material is positive with lipid stains
- Granular podocyte inclusions stain with toluidine blue in osmicated 1 micron sections (Fig. 12.10)
- In advanced lesions, focal and segmental and global glomerulosclerosis obscure classical features
- Distal tubules can show finely vacuolated cytoplasm
- Small interlobular arteries and arterioles show focal endothelial and smooth muscle vacuolization
- Interstitial foam cells and foci of interstitial fibrosis and tubular atrophy and arteriosclerosis develop with chronic lesions.

Electron Microscopy[8]

- Lamellated myelin inclusions with concentric layers (3–5 nm) and striped inclusions (zebra bodies) are found mainly in podocytes (Fig. 12.11)
- Sparse inclusions in glomerular capillary endothelial cells and mesangial or parietal cells.

Heredofamilial Glomerulopathies

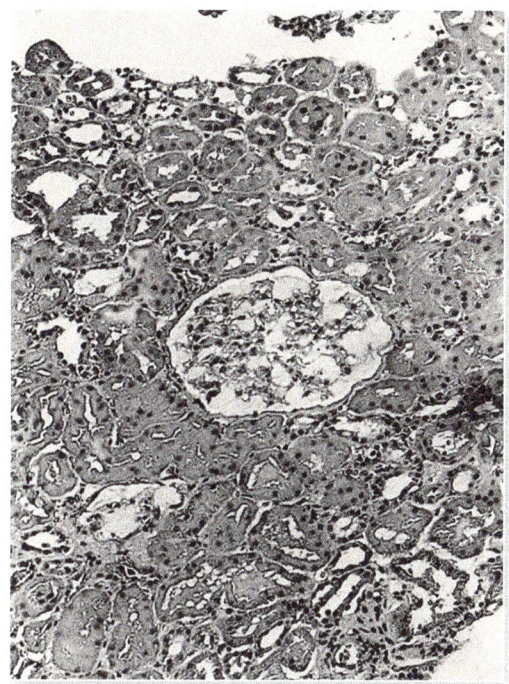

Figure 12.9: Foamy vacuolization of podocytes (H & E x 100)

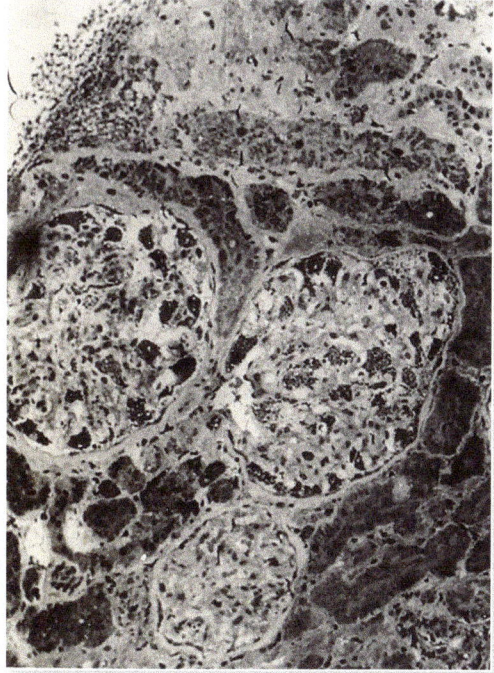

Figure 12.10: Granular inclusions in podocytes (Toluidine blue x 200)

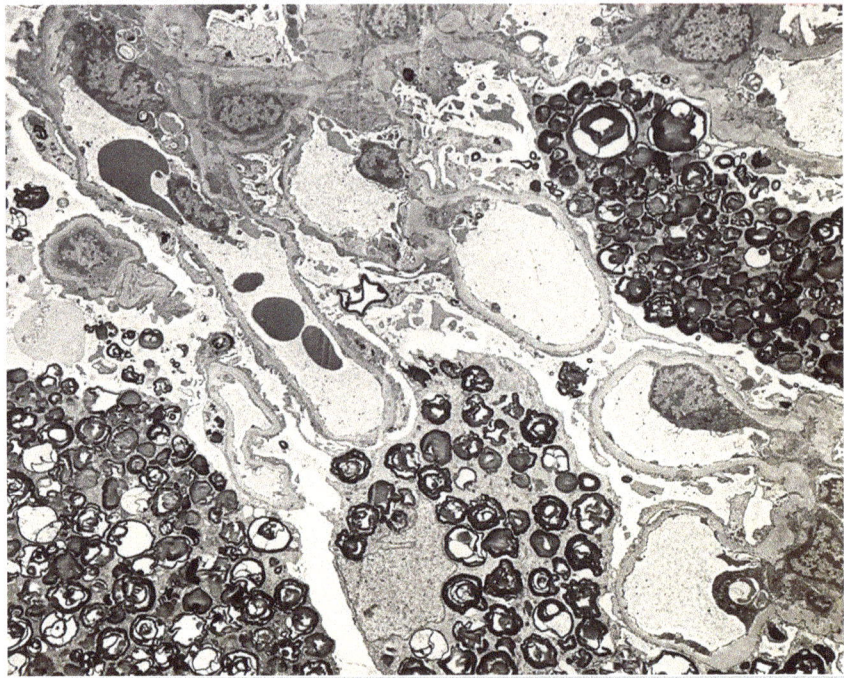

Figure 12.11: Lamellated myelin inclusions in podocytes (EM)

Differential Diagnosis

1. **Mucolipidosis, type 2 (I cell disease):** Vacuolated podocytes, when present, are positive for Alcian blue-PAS. Empty membrane bound intracellular vesicles within the podocyte cytoplasm are found on EM.
2. **Hurler syndrome (Mucopolysaccharidosis type I):** Intracellular vacuoles in podocytes rarely contain granular material, lacking in myelin inclusions, on EM.
3. **Gaucher syndrome:** Glomerular endocapillary cells and interstitial cells with pale, wrinkled cytoplasm are rarely present.

Course and Prognosis

Renal transplantation corrects enzyme deficiency in end-stage renal Fabry's disease with good survival and renal function, in our experience in CMC.[1] Enzyme replacement therapy slows progression of Fabry nephropathy by decreasing the glycosphingolipid deposits. Chronic glomerular and interstitial lesions can develop early in the course of the disease prior to clinical signs of CKD. A scoring system for the extent of lipid storage inclusions, glomerular sclerosis and interstitial fibrosis has been utilized by the International Study Group of Fabry Nephropathy, for the assessment of prognosis and response to therapy.[10] Graft recurrences are uncommon and have been reported to occur in transplants from live related asymptomatic female heterozygotes and associated with undetected or retrospective diagnosis of Fabry's disease in native kidneys after transplantation. A favorable outcome is limited by extrarenal involvement, infections and graft recurrences.[1]

FAMILIAL LECITHIN CHOLESTEROL ACYLTRANSFERASE DEFICIENCY

Familial lecithin cholesterol acyltransferase (LCAT) deficiency is an extremely rare autosomal recessive disorder caused by *LCAT* gene mutation on chromosome 16q21-q22. The LCAT enzyme catalyzes the formation of cholesterol esters in lipoproteins. LCAT deficiency is associated with reduction in plasma HDL cholesterol, lipid deposition in various organs including kidneys with proteinuria and renal failure, corneal opacities, hemolytic anemia and atherosclerosis.[11-15]

Microscopic Features

Light Microscopy[11]

- Glomerular mesangial expansion with mild hypercellularity and foam cells
- Capillary wall thickening and reduplication with interposition of foamy lipid material
- Foci of segmental sclerosis and global sclerosis of the tufts in advanced lesions
- Interstitial fibrosis with tubular atrophy and foam cells
- Arteriosclerosis with lipid deposits in vascular walls.

Immunofluorescence

Negative.

Electron Microscopy[11,14,15]

- Subepithelial and intramembranous lipid deposits
- Deposits contain osmiophilic curvilinear serpiginous and lamellar structures (Fig. 12.12)

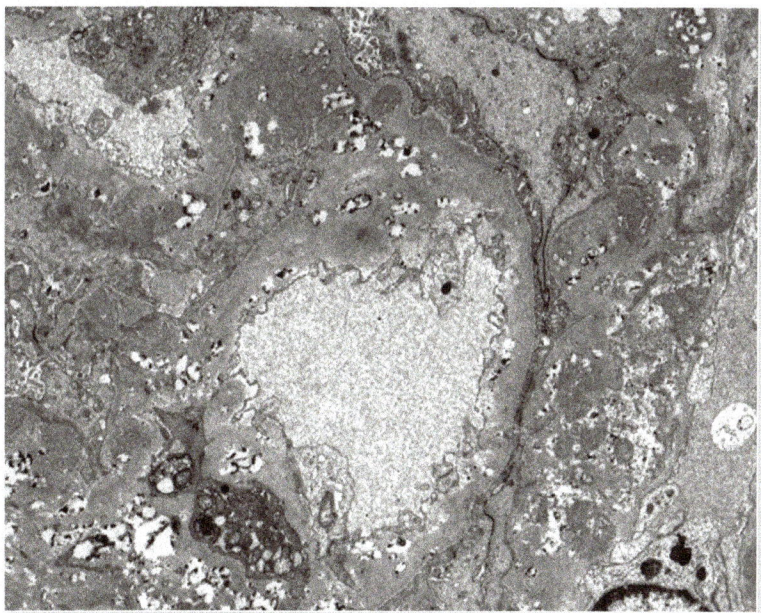

Figure 12.12: LCAT deficiency with electrolucent intramembranous and mesangial lipid deposits with osmophilic inclusions (EM)

Renal Biopsy Interpretation

- Subendothelial granular densities in lipid material are also present
- Mesangial lipid material contains large electron dense deposits with increased matrix.

Course and Prognosis

Proteinuria with renal failure is slowly progressive from onset in childhood and recurs in renal transplants. Concomitant membranous nephropathy has been reported recently with inhibitory anti-LCAT antibody and glomerular features similar to LCAT disease, detected by immunohistochemistry and immunofluorescence.[16]

LIPOPROTEIN GLOMERULOPATHY

Lipoprotein glomerulopathy is an autosomal recessive disorder of lipoprotein metabolism caused by mutations and deletions of *Apolipoprotein E* gene on chromosome 19q13.2 with its alleles associated with abnormal isoforms of this apolipoprotein. The disease predominantly occurs in Asians and mainly, the Japanese with hyperlipoproteinemia, steroid resistant nephrotic syndrome and late onset renal failure.[17-20]

Microscopic Features

Light Microscopy

- Enlarged glomeruli with capillary ectasia by pale laminated, vacuolated thrombi (Fig. 12.13)
- Thrombi are sudanophilic and stain with Oil-red O on frozen sections
- Mesangiolysis with attenuation of capillary walls is seen
- Duplication of capillary walls occurs later with mesangial sclerosis, hyalinosis and global sclerosis.

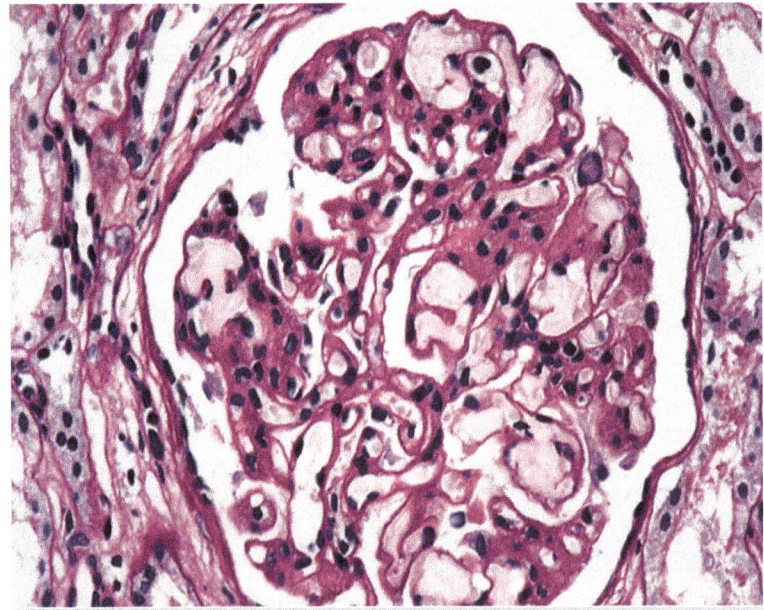

Figure 12.13: Lipoprotein glomerulopathy (PAS x 400) (Internet Resource)

Immunofluorescence
Negative.

Electron Microscopy
- Glomerular capillary lumina contain concentrically laminated, finely vacuolated thrombi
- Mesangial matrix increase with hypercellularity
- Segmental mesangial interposition with focal capillary wall thickening and reduplication of GBM.

Renal involvement by other lysosomal storage diseases is extremely rare and are not associated with significant impairment of renal function and include nephrosialidosis, sphingolipidoses (Niemann-Pick disease and gangliosidosis), mucolipidosis (I-cell Disease). Mucopolysaccharidosis, Farber's disease and glycoproteinoses (Fucosidosis). Cytoplasmic vacuoles containing sparse granular material with lipid lamellae or fibrillo-granular/lamellar inclusions can be found variably in podocytes, mesangial cells and endothelial cells or in tubular epithelial cells and interstitial macrophages on electron microscopy in these disorders.

REFERENCES

1. Branton MH, Schiffmann R, Sabnis SG, et al. Natural history of Fabryrenal disease: influence of alpha galactosidase A activity and genetic mutations on clinical course. Medicine (Baltimore). 2002;81:122-38.
2. Rao M, Jacob M, Korula A, Chandi SM, Jacob CK, Shastry JCM. Renal replacement therapy in Fabry's disease-A report of three cases and a review of the literature. JAPI. 1994;42(1):65-7.
3. Kotanko P, Kramar R, Devrnja D, Paschke E, Voigtländer T, Auinger M, et al. Results of a nationwide screening for Anderson-Fabry disease among dialysis patients. J Am Soc Nephrol. 2004;15(5):1323.
4. Tanaka M, Ohashi T, Kobayashi M, Eto Y, Miyamura N, Nishida K, et al. Identification of Fabry's disease by the screening of alpha-galactosidase A activity in male and female hemodialysis patients. Clin Nephrol. 2005;64(4):281-7.
5. Alroy J, Sabnis S, Kopp JB. Renal pathology in Fabry disease. J Am Soc Nephrol. 2002;13(Suppl 2):S134–S138.
6. Fischer EG, Moore MJ, Lager DJ. Fabry disease: a morphologic study of 11 cases. Mod Pathol. 2006;19:1295-301.
7. Tondel C, Bostad L, Hirth A, et al. Renal biopsy findings in children and adolescents with Fabry disease and minimal albuminuria. Am J Kidney Dis. 2008;51:767-76.
8. Sessa A, Toson A, Nebuloni M, et al. Renal ultrastructural findings in Anderson-Fabry disease. J Nephrol. 2002;15:109-12.
9. Sessa A, Meroni M, Battini G, et al. Renal pathological changes in Fabry disease. J Inherit Metab Dis. 2001;24 (Suppl 2):66-70.
10. Fogo AB, Bostad L, Scarstad E, et al. Scoring system for the renal pathology in Fabry disease: Report of the International Study Group of Fabry Nephropathy (ISFGN). Nephrol Dial Transplant. 2010;25:2168-77.
11. Papa V, et al. The role of ultrastructural examination in storage diseases ultrastructural pathology, iFirst:1–9, 2010DOI: 10.3109/01913121003780593.
12. Shoji K, Morita H, Ishigaki Y, et al. Lecithin-cholesterol acyltransferase (LCAT) deficiency without mutations in the coding sequence: a case report and literature review. Clin Nephrol. 2011;76(4):323-8.
13. Frasca GM, Sovereni L, Tampieri E, Franscechini G, Calabresi L, et al. A 33 year-old man with nephritic syndrome and Lecithin-Cholesterol Acyl Transferase (LCAT) deficiency. Description of two new mutations in the LCAT gene Nephrol Dial Transplant. 2004;19:1622-4.
14. Lager DJ, Rosenberg BF, Shapiro H, Bernstein J. Lecithin cholesterol acyl transferase deficiency: ultrastructural examination of sequential renal biopsies Mod Pathol. 1991;4(3):331-5.
15. Imbasciati E, Paties C, Scarpioni L, Mihatsch MJ. Renal lesions in familial lecithin-cholesterol acyl transferase deficiency. Ultrastructural heterogeneity of glomerular changes. Am J Nephrol. 1986;6(1):66-70.
16. Takahashi S, Hiromura K, Tsukida M, Ohishi Y. Nephrotic syndrome caused by immune-mediated LCAT deficiency. Am Soc Nephrol. 2013;24(8):1305-12.
17. Saito T, Sato H, Kudo K, Oikawa S, Shibata T, Hara Y, et al. Lipoprotein glomerulopathy: glomerular lipoprotein thrombi in a patient with hyperlipoproteinemia. Am J Kidney Dis.1989;13(2):148.
18. Saito T, Matsunaga A, Oikawa S. Impact of lipoprotein glomerulopathy on the relationship between lipids and renal diseases. Am J Kidney Dis. 2006;47(2):199.
19. Saito T, Oikawa S, Sato H, Sasaki J. Lipoprotein glomerulopathy: renal lipidosis induced by novel apolipoprotein E variants. Nephron.1999;83(3):193.
20. Saito T, Oikawa S, Sato H, Sato T, Ito S, SasakiJ. Lipoprotein glomerulopathy: significance of lipoprotein and ultrastructural features. Kidney Int Suppl. 1999;71:S37.

Congenital Nephrotic Syndrome and Podocytopathies

Nephrotic syndrome in the first year of life consists of two major groups, congenital and infantile nephrotic syndrome; the former detected in the first three months and the latter from 3 to 12 months of life respectively. The majority are caused **by genetic mutations encoding proteins that regulate the function of slit diaphragm or podocyte cytoskeleton, the glomerular basement membrane and mitochondria or transcription factors required for the development of the kidneys and the gonads.**

The major renal lesions associated with these hereditary forms of nephrotic syndrome are:
- Finnish type congenital nephrotic syndrome (FT-CNS)
- Diffuse mesangial sclerosis (DMS)
- Minimal change nephrotic syndrome (MCNS)
- Focal segmental, glomerular sclerosis (Familial FSGS I,II,III).

FINNISH TYPE CONGENITAL NEPHROTIC SYNDROME

Finnish type congenital nephrotic syndrome is an autosomal recessive disorder caused by mutation of the **nephrin gene, NPHS1** on 19q13.1 encoding for a transmembrane protein localized to the slit diaphragm. The disease predominantly occurs in Finland and rarely in other ethnic races worldwide and is associated with premature birth, low birthweight, enlarged placenta and nephrotic syndrome in utero.[1-3]

Microscopic Features

Light Microscopy

- Normal size glomeruli to persistence of fetal glomeruli
- Mild mesangial hypercellularity with mild increase in matrix (Fig. 12.14)
- Microcystic dilatation of Bowman's space
- Mesangial sclerosis with global glomerulosclerosis in advanced lesions
- Proximal tubular dilatation with microcysts
- Arteriolosclerosis and arteriosclerosis is noted with tubulointerstitial scarring.

Immunofluorescence

Negative for nephrin antisera.

Electron Microscopy

- Diffuse effacement of foot processes with absent slit diaphragms
- Thinner than normal GBM.

Course and Prognosis

Complications of nephrotic syndrome occur with infections and azotemia develops by 4 to 8 years of age. Recurrence of nephrotic syndrome after renal transplants is associated with anti-nephrin antibodies.

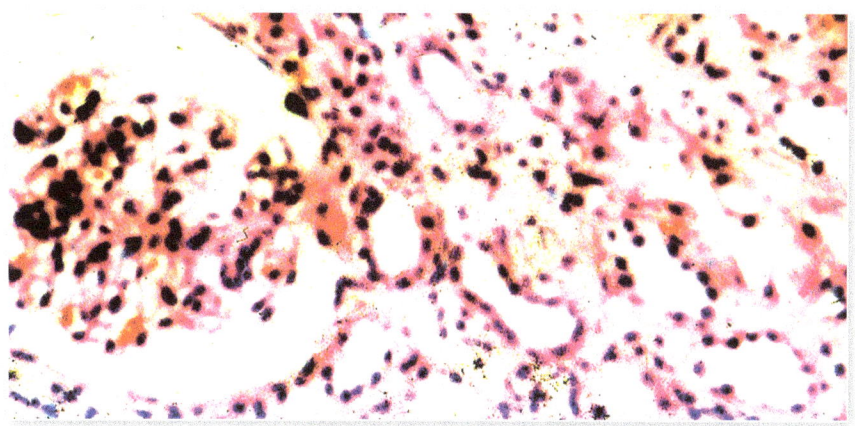

Figure 12.14: Congenital nephrotic syndrome: Finnish type (H & E x 200)

DIFFUSE MESANGIAL SCLEROSIS

Diffuse mesangial sclerosis has a broader range of presentation from birth to infancy and rapid rate of progression to renal failure. Isolated DMS occurs in the **non-syndromic form** and **syndromic forms** of the disease are associated with extrarenal manifestations. *WT1* gene mutations on chromosome 11p13 are found in both forms of the disease.[1-3]

Microscopic Features

Light Microscopy (Fig. 12.15)

- Mesangial matrix expansion with mild mesangial hypercellularity
- Mesangial sclerosis with marked hypertrophy of podocytes
- Large, vacuolated podocytes form a corona around sclerotic tufts
- Solid, retracted tufts with dilated Bowman's space.

Immunofluorescence

Nonspecific trapping of IgM and C3 in sclerotic tufts.

Immunohistochemistry

Nuclear expression of *WT-1* reduced or absent

Electron Microscopy

Irregular thickening and scalloping of GBM.

Course and Prognosis

End-stage renal disease develops by 3 to 4 years of age.

Syndromic forms of DMS include Denys-Drash syndrome and ocular renal syndromes (Pierson syndrome).

150 Renal Biopsy Interpretation

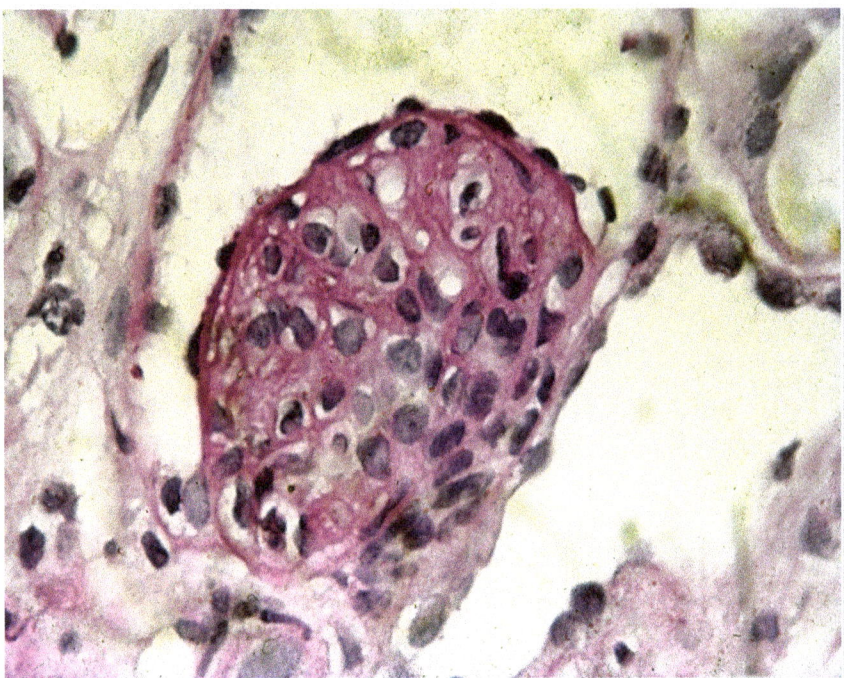

Figure 12.15: Diffuse mesangial sclerosis (PAS x 400)

Denys-Drash syndrome: It is the most important syndromic form which is an autosomal dominant triad of early onset nephrotic syndrome, Wilms syndrome and male pseudohermaphroditism associated with *WT1* gene mutation and diffuse mesangial sclerosis.

Pierson syndrome is an ocular renal syndrome associated with *LAMB2* gene mutation with loss of laminin beta2 protein expression of GBM, synaptic basal laminae and ocular basement membranes, resulting in irregular lamellation and attenuation of GBM and microcoria with pupil diameter of less than 2 mm. Diffuse mesangial sclerosis is seen with segmental and global glomerulosclerosis by light microscopy with attenuated GBM and crowding of podocytes on EM.

MINIMAL CHANGE NEPHROTIC SYNDROME

Inherited forms of MCNS that are steroid resistant have been reported with genetic mutations and include a non-syndromic type associated with the podocin (NPHS2) gene and a syndromic type with dysferlin (DYSF) gene of limb-girdle muscular dystrophy, 2B mutation.[1,4]

FOCAL SEGMENTAL GLOMERULOSCLEROSIS

Inherited non-syndromic forms of FSGS are associated with genetic mutations including NPHS1(nephrin), NPHS2 (podocin) and NPHS3 (phospholipase Cepsilon1) that are autosomal recessive; ACTN4 (alpha-actinin-4), TRPC-6 (Transient receptor potential cation channel-6), MYH9 (non-muscle myosin heavy chain protein) that are autosomal dominant mutations and CD2AP (CD2 receptor associated protein) that is either an autosomal recessive, or dominant mutation.[1,4,5]

Heredofamilial Glomerulopathies

Syndromic forms of genetically determined FSGS are associated with other organ abnormalities and include **Frasier syndrome** (WT-1 mutation with triad of nephrotic syndrome, male pseudohermaphroditism and gonadoblastoma), Nail-patella syndrome (*LMX1B* gene), Alport's syndrome (*COLA3, A4* and *A5* genes) and mitochondriopathies including COQ2 and COQ6 nephropathy (coenzyme Q2 and 6 synthetase) and mitochondrial tRNA mutations.

COLLAPSING GLOMERULOPATHY

Non-syndromic forms include COQ2 nephropathy and syndromic forms comprise action myoclonus renal failure (*SCARB2/Limp2* gene) and mandibuloacral dysplasia, associated with zinc metalloproteinase (*ZMPSTE24* gene).[1,6,7]

PODOCYTOPATHIES

Podocytopathies are proteinuric diseases resulting from intrinsic or extrinsic podocyte injury with alterations in the genotype or phenotype of podocytes and glomerular morphology. Podocytes are post-mitotic cells that regulate glomerular permselectivity; provide structural support along with mesangial cells to resist distension by intracapillary hydraulic pressure and are involved in remodeling of GBM and endocytosis of filtered proteins. The specialized architecture including the slit diaphragm complex, actin-based cytoskeleton with adhesion proteins, the adherent GBM and biochemical signals that maintain their differentiation, modulates their function.

The normal three-dimensional structure is lost in foot process effacement, associated with reorganization of the actin-based cytoskeleton and redistribution of slit diaphragm components to the cytoplasm. Irreversible podocyte effacement is often associated with genetic mutations and are steroid resistant.

Classification of Podocytopathies

Classification is based on histopathology, defined by podocyte number and four different morphological types and the etiology including idiopathic, genetic and reactive forms associated with podocyte injury.[6] Distinct pathways of podocyte injury and repair lead to four major morphologic patterns (Fig. 12.16). Causes of podocyte injury include intrinsic genetic mutations, involving nuclear transcription factors (WT1, PAX2 and LMX1B), actin based cytoskeleton (ACTN4 mutations), slit diaphragm complex (NPHS1, NPHS2 and CD2AP mutations) plasma membrane (TRPC6) mitochondria (tRNA,COQ2), metabolic enzymes (Fabry disease) and extracellular matrix (LAMB2) (Fig. 12.17).

1. **Minimal change nephropathy (MCN):** From mild podocyte injury with foot process effacement and normal podocyte number.
2. **Focal and segmental glomerulosclerosis (FSGS):** From severe podocyte injury, podocyte apoptosis/detachment and podocyte depletion with podocytopenia and segmental sclerosis.
3. **Diffuse mesangial sclerosis (DMS):** From developmental arrest and delayed cellular maturation with sclerosis of mesangial matrix and low rate of proliferation of podocytes.
4. **Collapsing glomerulopathy (CG):** From dysregulation of podocyte phenotype with dedifferentiation and exuberant proliferation with capillary collapse.

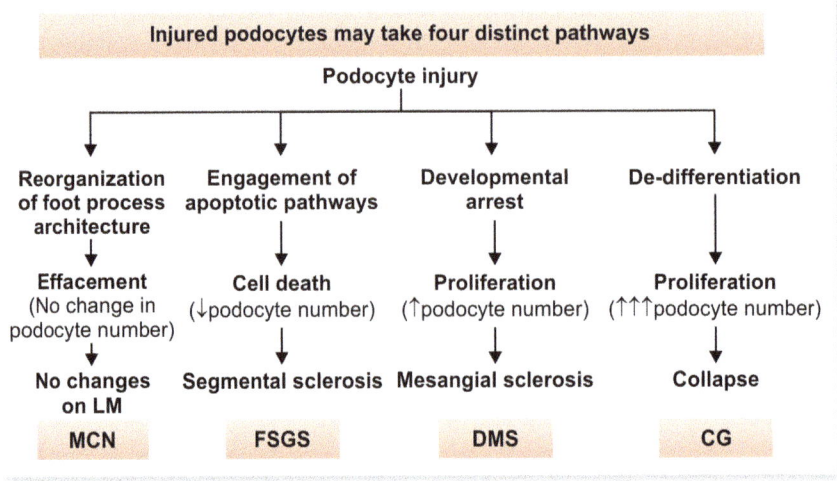

Figure 12.16: Distinct pathways of podocyte injury[6]
Source: CAJSN. 2007;2:529-42

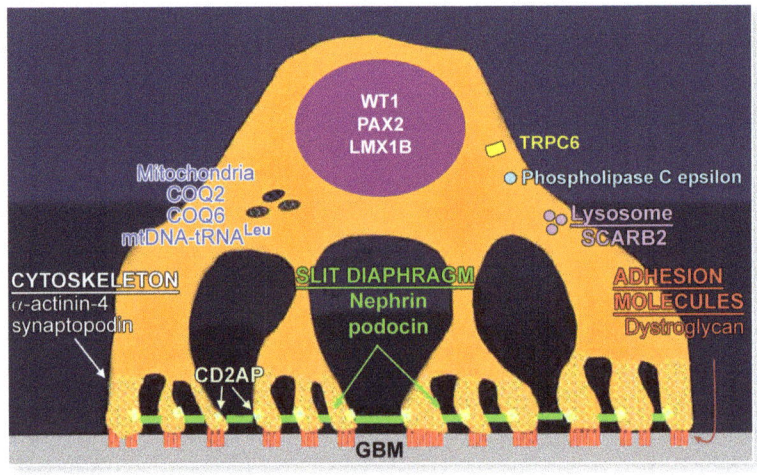

Figure 12.17: Sites of intrinsic podocyte genetic mutational injury (Internet Resource)

The extrinsic causes of podocyte injury with podocyte effacement include viral infections, toxins or medications, ischemia, immune complex deposition, mechanical forces and circulating lymphokines or FSGS permeability factor. The distinction between **genetic defects and these reactive etiological processes is crucial to the diagnosis of podocytopathies** and requires **molecular phenotypic markers and transcriptional profiling of RNA extracts from glomeruli.** Immunohistochemical expression of dystroglycans, an adhesion molecule, on the podocyte surface is reduced in steroid-sensitive MCN and **podocin expression is absent on immunofluorescence in steroid resistant genetic forms of MCN/FSGS.** In WT1 associated

DMS, there is **reduced expression of WT1 and increased expression of proliferation markers PAX2 and Ki-67. In collapsing glomerulopathy, there is loss of WT-1 and mature podocytic markers and increased Ki-67 with PAX2 and cytokeratin immunostaining of the immature, dedifferentiated podocytes.**[1,6,8,9]

REFERENCES

1. Lane JC, et al. Pediatric nephrotic syndrome: From the simple to the complex. Semin Nephrol. 2009;29:389-98.
2. Jalanko H. Congenital nephrotic syndrome. Pediatr Nephrol. 2009;24:2121-8.
3. Niaudet P. Congenital and infantile nephrotic syndrome. Current Paediatrics. 2006;16:262-8.
4. Caridi G, et al. Familial forms of nephrotic syndrome. Pediatr Nephrol. 2010;25:241-52L.
5. Tryggvason K, Patrakka J, Wartiovaara J. Hereditary proteinuria syndromes and mechanisms of proteinuria. N Engl J Med. 2006;354:1387-401.
6. Barisoni W, Schnapper J, Kopp. A proposed taxonomy for the podocytopathies: a reassessment of the primary nephrotic syndrome. CJASN. 2007;2(3):529-42.
7. Albaqumi M, Barisoni L. Current views on collapsing glomerulopathy. J Am Soc Nephrol. 2008;19(7):1276-81. Epub 2008 Feb 20.
8. Barisoni L, Schnapper W, Kopp J. Advances in the biology and genetics of the podocytopathies: implications for diagnosis and therapy. Arch. Pathol Lab Med. 2009;133:201-16.
9. Liapis H. Molecular pathology of nephrotic syndrome in childhood: a contemporary approach to diagnosis. Pediatr Devel Pathol. 2008;11:254-63.

CHAPTER 13

Tubulointerstitial Diseases

> **ABSTRACT**
> This chapter begins with the normal histology of the tubulointerstitial compartment for a comprehensive knowledge of non-neoplastic lesions including acute tubular necrosis, acute and chronic tubulointerstitial nephritis and specific forms of granulomatous interstitial nephritis with illustrations. IgG4-related tubulointerstitial nephropathy is detailed according to the consensus diagnostic criteria with pertinent microscopic and immunohistochemical features. Metabolic diseases, comprising primary oxalosis, Fanconi's syndrome, cystinosis, mitochondriopathies, hyperuricemic and hypercalcemic nephropathies are the rare entities encountered in our medical center. The subtypes of primary hyperoxaluria and their enzymatic defects and morphology of the oxalate deposits, course and prognosis are featured. A complete overview of the remaining crystallopathies is concisely featured for postgraduates trainees in nephropathology.

NORMAL STRUCTURE

The renal cortex is composed of the cortical labyrinth and the medullary rays. The former comprises the proximal and distal tubules, connecting tubules and initial portion of the collecting ducts. The tubules are closely packed with a scant interstitium that contains the peritubular capillary plexus and interstitial cells. The medullary rays contain the straight tubular segments of the proximal and distal tubules and the collecting ducts as they course from the cortex to and from the medulla. The medulla contains in addition the loops of Henle and collecting ducts with a wider interstitium. The proximal tubules are composed of cuboidal to columnar cells with granular eosinophilic cytoplasm with a prominent brush border and central round nucleus (Fig. 13.1). On electron microscopy, there are extensive basolateral invaginations with numerous mitochondria and luminal microvilli. The distal convoluted tubules are cuboidal cells with less eosinophilic cytoplasm and apical nuclei, lacking a brush border (Fig. 13.1). Basolateral invaginations and numerous elongated mitochondria are present (Fig. 13.1). The thin descending and ascending limbs of loop of Henle in the medulla have a flattened simple epithelium with attenuated cytoplasm devoid of a brush border, microvilli and basolateral invaginations with sparse mitochondria. Their nuclei bulge into the lumen, and the ascending thick limb has a similar structure to the distal convoluted tubule by light and electron microscopy (Fig. 13.2). Collecting tubules and cortical collecting ducts are lined by cuboidal to columnar cells respectively and the latter have a larger diameter with pale cytoplasm and central round nuclei with principal cells that have short microvilli and sparse organelles. The darker intercalated cells have many mitochondria, polyribosomes and membrane bound vesicles important for acid base homeostasis. The medullary collecting ducts contain mainly principal cells.

Tubulointerstitial Diseases

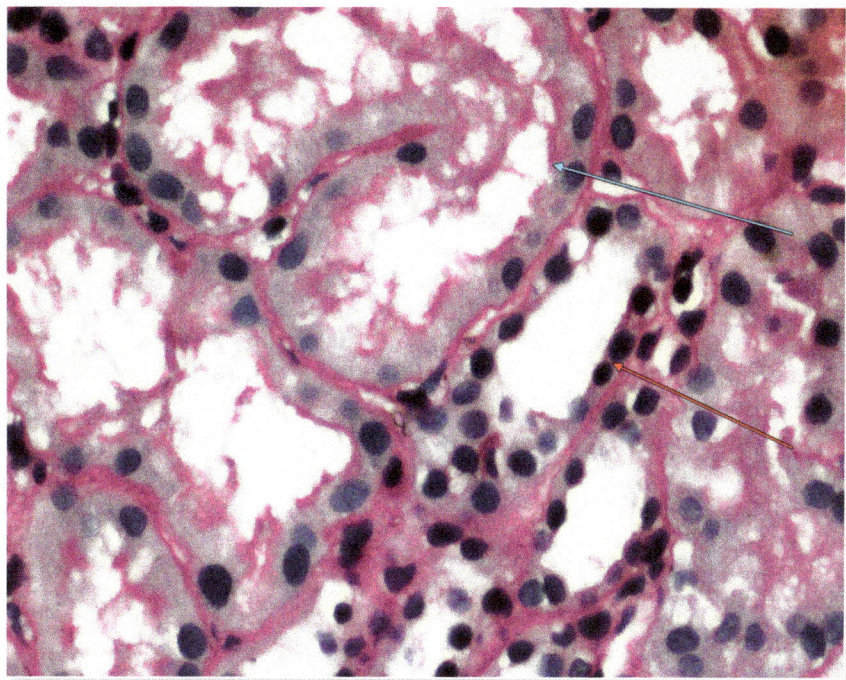

Figure 13.1: Proximal convoluted tubule with brush border (blue arrow) and distal tubule (red arrow) (PAS x 400)

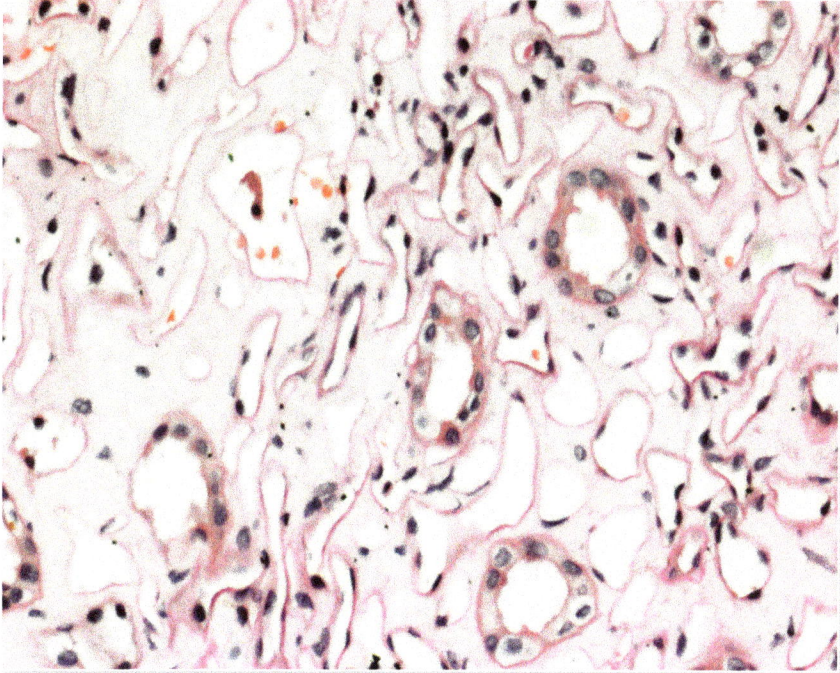

Figure 13.2: Renal medulla with collecting ducts and thin loops of Henle and vasa recta

ACUTE TUBULAR INJURY/NECROSIS

Acute tubular injury presents with varying degrees of acute renal failure defined by rise in serum creatinine, decreased GFR and reduced urinary output or anuria, resulting from acute ischemic or toxic injury.[1,2] Intrinsic acute renal failure is associated with intense and persistent renal vasoconstriction with marked reduction in renal blood flow. There is marked hypoperfusion of the outer medulla with consequent cellular injury, cell necrosis and apoptosis of susceptible tubular segments. Endothelial damage to peritubular capillaries with leukocyte aggregation, precedes tubular obstruction with cast formation, backleak and tubuloglomerular feedback with reduced ATP-dependent reabsorptive processes. Endothelial dysfunction lead to release of proinflammatory and chemotactic cytokines and inflammatory response.[2-8]

Acute ischemic tubular injury occurs in association with impairment of renal blood flow and caused by prolonged hypotension, major surgery, sepsis, concomitant chronic kidney disease and multiorgan dysfunction. This mainly involves the straight segments of proximal tubules and ascending limb of loop of Henle in foci.

Microscopic Features[2,3]

- Focal irregular tubular dilatation with flattening of lining epithelium
- Attenuation of brush border of proximal tubules (Fig. 13.3)
- Blebs of shed apical cell membrane or intact cells in the lumen
- Individual cell apoptosis with nuclear and cytoplasmic condensation
- Coagulation necrosis with pyknotic nuclei and disruption of basement membrane

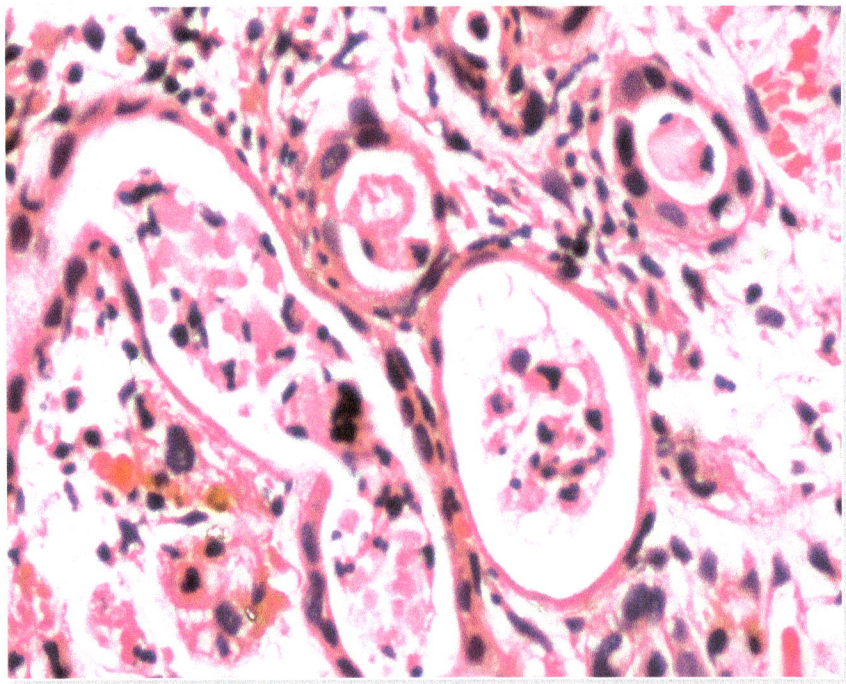

Figure 13.3: Acute tubular necrosis (H & E x 400)

Tubulointerstitial Diseases

- Distal tubules and collecting ducts contain a variety of hyaline, granular cellular, PAS positive proteinaceous casts
- Regeneration of tubular epithelial cells after 2 weeks with nuclear enlargement, hyperchromasia and mitoses
- Nucleated erythrocytes in peritubular capillaries of vasa recta of medulla
- Interstitial edema with focal neutrophilic infiltrates, admixed with lymphocytes and macrophages.

Electron Microscopy[3]

- Loss of brush border and blebs of apical cell membrane
- Desquamation of necrotic cells and condensation of cristae of mitochondria
- Individual cell apoptosis with nuclear fragmentation.

NEPHROTOXIC ACUTE TUBULAR NECROSIS

Nephrotoxic acute tubular necrosis (ATN) is associated with extensive involvement of proximal tubules resulting from nephrotoxic drugs such as antibiotics, antiviral and non-steroidal anti-inflammatory drugs (NSAIDs), immunosuppressive and cytotoxic chemotherapeutic agents, diuretics, anesthetics, herbal medicines, radiocontrast agents and heavy metals.[3] Mechanisms of renal failure include hemodynamic renal failure, with reduction of renal prostaglandins, due to cyclooxygenase inhibitors, mitochondrial DNA depletion with antiviral drugs, crystal deposition with sulfadiazine, acyclovir and indinavir or osmotic nephrosis with plasma expanders.[9,10]

Microscopic Features

Light Microscopy[3,10,11]

- Marked cytoplasmic swelling with vacuolization and loss of brush border
- Extensive necrosis with exfoliation of necrotic cells and attenuation of cytoplasm
- Intraluminal casts including heme casts from hemolysis and occasional oxalate crystals
- Intracellular inclusions or calcification and rarely tubular rupture in severe lesions.

Electron Microscopy

- Loss of microvilli, basolateral invaginations and cristae of mitochondria
- Lysosomal alterations, giant mitochondria and swelling/loss of cytoplasmic organelles.

Course and Prognosis

Ischemic acute tubular injury usually has a recovery phase after 2 weeks from the onset with stable renal functions. Renal failure can persist with other associated coexisting systemic complications and multiorgan involvement. The prognosis of nephrotoxic ATN is more variable depending on the extent, type and severity of the etiological agents.[2,3]

TUBULOINTERSTITIAL NEPHRITIS

There are two major forms of primary tubulointerstitial nephritis (TIN) with involvement of the tubules and interstitium by inflammatory cells. The acute form (acute TIN) is associated with a sudden onset and rapid deterioration of renal function with marked inflammation and interstitial edema. The chronic form (chronic TIN) has an insidious onset and slow progression of renal failure with interstitial fibrosis and less prominent inflammation. Acute TIN can be superimposed on chronic TIN (acute-on chronic TIN). In our case series of biopsy proven renal disease, interstitial nephritis had an incidence of 2.5%.[12] Interstitial nephritis can occur secondarily to glomerular or vascular diseases.

ACUTE TUBULOINTERSTITIAL NEPHRITIS

Acute tubulointerstitial nephritis is multifactorial in etiology, frequently with infections (bacterial, fungal, viral and protozoan) drugs (penicillins, NSAIDs, sulfonamides) or undetermined causes, presenting with microscopic hematuria, mild proteinuria and leukocyturia/eosinophiluria.[13-17]

Microscopic Features[15]

- Tubulointerstitial infiltrates with neutrophils, lymphocytes and macrophages
- Eosinophilic infiltrates and tubulitis (with lymphocytic infiltration of lining epithelium) in drug-induced TIN
- Interstitial expansion with edema
- Tubular dilatation with leukocytic casts and necrosis (Fig. 13.4)
- Microabscesses centered around necrotic tubules with bacterial infections.

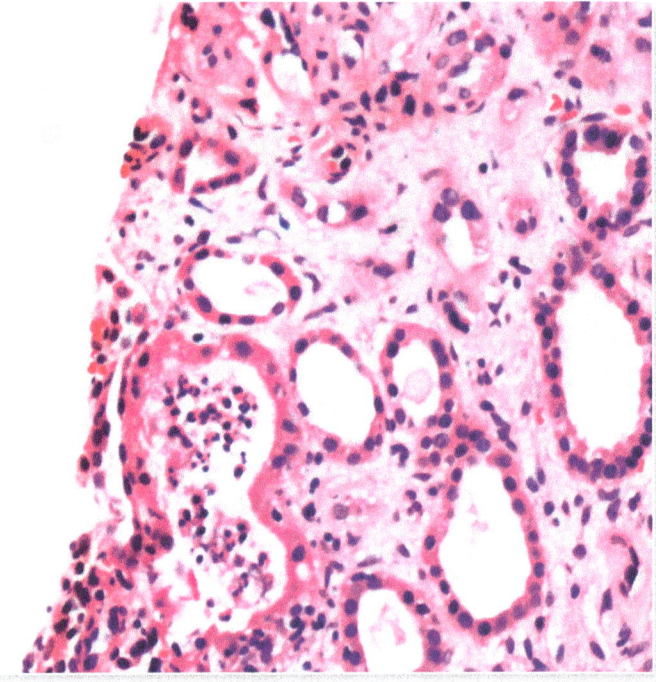

Figure 13.4: Acute tubulointerstitial nephritis (H & E x 200)

CHRONIC TUBULOINTERSTITIAL NEPHRITIS

Chronic tubulointerstitial nephritis is associated with:
- Infections
- Drug reactions
- Urinary tract obstruction
- Reflux nephropathy
- Immune-mediated primary and systemic auto-immune diseases (Sjogren syndrome/ antitubular basement membrane disease)
- Plasma cell dyscrasias, monoclonal gammopathy, light chain cast nephropathy
- Metabolic disorders (gout, hypercalcemia and hypokalemia)
- Inherited diseases (cystinosis, hyperoxaluria, Wilson's disease)
- Miscellaneous (Balkan nephropathy).

Microscopic Features

- Diffuse interstitial fibrosis with infiltrates/aggregates of lymphocytes, plasma cells and histiocytes with lymphoid follicle formation (Fig. 13.5)
- Tubular atrophy with thickened, lamellated basement membranes is noted
- Inspissated colloid casts in dilated tubules with flattened lining epithelium (in pyelonephritic scars)
- Hypertrophy of intervening tubules with tall columnar epithelium is seen
- Glomerular tuft atrophy with capsular fibrosis, pericapsular fibrosis and arteriosclerosis.

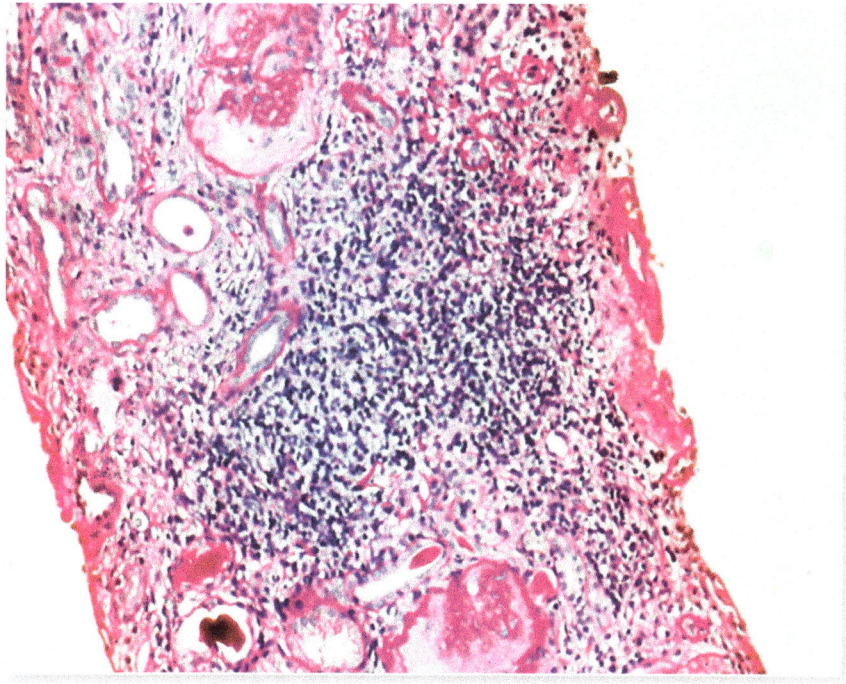

Figure 13.5: Chronic tubulointerstitial nephritis (H & E x 100)

GRANULOMATOUS INTERSTITIAL NEPHRITIS

Granulomatous interstitial nephritis is caused by the following etiological factors[18-26]
- *Infections*:
  - Tuberculosis
  - Fungi (Cryptococcosis, Candidiasis, Histoplasmosis, Zygomycosis)
  - Brucellosis
  - Parasitic
- *Drugs*: Penicillins, sulfonamides, gentamicin, nitrofurantoin, NSAIDs, diuretics, allopurinol, carbamazepine, diphenylhydantoin
- Sarcoidosis
- *Metabolic disorders*: Gout and oxalosis
- Wegener's granulomatous vasculitis
- Cholesterol granulomas
- Tubulointerstitial nephritis and uveitis syndrome
- Xanthogranulomatous pyelonephritis.

Microscopic Features

- Interstitial expansion by histiocytes, including epithelioid histiocytes, multinucleate giant cells forming non-caseating granulomata with lymphocytes and plasma cells and scattered eosinophils
- Acid fast stains for mycobacteria routinely done, if negative, does not exclude tuberculosis
- Fungal stains reveal causative microorganisms (Fig. 13.6) and are associated with necrotizing granulomas in diabetics, or with immunosuppression, in allografts or immunocompromised hosts

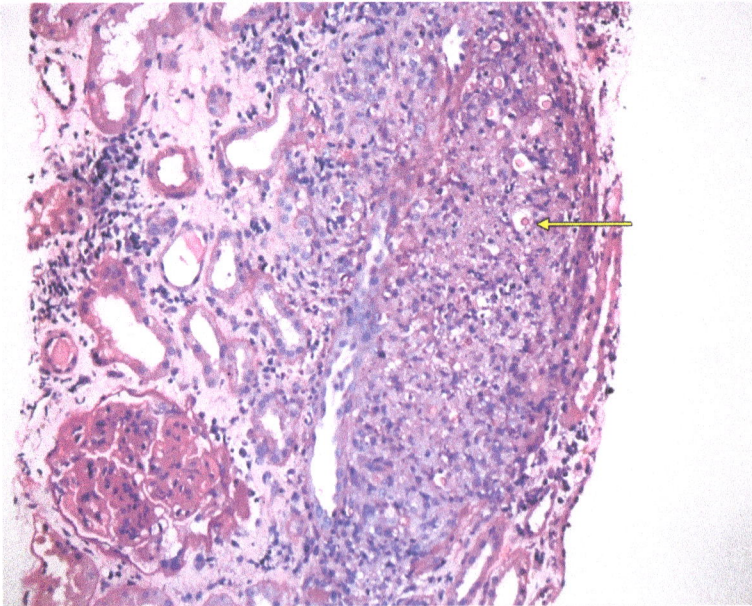

Figure 13.6: Cryptococcal granulomatous interstitial nephritis (arrow) with concomitant diffuse proliferative lupus nephritis (PAS x 200)

- Xanthogranulomatous pyelonephritis contains sheets of foamy histiocytes with or without giant cells and is associated with staghorn renal calculi and *Proteus mirabilis* or *Escherichia coli*, Pseudomonas, *Enterococcus faecalis* and Klebsiella infection.

IgG4-RELATED TUBULOINTERSTITIAL NEPHROPATHY

IgG4-related tubulointerstitial nephropathy is a manifestation of a multisystem autoimmune disease associated with IgG4 positive plasma cells infiltrating the parenchyma of various organs leading to pancreatitis, sialadenitis, chronic sclerosing cholangitis, interstitial pneumonitis retroperitoneal fibrosis and periaortitis. Renal involvement presents with acute/chronic progressive renal failure, radiological evidence and markedly elevated serum IgG and/or IgG4 levels or hypergammaglobulinemia.[27] Concomitant membranous nephropathy can occur. The diagnostic criteria proposed by Mayoclinic Nephropathologists and American collaborators comprise major histologic features of plasma cell-rich TIN, supported by tubular basement membrane complex deposits by IF, IHC and/or electron microscopy, with at least one other feature from the categories of "imaging", "serology"or other organ involvement.[28] The disease is extremely rare and to our knowledge, the first Indian case report has been currently published from our medical center[29] associated with interstitial pneumonia, serum IgG level of 7000 mg/dL and IgG4 of 747 mg/dL.

Microscopic Features[30-34]

- Plasma cell rich interstitial infiltrate admixed with lymphocytes with scattered eosinophils (Fig. 13.7)
- Expansile or whirling/storiform fibrosis with tubular loss and atrophy and thickened basement membranes
- Global glomerulosclerosis with glomerular atrophy and arteriosclerosis.

Immunofluorescence

Diffuse, granular IgG staining of tubular basement membranes.

Immunohistochemistry[32,33] (Figs 13.8 and 13.9)

- Moderate to marked increase in IgG4 positive plasma cells, >10/hpf in densely cellular area. Ratio of IgG4 to IgG varies depending on density of inflammation in renal biopsy sample and can exceed 40–50%
- Diagnostic utility of IgG4 immunostaining had 100% sensitivity and 92% specificity in IgG4-related TIN on exclusion of pauci-immune GN in a case series from Mayo clinic.[27]

Electron Microscopy

Electron dense immune deposits on thickened tubular basement membranes.

Differential Diagnosis[28]

Autoimmune tubulointerstitial diseases including SLE and Sjogren syndrome are associated with lymphoplasmacytic infiltrates and infrequently associated with a mild increase of IgG4

162 Renal Biopsy Interpretation

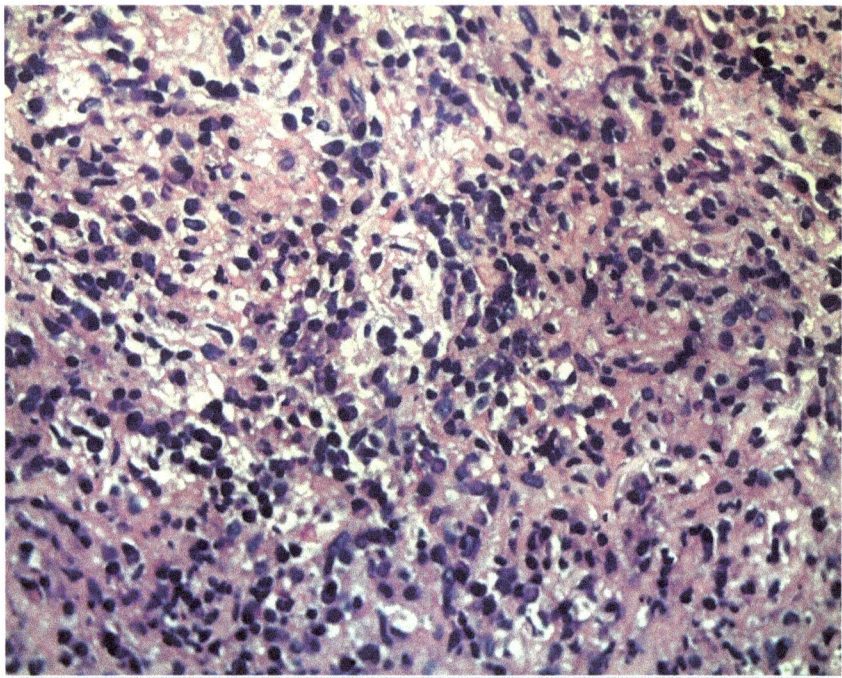

Figure 13.7: IgG4-related sclerosing tubulointerstitial nephropathy with lymphoplasmacytic infiltrate (H & E x 400)

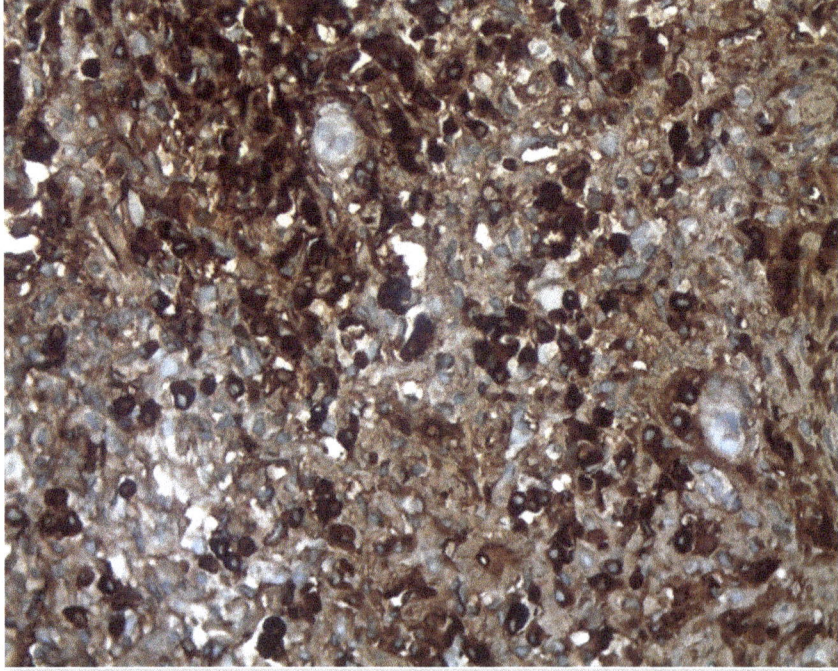

Figure 13.8: IgG positive plasma cells (IHC x 400)

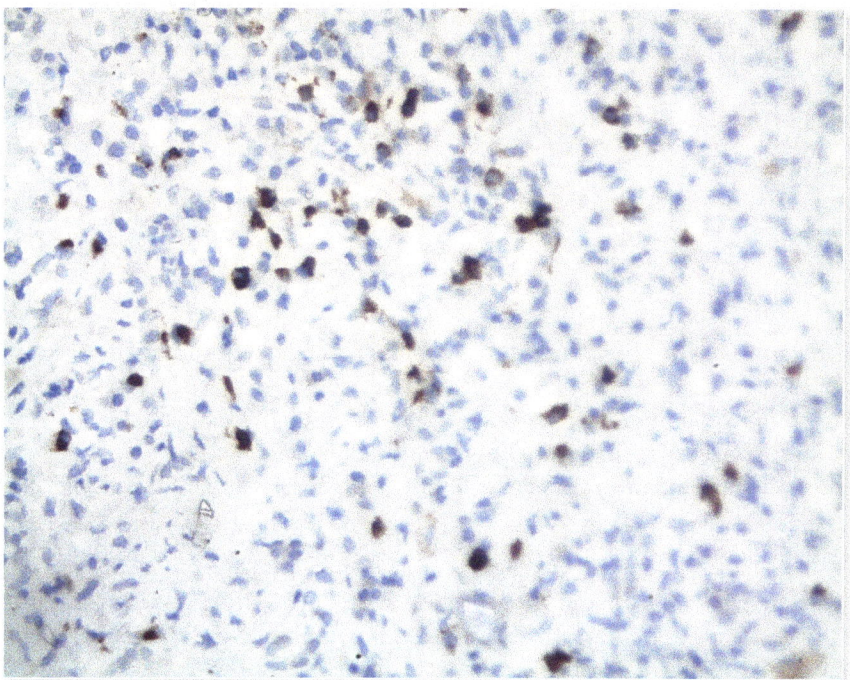

Figure 13.9: IgG4 positive plasma cells (25 per HPF) on IHC x 400

positive plasma cells. The diagnostic histopathologic criteria of IgG4-TIN with IHC, combined with clinical, radiological and serological findings can exclude other forms of TIN.

Multiple myeloma/monoclonal gammopathy is associated with plasma cell infiltrates in renal parenchyma and monoclonal light chain restriction for either kappa or lambda light chains.

Course and Prognosis

Responsiveness to steroids has been documented in the literature, including our center, for the TIN as also for the IgG4-related systemic disease.[28-37]

METABOLIC DISORDERS (CRYSTALLOPATHIES)

Primary Hyperoxaluria (PH)

It is an autosomal recessive inherited peroxisomal disorder has two subtypes:
- **Type I PH** is more common and occurs mainly in infants associated with mutations in the *AGXT* gene on chromosome 2q37.3 with deficiency of the hepatic enzyme alanine glyoxylate aminotransferase (AGT) that transaminates glyoxylate to glycine. Glyoxylate is oxidized to oxalate and further reduced to glycolic acid. The oxalate deposits in the kidneys lead to chronic tubulointerstitial nephritis and calcium oxalate lithiasis and chronic renal failure. A severe infantile form is seen in 10% of cases manifesting with metabolic acidosis, failure to thrive, anemia and progressive parenchymal disease with systemic oxalosis, hyperoxaluria and glycolicaciduria. Renal involvement in adults is seen in the fourth or fifth decade.[38-45]

164 Renal Biopsy Interpretation

- **Type II PH** is associated with defective cytosolic D-glycerate dehydrogenase-glyoxylate reductase and primarily oxalate lithiasis with no evidence of renal failure.[44,45]

Secondary or Acquired Oxalosis

Secondary or acquired oxalosis can occur at any age due to excessive dietary ingestion of oxalate or its precursors, increased intestinal absorption or decreased excretion as in chronic renal failure.[38,39]

Microscopic Features

- Birefringent polyhedral or rhomboidal oxalate crystals with radial striations in tubules (Fig. 13.10)
- Marked tubular dilatation with flattening of lining epithelium and necrosis
- Interstitial deposits of oxalate with foreign body giant cell reaction
- Chronic interstitial inflammatory cell infiltrates with fibrosis and diffuse glomerulosclerosis.

Course and Prognosis

Effective reduction in urinary oxalate by activation of AGT by pyridoxine is seen only in a minority of patients with Type I PH. Enzyme replacement by combined liver and renal transplantation has an improved long-term prognosis.[46,47]

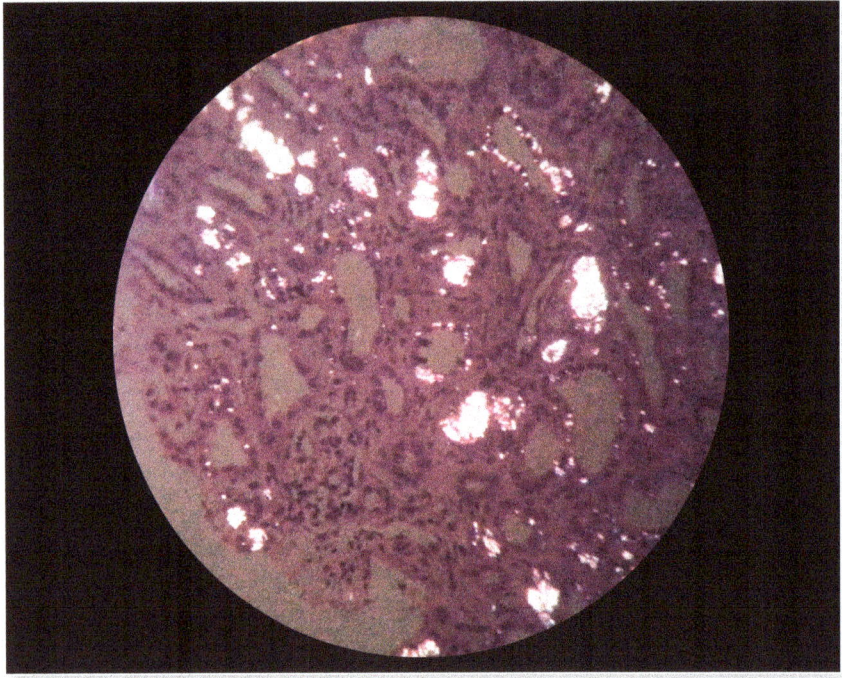

Figure 13.10: Intratubular oxalate crystals with polarized light × 100

Fanconi's Syndrome

Fanconi's syndrome is defined as a proximal tubular dysfunction leading to aminoaciduria, glucosuria and phosphaturia together with impaired reabsorption of bicarbonates, urate, calcium and low molecular weight proteins. Reabsorption of low molecular weight proteins in the proximal tubule occurs via luminal receptors with endocytosis and endosomal acidification by recycling of receptors back to the brush border and of ligand into lysosomes for processing. Reabsorption of many solutes occurs via luminal surface transporters driven by gradients generated by Na/K ATPase and dependent on intracellular energy. Energy depletion in mitochondriopathies, cystinosis, genetic enzymatic defects involved in oxidative phosphorylation and drug/chemical/toxic injury can cause Fanconi's syndrome. Therefore, hereditary and acquired forms of this syndrome occur, manifesting in children with proximal renal tubular acidosis, polyuria, polydipsia and failure to thrive and vitamin-D resistant rickets.[48-52] Acquired Fanconi's syndrome is primarily an adult disease associated with toxic or immunologic injury including drug and heavy metal toxicity, multiple myeloma, dysproteinemias, and antitubular basement membrane antibodies.[53-55]

Microscopic Features

Microscopic features are nonspecific and are related to the underlying cause, with loss of the brush border, tubular necrosis with toxic injury, progressing to interstitial fibrosis with tubular atrophy and glomerulosclerosis in the chronic stages.

CYSTINOSIS

Cystinosis is a rare multisystem autosomal recessive lysosomal transport disorder due to mutations in CTNS gene on 17p13 chromosome encoding cystinosin, a transmembrane protein and is one of the most common causes of Fanconi's syndrome. The disease predominantly involves the European race but has been reported in Hispanics and Africans. The severe early infantile form is associated with nephropathy progessing to endstage renal disease in the first year of life. The late onset indolent adolescent form eventually progresses with deterioration of renal function. The adult form mainly has ocular manifestations with corneal crystalline deposits. Oral cysteamine and renal transplantation has prolonged survival and life span in the infantile form.[56-58]

Microscopic Features

- Proximal tubular atrophy with narrowing of the postglomerular segment (swan-neck deformity)
- Interstitial fibrosis with variable inflammation and glomerular solidification
- Refractile rectangular/hexagonal crystals in interstitium, cortical tubular lumina and occasional tubular and glomerular epithelial cells with mulinucleation of podocytes (Fig. 13.11).

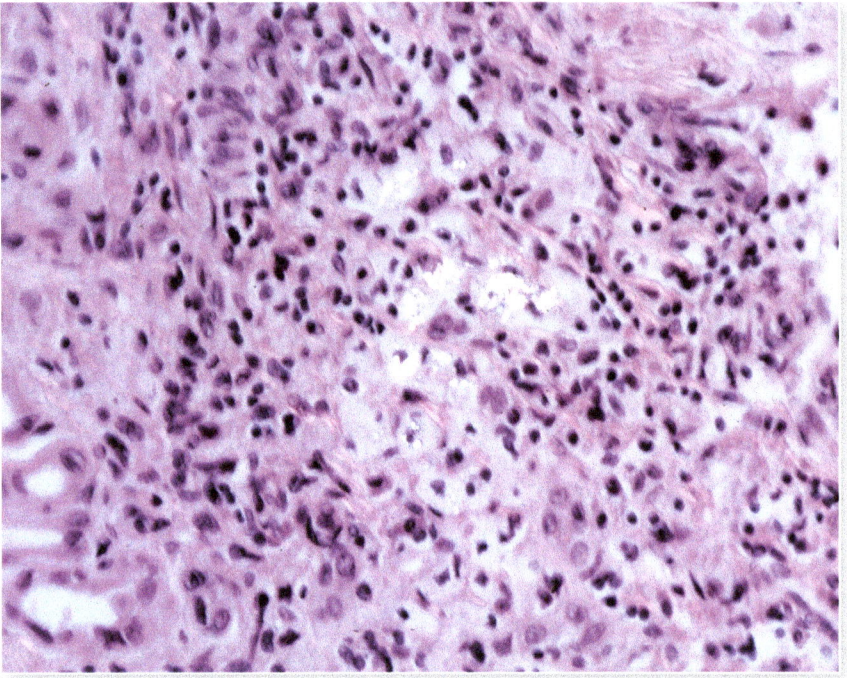

Figure 13.11: Cystine crystals in interstitium (H & E x 100)

MITOCHONDRIOPATHIES

These are extremely rare, associated with proximal tubulopathy and Fanconi's syndrome, presenting with a mulisystem disorder involving mainly the neuromuscular system.

Microscopic Features[59,60]

- Tubular dilatation with casts and granular epithelial cells with giant mitochondria displaying paracrystalline arrays or dense circular or deficient/aberrant cristae on EM
- Focal and segmental sclerosis including the collapsing variant of FSGS occurs with mitochondrial tRNA and nuclear DNA mutations, respectively.

HYPERURICEMIA AND URATE NEPHROPATHY

Hyperuricemia and urate nephropathy are associated with inherited aberration of purine metabolism due to enzymatic defects,[61] with complete absence or decreased hypoxanthinineguanine phosphoribosyl transferase (HGPRT), raised activity of PB-ribose-P synthetase and deficiency of glucose 6-phosphatase (glycogen storage disease I). Reduced excretion or increased reabsorption of uric acid occurs in chronic lead toxicity, purine rich diet and increased production during treatment of leukemias and lymphomas or myeloproliferative disorders in tumor lysis syndrome. Acute uric acid nephropathy presents with acute oliguric or anuric renal failure.

Tubulointerstitial Diseases

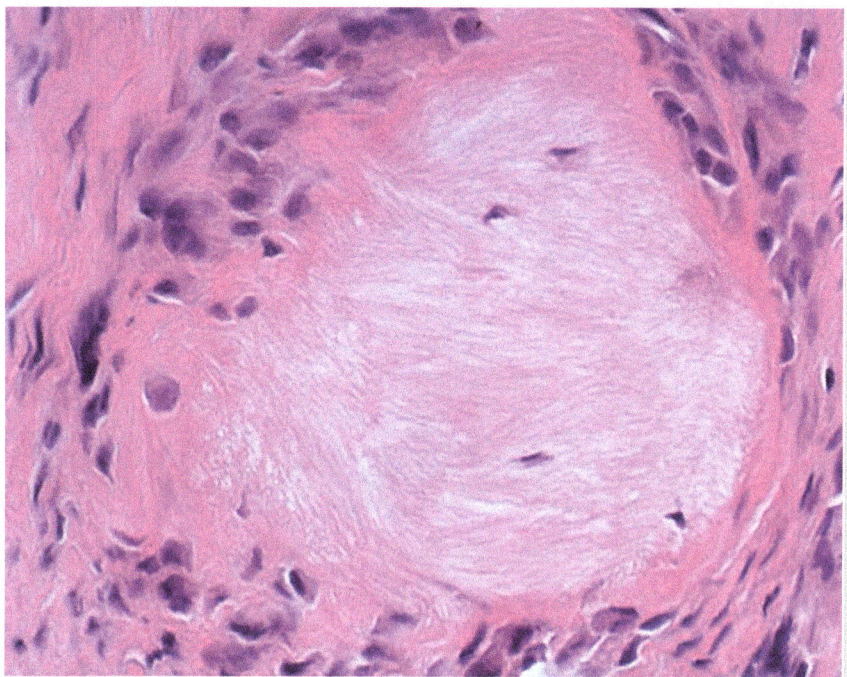

Figure 13.12: Chronic urate nephropathy (H & E x 400) (Internet Resource)

Chronic urate nephropathy can present with proteinuria, hypertension and renal failure, but its incidence has decreased with effective treatment for gout with uricosuric agents and allopurinol.

Microscopic Features

- Birefringent elongated needle-shaped crystalline deposits are found in the loops of Henle and collecting ducts
- Amorphous monosodium urate deposits in the interstitium forming gouty tophi with granulomatous reaction (Fig. 13.12)
- Interstitial fibrosis with tubular atrophy, arteriosclerosis and glomerulosclerosis seen in the chronic phase.

HYPERCALCEMIC NEPHROPATHY

Hypercalcemic nephropathy is associated with hypercalcemia and hypercalciuria in primary hyperparathyroidism, other diseases involving calcium and phosphate metabolism and distal renal tubular acidosis.

Microscopic Features

- Tubular luminal concretions of calcium salts with tubular basement membrane and interstitial deposits (Fig. 13.13)

168 Renal Biopsy Interpretation

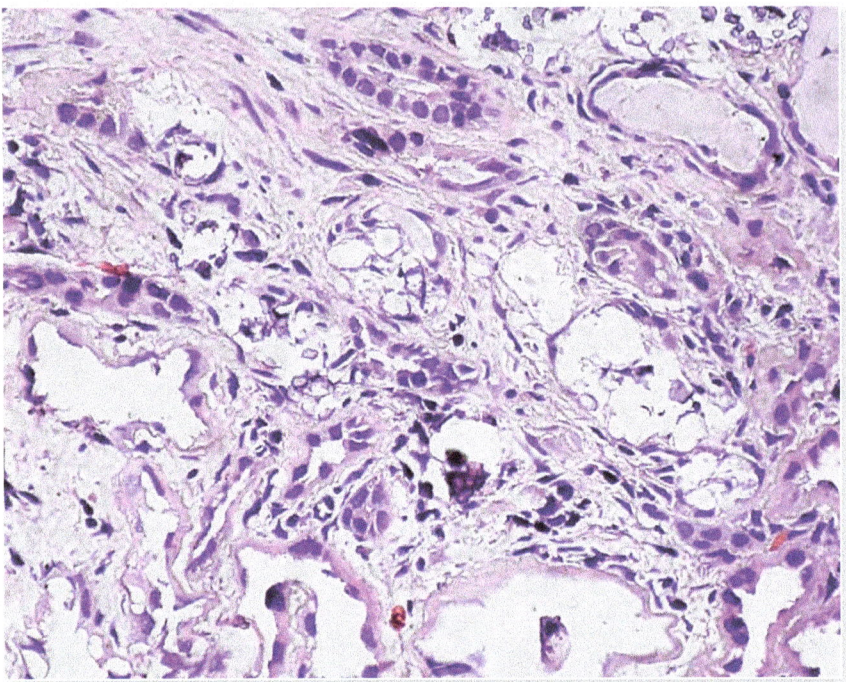

Figure 13.13: Hypercalcemic nephropathy (H & E x 200)

- Calcium deposits stain bluish-purple on H & E, positive for Alizarin Red S in renal cortex and medulla
- Calcium phosphate deposits stain black with vonKossa and are **refractile but not birefringent.**

REFERENCES

1. Munshi R, Hsu C, Himmelfarb J. Advances In understanding ischemic acute kidney Injury. BMC Medicine. 2011;9(11):1-6 doi:10.1186/1741-7015-9-11.
2. Devarajan P. Update on mechanisms of ischemic acute kidney injury. J Am Soc Nephrol. 2006;17:1503-20, 2006. doi: 10.1681/ASN.2006010017.
3. Racusen L, Kashgarian M. Ischemic and toxic acute tubular injury and other ischemic renal injury. In: Jennette JC, Olson JL, Schwartz MM, Silva FG (Eds). Pathology of the Kidney, 6th edition. Philadelphia: Lippincott Williams, Wilkins; 2007.pp.1139-98.
4. Bonventre JV, Weinberg JM. Recent advances in the pathophysiology of ischemic acute renal failure. JASN. 2003;14(8):2199-2210.
5. Bonventre JV, Zuk A. Ischemic acute renal failure: an inflammatory disease? Kidney Int. 2004;66:480-5.
6. Friedewald JJ, Rabb H. Inflammatory cells in ischemic acute renal failure. Kidney Int. 2004; 66:486-90.
7. Molitoris BA, Sutton TA. Endothelial injury and dysfunction: role in the extension phase of acute renal failure. Kidney Int. 2004;66:496-9.
8. Ramesh G, Reeves WB. Inflammatory cytokines in acute renal failure. Kidney Int Suppl. 2004;66(91):S56-S61.
9. Perazella MA. Drug-induced renal failure: uptodate on new medications and unique mechanisms of nephrotoxicity. American Journal of Medical Sciences. 2003;325:349-62.
10. Van Vleet TR, Schnellmann RG. Toxic nephropathy: environmental chemicals. Semin Nephrol. 2003;23:500-8.

11. Cronin RE, Henrich WL. Toxic nephropathies. In: Brenner BM (Ed). The Kidney, 6th ed. Philadelphia: WB Saunders, 2000. p.563.
12. Narasimhan B, Chacko B, John GT, Korula A, Kirubakaran MG, Jacob CK. Characterization of kidney lesions in Indian adults: towards a renal biopsy registry. J Nephrol. 2006;19:205-10.
13. Baker RJ, Pusey CD. The changing profile of acute tubulointerstitial nephritis. Nephrol Dial Transplant. 2004;19:8-11.
14. Distler A, Keller F, Kunzendorf U, et al. The outcome of acute interstitial nephritis: risk factors for the transition from acute to chronic interstitial nephritis. Clin Nephrol. 2003;59:65.
15. Buysen JG, Houthoff HJ, Krediet RT, Arisz L. Acute interstitial nephritis: a clinical and morphological study in 27 patients. Nephrol Dial Transplant. 1990;5:94-9.
16. Rossert J. Drug-induced acute interstitial nephritis. Kidney Int. 2001;60:804-17.
17. Braden GL, O'Shea MH, Mulhern JG. Tubulointerstitial diseases. AmJ Kidney Dis. 2005;46(3):560-72.
18. Viero RM, Cavallo T. Granulomatous interstitial nephritis. Hum Pathol. 1995;26:1347-53.
19. Joss N, Morris S, Young B, Geddes C. Granulomatousinterstitial nephritis Clin J Am Soc Nephrol. 2007;2: 222-230
20. Mallinson WJ, Fuller RW, Levinson DA, et al. Diffuse interstitial tuberculosis an unusual cause of renal failure. Q J Med.1981;57:31-5.
21. Sampathkumar K, Sooraj YS, Mahaldar AR, et al. Granulomatous interstitial nephritis due to tuberculosis-a rare presentation. Saudi J Kidney Dis Transpl. 2009;20:842-5.
22. Kaul A, Sharma RK, Krishnasamy J, Ruhela V, Kumari N. Rapidly progressive renal failure—a rare presentation of granulomatous interstitial nephritis due to tuberculosis—case report and review of literature NDT Plus. 2011;4: 383-5 doi: 10.1093/ndtplus/sfr067.
23. Mignon F, Mery JP, Mougenot B, et al. Granulomatous interstitial nephritis. Adv Nephrol Necker Hosp.1984;13: 219-45.
24. Benn JJ, Scoble JE, Thomas AC, et al. Cryptogenic tuberculosis as a preventable cause of end-stage renal failure. Am J Nephrol. 1988;8:306-8.
25. O'Riordan E, Willert RP, Reeve R, Kalra PA, O'Donoghue DJ, Foley RN, et al. Isolated sarcoid granulomatous interstitial nephritis: review of five cases at one center. Clin Nephrol. 2001;55(4):297-302.
26. David VG, Korula A, Choudhrie L, Michael JS, Jacob S, Jacob CK, et al. Cryptococcal granulomatous interstitial nephritis and dissemination in a patient with untreated lupus nephritis. Nephrol Dial Transplant. 2009;24:3243-5. doi: 10.1093/ndt/gfp293.
27. Rudmik L, Trpkov K, Nash C, Kinnear S, Falck V, Dushinski J, et al. Autoimmune pancreatitis associated with renal lesions mimicking metastatic tumours. CMAJ. 2006;175(4):367-9.
28. Raissian Y, Nasr SH, Larsen CP, Colvin RB, Smyrk TC, Takahashi N, et al. Diagnosis of IgG4-related tubulointerstitial Nephritis. J Am Soc Nephrol. 2011;22:1343-52.
29. Saravanan M, Alexander S, Matthai SM, Korula A, Varughese S, Tamilarasi V. Immunoglobulin G4-related tubulointerstitial nephritis associated with interstitial pulmonary disease: report of a case with review of literature. Indian J Nephrol. 2015;25(2):113–6. DIO: 10.4103/0971–4065.136886.
30. Murashima M, Tomaszewski J, Glickman JD. Chronic tubulointerstitial nephritis presenting as multiple renal nodules and pancreatic insufficiency. Am J Kidney Dis. 2007;49(1):e7.
31. Saeki T, Nishi S, Imai N, Ito T, Yamazaki h, Kawano M. Clinicopathological characteristics of patients with IgG4-related tubulointerstitial nephritis KidneyInt. 2010;78:1016-23 | doi:10.1038/ki.2010.271
32. Deshpande V, Zen Y, Chan JKC, YI EE, SatoY, Yoshino T. Consensus statement on the pathology of IgG4-related disease. ModPathol. 2012;25:1181-1192 doi:10.1038/Mod Pathol.2012.72.
33. Kawano M, Mizushima I, Yamaguchi Y, Imai N, Nakashima H, Nishi S. Immunohistochemical characteristics of IgG4-related tubulointerstitial Nephritis: Detailed Analysis of 20 Japanese Cases. International Journal of Rheumatology Volume 2012, Article ID 609795, 9pagesdoi:10.1155/2012/609795.
34. Yamaguchi Y, Kanetsuna Y, Honda K, Yamanaka N, Kawano M, Nagata M. Characteristic tubulointerstitial nephritis in IgG4-related disease, Human Pathology. 2012;43(.4):536-49.
35. Alexander MP, Larsen CP, Gibson IW, Nasr SH, Sethi S, Fidler ME, et al. Membranous glomerulonephritis is a manifestation of IgG4-related disease. Kidney Int. 2013;83(3):455-62.
36. Watson SJ, Jenkins DA, Bellamy CO. Nephropathy in IgG4-related systemic disease. Am J Surg Pathol. 2006;30(11):1472-7.
37. Deshpande V. The pathology of IgG4 related disease. Seminars in Diagnostic Pathology. 2012;29:191-6.

38. Reginato AJ, Kurnik B. Calcium oxalate and other crystals associated with kidney diseases and arthritis. Semin Arthritis Rheum. 1989;18:198-210.
39. Wandzilak TR, Williams HE. The hyperoxaluric syndromes. Endocrinal Metab Clin North Am. 1990;19:851-67.
40. Leumann E, Hoppe B. The primary hyperoxalurias. J Am Soc Nephrol. 2001;12:1986-93.
41. Coulter-Mackie MB, Rumsby G. Genetic heterogeneity in primary hyperoxaluria type1: impact on diagnosis. Mol Genet Metab. 2004;83:38-46.
42. Danpure CJ. Molecular aetiology of primary hyperoxaluria type 1. Nephron Exp Nephrol. 2004;98:e39.
43. Pirulli D, Marangella M, Amoroso A. Primary hyperoxaluria: Genotype-phenotype correlation. J Nephrol. 2003;16:297-309.
44. Milliner DS, Wilson DM, Smith LH. Phenotypic expression of primary hyperoxaluria: comparative features of types I and II. Kidney Int. 2001;59:31-6.
45. Johnson SA, Rumsby G, Cregeen D, Hulton SA. Primary hyperoxaluria type 2 in children. Pediatr Nephrol. 2002;17:597-601.
46. Gagnadoux MF, Lacaille F, Niaudet P, et al. Long term results of liver-kidney transplantation in children with primary hyperoxaluria. Pediatr Nephrol. 2001;16:946-50.
47. Cibrik DM, Kaplan B, Arndorfer JA, Meier-Kriesche HU. Renal allograft survival in patients with oxalosis. Transplantation. 2002;74:707-10.
48. Katzir Z, Dinour D, Reznik-Wolf H, Nissenkorn A, Holtzman E. Familial pure proximal renal tubular acidosis: a clinical and genetic study. Nephrol Dial Transplant. 2008;23:1211-5.
49. Alper SL. Familial renal tubular acidosis. J Nephrol. 2010;23:S57-S76.
50. Izzedine H, Launay-Vacher V, Isnard-Bagnis C, Deray G. Drug-induced Fanconis syndrome. Am J Kidney Dis. 2003; 41:292-309.
51. Quigley R. Proximal renal tubular acidosis. J Nephro. 2006;19:S41-S45.
52. Batlle D, Haque SK. Genetic causes and mechanisms of distalrenal tubular acidosis. Nephrol Dial Transplant. 2012; 27:3691-704.
53. Messiaen T, Deret S, Mougenot B, et al. Adult Fanconi syndrome secondary to light chain gammopathy. Clinicopathologic heterogeneity and unusual features in 11 patients. Medicine (Baltimore). 2000;79:135-54.
54. Maldonado JE, Velosa JA, Kyle RA, Wagoner RD, Holley KE, Salassa RM. Fanconi syndrome in adults. A manifestation of a latent form of myeloma. Am J Med. 1975;58:354-64.
55. Bridoux F, Sirac C, Hugue V, et al. Fanconi's syndrome induced by a monoclonal Vkappa3 light chain in Waldenstrom's macroglobulinemia. Am J Kidney Dis. 2005;45:749-57.
56. Nesterova G, Gahl W. Nephropathic cystinosis: late complications of a multisystemic disease. Pediatr Nephrol Jun. 2008;23(6):863-78.
57. Chevalier RL, Forbes MS. Generation and evolution of atubular glomeruli in the progression of renal disorders. J Am Soc Nephrol. 2008;19(2):197-206.
58. Almond PS, Matas AJ, Nakhleh RE. Renal transplantation for infantile cystinosis: long-term follow-up. J Pediatr Surg. 1993;28(2):232-8.
59. Barisoni L, Diomedi-Camassei F, Santorelli FM, Caridi G, Thomas DB, Emma F, et al. Collapsing glomerulopathy associated with inherited mitochondrial injury. Kidney Int. 2008;74:237-43.
60. Santorelli FM, Caridi G, Piemonte F, Montini G, Giovanni M, Ghiggeri GM, et al. COQ2 Nephropathy: A newly described inherited mitochondriopathy with primary renal involvement. JASN. 2007;18(10):2773-80.
61. Cameron JS, Simmonds HA. Hereditary hyperuricemia and renal disease. Seminars in Nephrol. 2005;25(1):9-18.

CHAPTER **14**

Vascular Renal Diseases

ABSTRACT

The normal histology of the renal vasculature is detailed as the basis for various pathologic lesions involving mainly the arterioles, interlobular and arcuate arteries in a renal biopsy.

The vascular and glomerular lesions of benign and malignant forms of hypertensive arterionephrosclerosis are highlighted with their differential diagnosis, course and prognosis.

Thrombotic microangiopathy and the major manifestations of the hemolytic uremic syndrome (HUS), thrombotic thrombocytopenic purpura and disseminated intravascular coagulation are dealt with clarity and expertise including excellent illustrations of the typical forms of HUS from our medical center. Atypical HUS and other thrombotic vasculopathies presenting with the phospholipid antibody syndrome and their complications are also detailed in the interests of postgraduates and nephropathologists.

Pre-eclamptic toxemia and eclampsia with the pathognomonic features are clearly depicted with the differential diagnosis and selected references for further information.

NORMAL STRUCTURE OF RENAL VASCULATURE

The main renal artery on each side divides to form the anterior and posterior branches with their superior and inferior segmental arteries respectively. The segmental arteries then form the interlobar arteries as they enter the renal sinus. Each interlobar artery branches to form 6 to 8 arcuate arteries as it courses between the renal pyramid and the column of Bertin. The arcuate arteries ascend the lateral surface of the pyramid and across the corticomedullary junction to form the interlobular arteries as perpendicular branches. The interlobular arteries are seen in the cortical parenchyma, coursing between the medullary rays and branching to form the afferent arteriole that enters the glomerular tufts. The arterial vasculature comprises end arteries with no collateral blood flow. Therefore, parenchymal infarction can occur with occlusion of the segmental renal arteries or their sequential branches. Microscopically, the largest arteries including the interlobar and arcuate arteries have an internal and external elastic lamina demarcating the media, whereas the interlobular arteries have only an internal elastic lamina and the arterioles are devoid of both elastic lamina. The afferent arterioles are lined by nonfenestrated endothelium, have a thicker media with one to three layers of medial smooth muscle cells and the efferent arterioles have a single layer of smooth muscle. The latter branch to form the peritubular capillary plexus in the cortex and the descending vasa recta in the medulla, with decreased to absent smooth muscle, in the ascending portion and a thin fenestrated endothelial lining. The interlobular, arcuate and intralobar veins, course parallel to the arteries and the intralobar veins converge to form the main renal vein, anterior to the renal pelvis. The cortical veins have a thin to attenuated smooth muscle media and the medullary veins increase in caliber with a continuous thicker media.

JUXTAGLOMERULAR APPARATUS

Juxtaglomerular apparatus (JGA) is composed of specialized epithelial cells known as the macula densa, vascular components in the walls of afferent and efferent arterioles and extraglomerular mesangial lacis cells and matrix. The macula densa is a plaque of specialized tubular epithelial cells, that are low columnar with apical nuclei and short surface microvilli devoid of lateral interdigitations. In the wall of the afferent arterioles are clusters of granular modified smooth muscle cells producing renin and angiotensin II. The JGA regulates haemodynamics in response to hematogenous influences and composition of tubular fluid.

The vascular lesions comprise benign and malignant nephrosclerosis, thrombotic microangiopathies (including Classical and Atypical Hemolytic Uremic Syndrome, Thrombotic Thrombocytopenic Purpura and Disseminated Intravascular Coagulation) and other thrombotic vasculopathies of antiphospholipid antibody syndrome, pre-eclamptic toxemia and eclampsia.

Arterionephrosclerosis includes vascular and parenchymal lesions that are associated with arterial sclerosis, caused by mild to moderate hypertension, known as **benign nephrosclerosis**.[1-6]

Microscopic Features

Light Microscopy

Vascular lesions:
- Arteriolar hyalinosis associated with eosinophilic hyaline material in the intima (Fig. 14.1)
- Periodic acid schiff (PAS) positive and fuschinophilic on the Masson trichrome stain
- Atrophy of the muscular layer
- Intimal fibrosis of arcuate artery and interlobular arteries
- Myofibroblastic and fibroblastic intimal proliferation
- Deposition of concentric layers of collagen with narrowing of the lumen
- Medial hyperplasia with fibrosis and foci of atrophy are seen.

Glomerular lesions:
- Glomeruli display wrinkling and thickening and replication of GBM (Fig. 14.2)
- Mesangial matrix expansion and collagenization, internal to Bowman's capsule
- Foci of ischemic atrophy and global solidification of the tufts
- Foci of interstitial fibrosis with tubular atrophy and mononuclear cell infiltrates
- Foci of secondary peri-hilar segmental glomerulosclerosis and hyalinosis.

Immunofluorescence:
Nonspecific trapping of IgM and C3 in areas of sclerosis.

Electron Microscopy

- Wrinkling and thickening of capillary walls and paramesangial GBM
- Granular to amorphous electron dense hyaline material subjacent to endothelium.

Vascular Renal Diseases

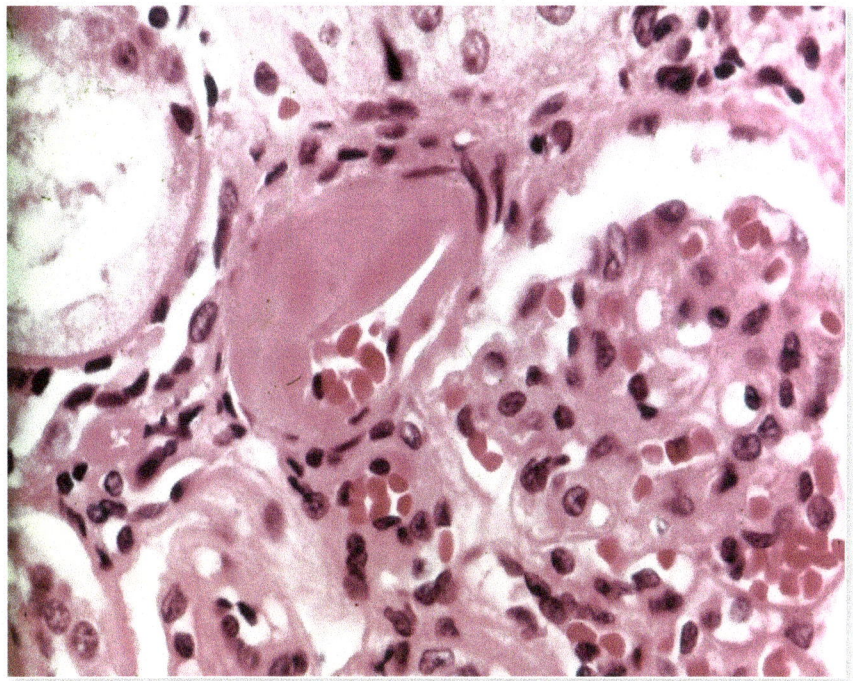

Figure 14.1: Benign arteriolonephrosclerosis (H & E x 200)

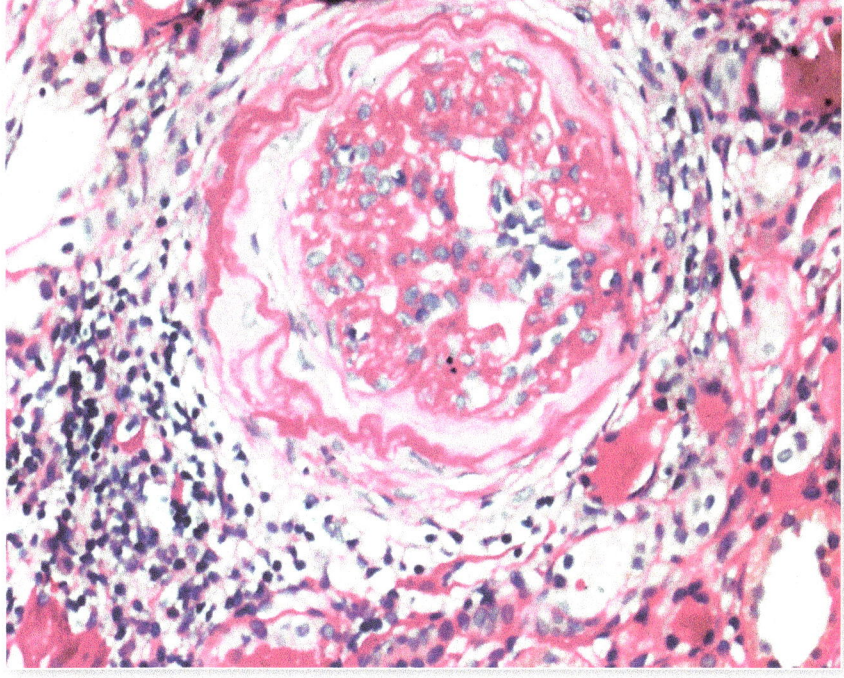

Figure 14.2: Ischemic glomerulosclerosis (H & E x 400)

Differential Diagnosis

Chronic ischemic nephropathy secondary to:
- **Chronic thrombotic microangiopathy:** Sclerotic tuft is seen with replication of GBM and no retraction
- **Chronic tubulointerstitial nephritis:** Inflammatory component is more severe than is seen with hypertension
- **Renal artery stenosis:** Glomeruli are crowded together and atrophic tubules with inapparent lumina are seen.

MALIGNANT HYPERTENSIVE NEPHROSCLEROSIS

Malignant hypertensive nephrosclerosis is defined as severe hypertension in the range of 210/130 mmHg, that can be associated with retinal vascular hemorrhages and papilledema, renal functional impairment and target organ damage. In primary malignant hypertension, acute necrotizing lesions precede the hypertension and are a form of thrombotic microangiopathy, presenting with hemolytic uremic syndrome. Longstanding accelerated hypertension is considered secondary malignant hypertension, resulting in chronic or acute-on-chronic morphologic vascular lesions.[7,8]

Microscopic Features

- **Acute lesions** consist of focal segmental fibrinoid glomerular tuft necrosis with karyorrhexis
- Disruption of GBM and associated mesangiolysis
- Other glomeruli with markedly dilated and congested capillary lumina
- Platelet fibrin thrombi and fragmented erythrocytes in engorged capillaries
- Afferent arteriolar fibrinoid necrosis.

Chronic Lesions

- Ischemic wrinkling of glomerular capillary walls with atrophy of the tufts
- Subendothelial expansion with reduplication of capillary walls on the JMS stain
- Secondary focal and segmental sclerosis and global solidification of glomerular tuft
- Tubulointerstitial compartment displays thickening of tubular basement membranes
- Interstitial fibrosis with scattered lymphocytes
- Focal tubular necrosis and cortical infarcts.

Extraglomerular Blood Vessels

- Interlobular arteries with fibrinoid necrosis and schistocytes in the wall (Fig. 14.3)
- Concentric intimal fibrosis with luminal narrowing ("onion-skin" thickening) (Fig. 14.4)
- Splitting and reduplication of internal elastic lamina on JMS and elastic stains
- Basophilic intimal thickening and medial hyperplasia of medium sized arteries.

Immunofluorescence: Nonspecific trapping of IgM and C3 in walls of arterioles.

Vascular Renal Diseases 175

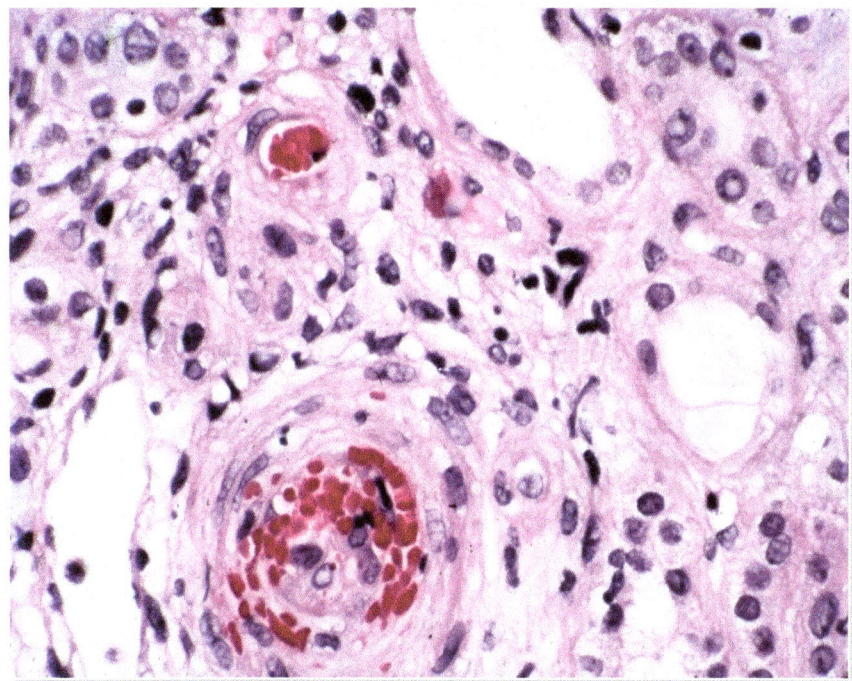

Figure 14.3: Malignant hypertension: Arterial fibrinoid necrosis with schistocytes (H & E x 200)

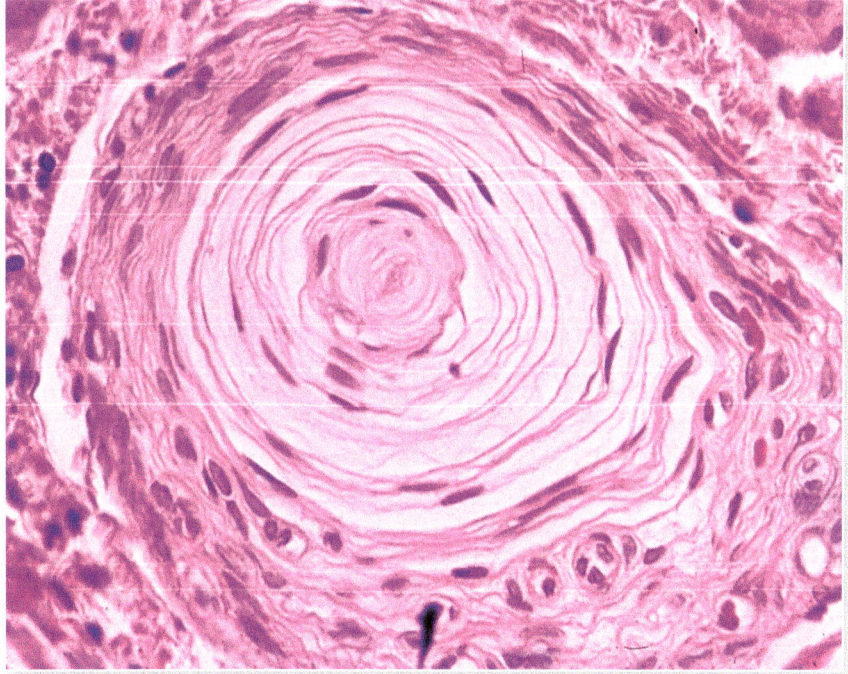

Figure 14.4: Arterial concentric intimal fibrosis (onion-skin) (H & E x 400)

Electron Microscopy

- Subendothelial electrolucent expansion of glomeruli with fibrin tactoids, luminal platelets and fragmented erythrocytes
- Lucent areas in foci of mesangiolysis can be present
- Electron dense or amorphous material in the foci of fibrinoid necrosis.

Differential Diagnosis

Thrombotic microangiopathy secondary to:
- Hemolytic uremic syndrome
- Thrombotic thrombocytopenic purpura
- Systemic sclerosis renal crisis
- Antiphospholipid antibody syndrome
- Acute postpartum renal failure
- Cyclosporine and mitomycin drug toxicity
- Bone marrow and stem cell transplantation.

Course and Prognosis

Optimal blood pressure regulation with appropriate and effective antihypertensive medication reverses and halts the progression of hypertensive nephrosclerosis. The diastolic blood pressure is a predictor of progression of renal hypertensive disease. Concomitant risk factors include age, diabetes mellitus, male gender, ethnic race, genetic polymorphisms, obesity with triglyceridemia and uric acid levels. There is a genetic susceptibility to the progression of hypertensive nephrosclerosis in African-Americans, when compared to Caucasians.[1-3]

THROMBOTIC MICROANGIOPATHY

Thrombotic microangiopathy is defined as a spectrum of disorders characterized morphologically by microvascular thrombosis and a specific angiopathy with an overlap of clinical manifestations. The three major categories are hemolytic uremic syndrome, thrombotic thrombocytopenic purpura and disseminated intravascular coagulation.

Hemolytic Uremic Syndrome

Hemolytic uremic syndrome (HUS) is characterized by the clinical triad of microangiopathic hemolytic anemia, thrombocytopenia and acute renal failure, with diffuse endothelial injury and associated microvascular capillary thrombosis. The classical form occurs mainly in infants and children with prodromal diarrhea, referred to as D+ HUS, caused by verotoxin producing *Escherichia coli* (VETC, serotype 157:H7) in North America and Europe.[9-11] In developing countries, the *Shiga toxin of Shigella* dysenteriae type I has been implicated in epidemics, previously from India including Vellore, Tamil Nadu[12] and other parts of Asia and Africa.

Microscopic Features

Acute Phase
- Glomerular endothelial swelling with subendothelial expansion and thickening of capillary walls
- Closure of capillary lumina with focal fibrin thrombi
- Focal mesangiolysis with dissolution of matrix
- Glomerular capillary ectasia with schistocytes in capillary lumina
- Focal glomerular infarcts or segmental fibrinoid necrosis (Figs 14.5 and 14.6)
- Global coagulative glomerular necrosis in foci of cortical parenchymal necrosis
- Fibrinoid necrosis of hilar arterioles and interlobular arteries with fibrin thrombi
- Basophilic intimal thickening of arcuate and interlobar arteries
- Foci of tubular necrosis and interstitial edema with neutrophilic infiltrates (Fig. 14.7).

Chronic Phase
- Mesangial cytoplasmic interposition in expanded subendothelial zones
- Neo-basement membrane material formation with reduplication of capillary walls
- Wrinkling of glomerular capillary walls with ischemia
- Segmental mesangial or global glomerulosclerosis
- Arteriolar intimal proliferation with organizing thrombi
- Arteriolosclerosis with concentric intimal arterial fibrosis.

Immunofluorescence
Fibrin or fibrinogen in thrombi and nonspecific trapping of IgM and C3 in vascular walls/glomeruli.

Electron microscopy (Figs 14.8A to C)
- Subendothelial expansion with fluffy or fibrillar material in electrolucent zones
- Fibrin-platelet luminal thrombi and angulated fibrin tactoids in the walls of glomeruli and arteries
- Extension of electrolucent zones into mesangium with lysis, under paramesangial BM
- Detachment of paramesangial BM with aneurysmal dilatation of capillary lumen
- Mesangial interposition with matrix deposition and condensation in chronic phase
- Focal foot process effacement.

Atypical HUS

Atypical HUS accounts for 5–12% of HUS, that is not preceded by Diarrhea (D-HUS) and is often sporadic in occurrence with recurrences, in children and adults. Primary atypical HUS is associated with complement deregulation and secondary forms are precipitated by bacterial (Streptococcal pneumonia), viral infections, vasculo-toxic drugs, autoimmune diseases, pregnancy, malignancy, transplants and metabolic disorders.[13-19]

The *familial or genetic* type is associated with mutations in regulatory factors of the alternate complement pathway: Complement factor H (25%), complement factor I (5–10%), membrane cofactor protein, CD46 (10%), complement components: C3 (2–10%) and complement factor

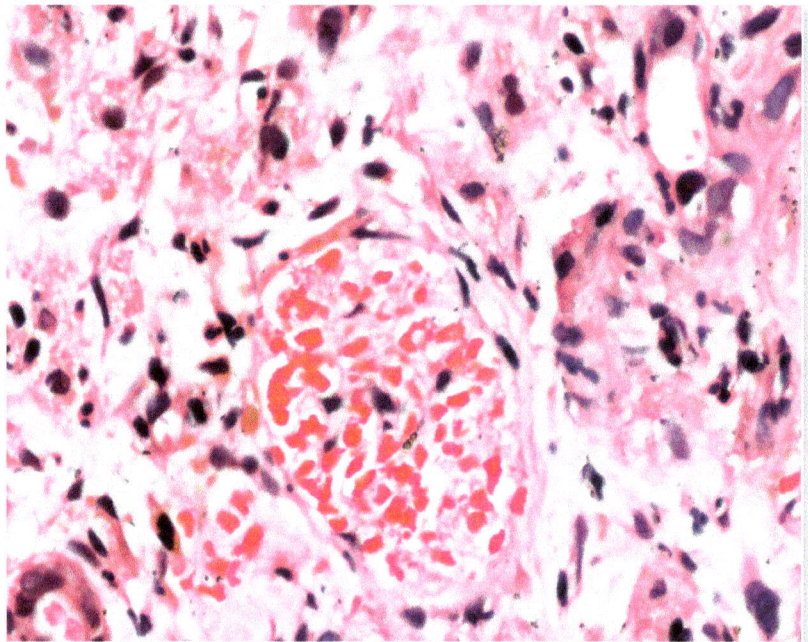

Figure 14.5: Glomerular infarct in pediatric HUS (H & E x 20X)

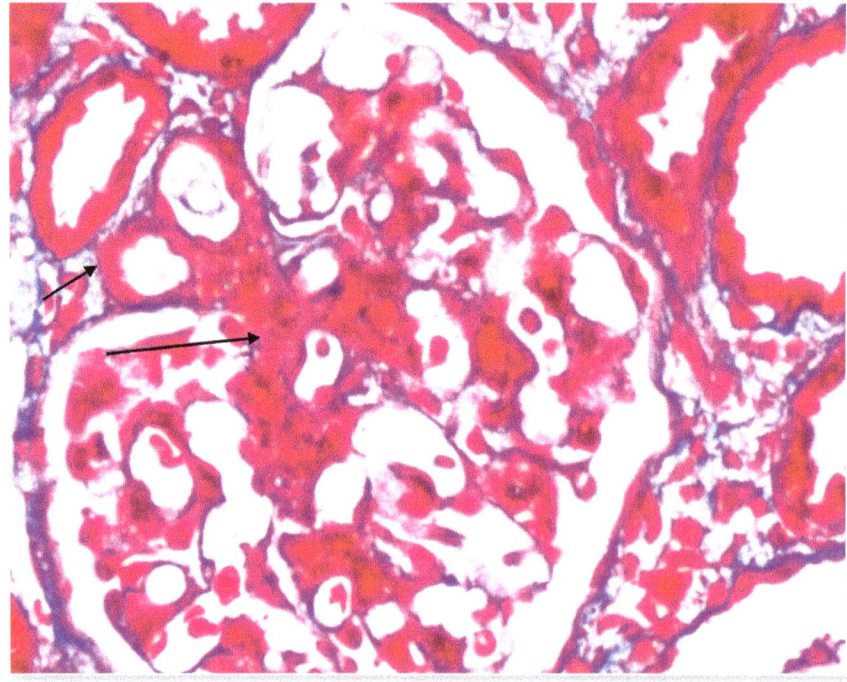

Figure 14.6: Fibrinoid necrosis of preglomerular arterioles (short arrow) and capillary tuft (long arrow) (Masson Trichrome x 400)

Vascular Renal Diseases

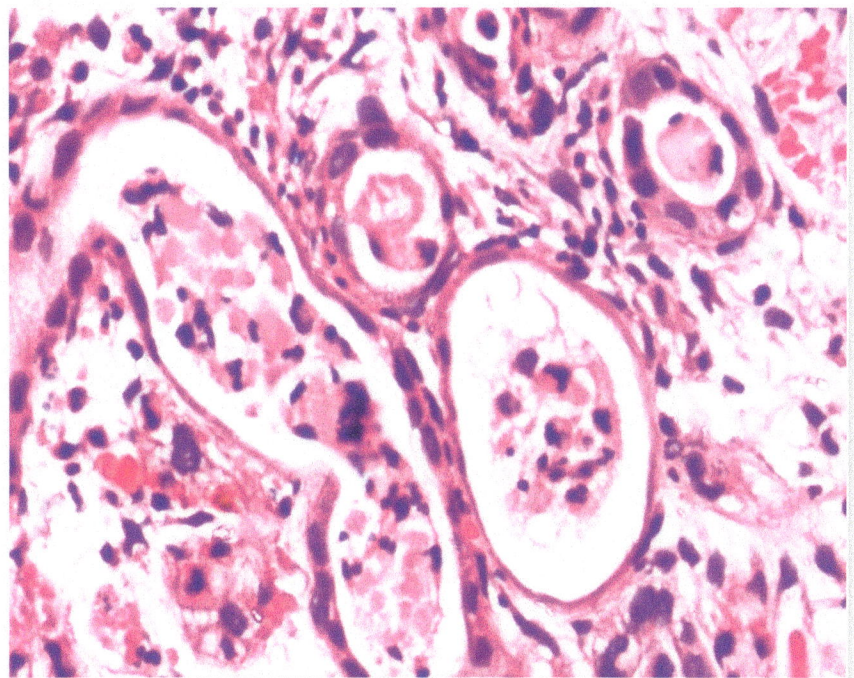

Figure 14.7: Acute tubular necrosis (H & E x 100)

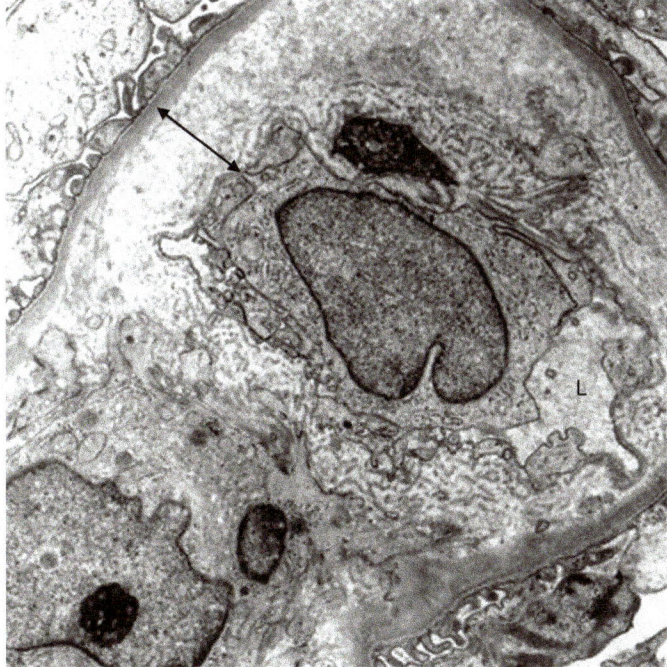

Figure 14.8A: Electrolucent expansion of subendothelial region (EM) (Internet Resource)

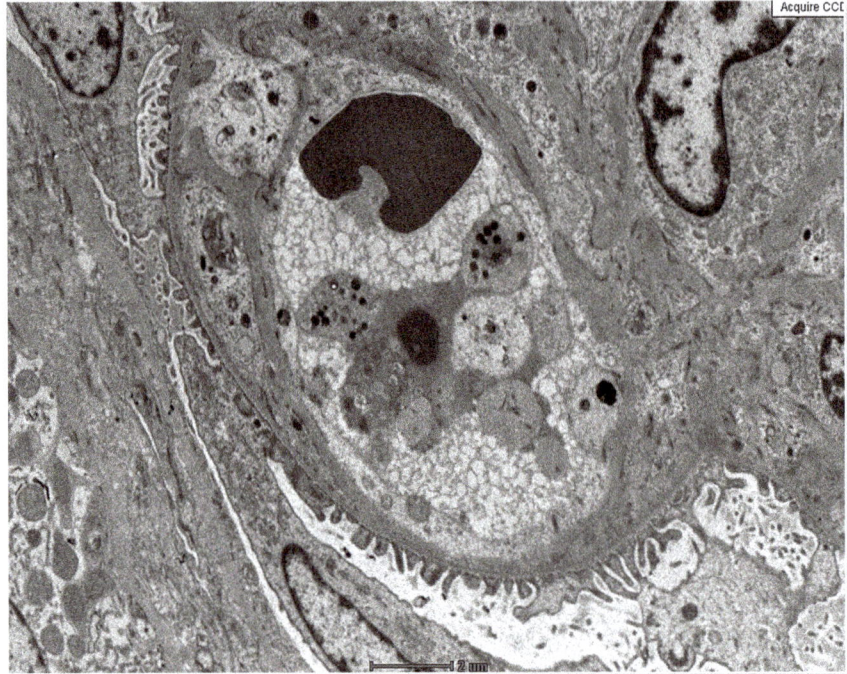

Figure 14.8B: Platelet aggregate and fragmented RBC in glomerular capillary lumen with mesangial cell interposition of GBM (tem: 4200 X)

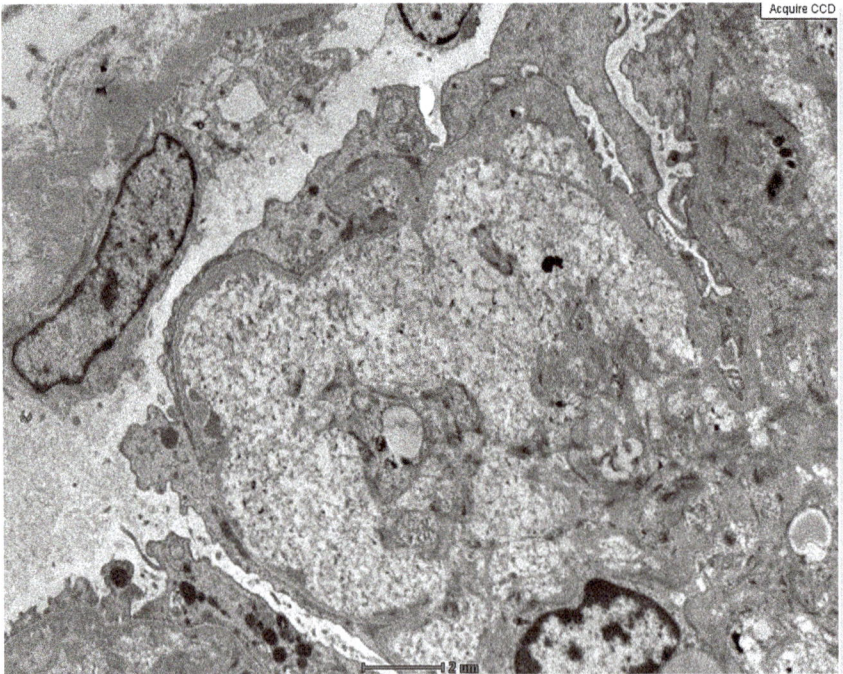

Figure 14.8C: Rarefaction of lamina rara interna with flocculent debris in TMA (tem x 4200)

B mutations. Autoantibodies to CFH or CFI and genetic polymorphisms in CFH have also been reported. The microscopic features are similar to D+ HUS with capillary thrombosis and variable early arterial involvement with glomerular capillary immunoglobulin and complement deposits.

Course and Prognosis

Pediatric (D+) HUS presenting with hematuria, proteinuria and oliguria and predominant glomerular lesions have a better prognosis responding to dialysis and supportive treatment. Adult cases of atypical HUS with heterogeneous causes and arterial involvement or cortical parenchymal necrosis have an increased (10–30%) mortality and progress to end-stage renal disease. Plasma exchange and eculizumab, a monoclonal antibody against the effector components of C5 are current modalities of treatment of atypical HUS with genetic defects in the complement system.

Other types of HUS include iatrogenic HUS (drug induced and bone marrow transplantation), systemic sclerosis renal crisis, postpartum HUS, malignant hypertensive nephropathy, radiation nephritis and idiopathic HUS with similar microscopic features.

Thrombotic Thrombocytopenic Purpura

Thrombotic thrombocytopenic purpura is defined by a clinical pentad of fever, microangiopathic hemolytic anemia, thrombocytopenia, fluctuating neurologic dysfunction and later onset of mild renal failure associated with multifocal platelet rich thrombi in various organs including adrenal cortex, pancreas and thyroid. There is an associated dysfunction of von Willebrand factor with circulating larger multimeric forms of vWF and their defective cleavage by metalloproteinase ADAMTS13 with microvascular thrombosis.[9,16]

Microscopic Features

- Glomerular capillary and eccentric arteriolar granular, amorphous platelet-fibrin thrombi
- Mild endothelial swelling and no subendothelial expansion
- No evidence of mural fibrinoid necrosis
- Organization of thrombi with endothelial proliferation forming "glomeruloid bodies"
- Acute tubular necrosis and interstitial hemorrhage.

Immunofluorescence

- Thrombi stain for fibrinogen and fibrin
- Negative for complement components.

Electron Microscopy

- Microvascular thrombi with mainly platelet aggregates admixed with less fibrin
- Subendothelial electron dense material devoid of electrolucent lesions.

Prognosis

The high mortality rates have improved after plasma exchange with fresh frozen plasma and removal of vWF cleaving protease inhibitors and replacement of vWF cleaving proteases.

Disseminated Intravascular Coagulation

Disseminated intravascular coagulation is a consumptive coagulopathy with depletion of coagulation factors and platelets and activated fibrinolysis. There is associated multifocal petechial, purpuric hemorrhage and multiorgan failure with schistocytes, fibrin split products and thrombocytopenia. The causes include gram negative bacterial infections, viral hemorrhagic fever (Dengue), pregnancy-induced complications, malignancy and trauma.[20,21]

Microscopic Features

- Fibrin rich thrombi in glomerular capillaries, arterioles and venules
- Organized thrombi less frequent
- PTAH positive fibrin strands seen.

Immunofluorescence
Positive for fibrin and fibrinogen, negative for immunoglobulins/complement.

Electron Microscopy
Vascular occlusive fibrin thrombi are seen with no subendothelial expansion.

Prognosis

Prognosis depends on the underlying cause and severity of multiorgan failure and efficacy of supportive treatment by blood products, heparin and dialysis.

ANTIPHOSPHOLIPID ANTIBODY SYNDROME

Antiphospholipid antibody syndrome (APS) is characterized by circulating antiphospholipid antibodies with venous, arterial, arteriolar or capillary venous thrombosis and/or pregnancy loss. This occurs as a primary idiopathic form or secondary to systemic autoimmune diseases such as SLE and rheumatoid arthritis. The antiphospholipid antibodies include lupus anticoagulant and anticardiolipin. Both laboratory tests are required for a diagnosis as only 50% of cases are positive for one or the other. At least one clinical criterion has to be present, for a diagnosis.[22]

Microscopic Features

Primary APS

- Fibrotic intimal thickening of interlobular and arcuate arteries
- Acute necrotizing and thrombotic glomerular and arteriolar lesions, similar to HUS
- Focal infarction caused by thrombosis of main renal artery
- GBM reduplication in reparative phase, with scarring and ischemic atrophy of tufts
- Organized and recanalized thrombi in arterioles and arteries.

Secondary APS

Microscopic features of APS with concomitant underlying lupus nephritis or lupus like glomerulonephritis are present.

Vascular Renal Diseases

Immunofluorescence

It is positive for fibrin and fibrinogen, nonspecific trapping of IgM and C3 in sclerotic foci. In secondary APS, "full house pattern" with immunoglobulins and C1q and C4 are present in lupus nephritis.

Electron Microscopy

Features are similar to hemolytic uremic syndrome (HUS).

Course and Prognosis

The ischemic complications of cerebral arterial thrombosis and deep venous thrombosis with thromboembolism in Primary APS and renal manifestations leading to endstage renal disease, particularly in secondary APS, have a dismal prognosis and high recurrence rate.

PRE-ECLAMPTIC TOXEMIA AND ECLAMPSIA

Pre-eclampsia is characterized by the occurrence of hypertension (>140/90 mm Hg), proteinuria, edema and renal insufficiency, usually after 20 weeks of pregnancy, due to abnormal placentation and release of toxic factors and trophoblastic material into the maternal circulation. Eclampsia is associated with convulsions in a patient with pre-eclampsia. Molar pregnancy can be associated with pre-eclamptic toxemia (PET) prior to 20 weeks' gestation. PET/Eclampsia can supervene with pre-existent chronic hypertensive disease.[23,24]

Microscopic Features

Light Microscopy

- Glomeruli are enlarged with diffuse endothelial swelling and narrowing of capillary lumina (Fig. 14.9)
- Marked endotheliosis and apparent solidification of the tuft (bloodless glomeruli) (Fig. 14.9)
- Mild mesangial expansion with mild hypercellularity
- Elongation and dilatation of glomerular tip with herniation into proximal tubule
- Replication of GBM subjacent to and around endothelial cells (seen on JMS stain), within a week
- Focal adhesions of glomerular tip with Bowman's capsule
- Secondary focal and segmental sclerosis is rarely seen
- Arteriolar and arterial lesions present suggest pre-existent hypertensive disease.

Immunofluorescence

Nonspecific trapping of IgM and C3 in glomerular tufts.

Electron Microscopy

Pathognomonic features:
- Marked endotheliosis with apparent occlusion of glomerular capillary lumen
- Foamy vacuolization of endothelial cells

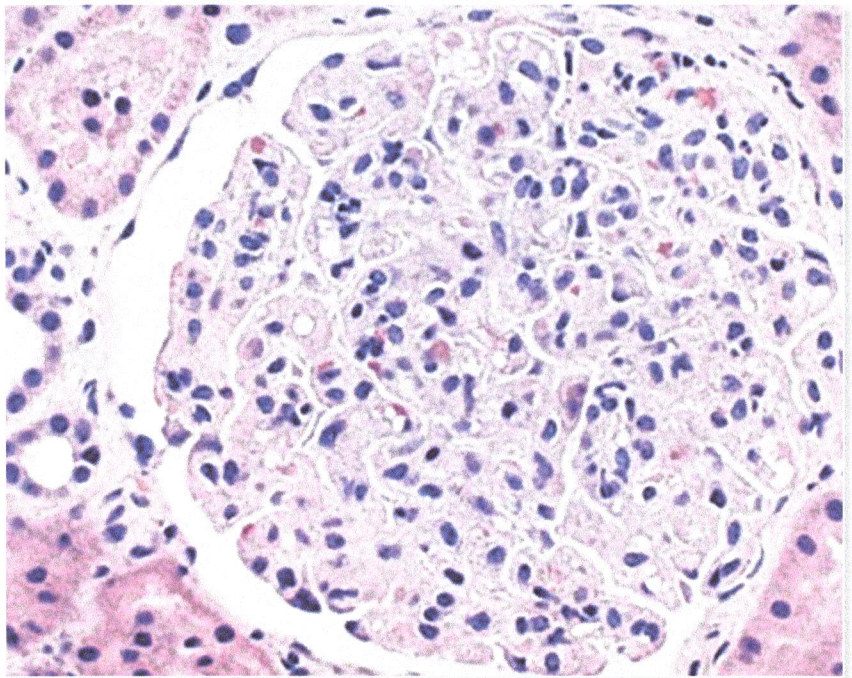

Figure 14.9: Diffuse endothelial enlargement with luminal occlusion (H & E x 400)

- Extensions of endothelial cytoplasm into the lumen and subendothelial space
- Electron dense insudated plasmatic material and replicated GBM around endothelial cells.

Differential Diagnosis

1. **Hemolytic uremic syndrome:** It is associated with the distinctive features of segmental glomerular and afferent arteriolar fibrinoid necrosis with subendothelial expansion and schistocytes on glomerular capillary walls in the acute phase and GBM reduplication in the reparative phase.
2. **Thrombotic thrombocytopenic purpura**: It is differentiated by the presence of platelet thrombi in glomerular capillaries and small vessels, devoid of underlying fibrinoid necrosis.
3. **Disseminated intravascular coagulation:** Features occlusive microvascular fibrin thrombi and no evidence of mural fibrinoid necrosis.
4. **Tip lesion variant of FSGS**: The consolidation of the herniated tip segments of glomeruli into the proximal tubule is not associated with endotheliosis of the remainder of the tufts as in PET.

Course and Prognosis

The clinical features of PET/Eclampsia subside within 24 hours of delivery. The glomerular capillary endotheliosis is reversible and resolves within 2 weeks of delivery. Persistent proteinuria, hypertension and renal failure is associated with other chronic underlying diseases, including focal and segmental glomerulosclerosis.

REFERENCES

1. Marcantoni C, Fogo AB. A perspective on arterionephrosclerosis: from pathology to potential pathogenesis. J Nephrol. 2007;20(5):518-24.
2. Dasgupta I, Porter C, Innes A, Burden A. Benign hypertensive nephrosclerosis. Q J Med. 2007;100;113-9.
3. Vikse BE, Aasarod K, Bostad L, Iverson BM. Clinical prognostic factors in biopsy proven benign nephrosclerosis. Nephrol Dial Transplant. 2003;18:517-23.
4. Fogo AB. Mechanisms in nephrosclerosis and hypertension-beyond hemodynamics. J Nephrol. 2001;14 (Suppl 4) :S63-9.
5. Hill GS. Hypertensive nephrosclerosis. Curr Opin Nephrol Hypertens. 2008;17(3):266-70. doi: 10.1097/MNH.0b013e3282f88a1f.
6. Fogo A, Ichikawa I. Evidence for a pathogenic linkage between glomerular hypertrophy and sclerosis. Am J Kidney Dis. 1991;17(6):666-9.
7. Van den Born BJH, Honnebier UPF, Koopmans RP, Van Montfran GA. Microangiopathic hemolysis and renal failure in malignant hypertension. Hypertension. 2005;45:246-51.
8. Thachil J. The malignant hypertension-thrombotic microangiopathy link. Hypertension. 2008;52:e32.
9. Ruggenenti P, Noris M, Remuzzi G. Thrombotic microangiopathy, hemolytic uremic syndrome, and thrombotic thrombocytopenic purpura. Kidney Int. 2001;60:831-46; doi:10. 1046/j. 1523-1755. 2001. 060003831.
10. Remuzzi G, Ruggenenti P. The hemolytic uremic syndrome. Kidney Int. 1995;47:2-19.
11. Siegler RL. The hemolytic uremic syndrome. Pediatr Clin North Am. 1995;42(6):1505-29.
12. Date A, Raghupathy P, Shastry J CM. Nephron injury in the hemolytic-uraemic syndrome complicating bacillary dysentery. J Pathology. 1981;133:1-16.
13. Fitzpatrick MM, Walters MD, Trompeter RS, Dillon MJ, Barratt TM. A typical (non-diarrhea-associated) hemolytic-uremic syndrome in childhood. J Pediatr. 1993;122:532-7.
14. Neuhaus TJ, Calonder S, Leumann EP. Heterogeneity of atypical haemolytic uraemic syndromes. Archives of Disease in Childhood. 1997;76:518-21.
15. Kavanagh D, Goodship TH, Richards A. Atypical hemolytic uremic syndrome seminars nephral. 2013;33(6): 508-30.
16. Besbas N, Karpman D, Landau D, Loirat C, Proesmans W, Remuzzi G, et al. A classification of hemolytic uremic syndrome and thrombotic thrombocytopenic purpura and related disorders. Kidney Int. 2006;70: 423-31.
17. Constantinescu AR, Bitzan M, Weiss LS, Christen E, Kaplan BS, Cnaan A, et al. Non-enteropathic hemolytic uremic syndrome: causes and short-term course. Am J Kidney Dis. 2004;43:976-82.
18. Abarrategui-Garrido C, Melgosa M, Pena-Carrion A, de Jorge EG, de Cordoba SR, Lopez Trascasa M, et al. Mutations in proteins of the alternative pathway of complement and the pathogenesis of atypical hemolytic uremic syndrome. Am J Kidney Dis. 52. 2008;52:171-80.
19. Vaziri-Sani F, Holmberg L, Sjoholm AG, Kristoffersson AC, Manea M, Fremeaux-Bacchi V, et al. Phenotypic expression of factor H mutations in patients with atypical hemolytic uremic syndrome. Kidney Int. 2006;69:981-8.
20. Levi M, Ten Cate H. Disseminated intravascular coagulation. N Engl J Med. 1999;341(8):586-92.
21. Taylor FB Jr, Toh CH, Hoots WK, Wada H, Levi M. Towards definition, clinical and laboratory criteria, and a scoring system for disseminated intravascular coagulation. Thromb Haemost. 2001;86(5):1327-30.
22. Piette JC, Cacoub P, Wechsler B. Renal manifestations of the antiphospholipid syndrome. Semin Arthritis Rheum. 1994;23:357-66.
23. Karumanchi SA, Maynard SE, Stillman IE, et al. Preeclampsia: A renal perspective. Kidney Int. 2005;67:2101.
24. Lafayette R. The kidney in preeclampsia. Kidney Int. 2005;67:1194-1203.

CHAPTER 15

Renal Transplant Diseases

ABSTRACT

The causes of renal dysfunction that are detected on a renal biopsy with expertise are detailed in this chapter. The current update of Banff Classification of acute and chronic antibody mediated and cell mediated and vascular rejection with the microscopic features are primarily elucidated with excellent illustrations. The correlation of immunohistochemical positive C4d staining of peritubular and glomerular capillaries with presence of donor specific antibodies and morphological features and microvascular inflammation score with C4d negativity in antibody mediated rejection and transplant glomerulopathy are emphasized. Tubulointerstitial and vascular features of calcineurin inhibitor drug toxicity and their differential diagnosis are considered in depth. Infections in the allograft and cytopathic features and stages of polyoma virus nephropathy in particular are highlighted with other viral infections.

The frequent and rarer forms of recurrent glomerulonephritis are discussed in detail with appropriate photomicrographs. Post-transplant lymphoproliferative disorders in the allograft with early focal, polymorphous, monomorphic and rare forms of lymphomas are categorized and differentiated from severe cellular rejection.

Renal allograft biopsies are performed to detect the causes of graft dysfunction, to predict response to immunosuppression and to determine the long-term outcome. Rejection is the most common cause of graft failure resulting from humoral and cell mediated responses of the recipient to specific histocompatibility antigens in the donor kidney.

CAUSES OF GRAFT DYSFUNCTION

- Acute or chronic antibody/cell mediated rejection
- Drug toxicity
- Acute tubular/preservation injury
- Infection
- Recurrent/de novo glomerulonephritis
- Post-transplant lymphoproliferative disorder.

Revised Banff 2017 Classification of 2007 Diagnostic Categories[1,2]

Category 1: Normal Biopsy or Nonspecific Changes

Category 2: Antibody-mediated Changes

Renal Transplant Diseases

Active Antibody-mediated Rejection (ABMR); All 3 Criteria Must be Met for Diagnosis

1. Histologic evidence of acute tissue injury, including 1 or more of the following:
   - Microvascular inflammation (g > 0 and/or ptc > 0), in the absence of recurrent or de novo glomerulonephritis, although in the presence of acute t-cell mediated rejection (TCMR), borderline infiltrate, or infection, ptc ≥ 1 alone is not sufficient and g must be ≥ 1
   - Intimal or transmural arteritis (v > 0)
   - Acute thrombotic microangiopathy, in the absence of any other cause
   - Acute tubular injury, in the absence of any other apparent cause.
2. Evidence of current/recent antibody interaction with vascular endothelium, including 1 or more of the following:
   - Linear C4d staining in peritubular capillaries (C4d2 or C4d3 by IF on frozen sections, or C4d > 0 by IHC on paraffin sections)
   - At least moderate microvascular inflammation [(g + ptc ≥2)] in the absence of recurrent or de novo glomerulonephritis, although in the presence of acute TCMR, borderline infiltrate, or infection, ptc ≥ 2 alone is not sufficient and g must be ≥1
   - Increased expression of gene transcripts/classifiers in the biopsy tissue strongly associated with ABMR, if thoroughly validated.
3. Serologic evidence of donor- specific antibodies (DSA to HLA or other antigens). C4d staining or expression of validated transcripts/classifiers as noted above in criterion 2 may substitute for (DSA); however thorough DSA testing, including testing for non-HLA antibodies if HLA antibody testing is negative, is strongly advised whenever criteria 1 and 2 are met.

Chronic Active ABMR; All 3 Criteria Must be Met for Diagnosis

1. Morphologic evidence of chronic tissue injury, including 1 or more of the following:
   - Transplant glomerulopathy (cg >0) if no evidence of chronic TMA or chronic recurrent/de novo glomerulonephritis; includes changes evident by electron microscopy (EM) alone (cg1a)
   - Severe peritubular capillary basement membrane multilayering (requires EM)
   - Arterial intimal fibrosis of new onset, excluding other causes; leukocytes within the sclerotic intima favor chronic ABMR if there is no prior history of TCMR, but are not required.
2. Identical to criterion 2 for active ABMR, above
3. Identical to criterion 3 for active ABMR, above, including strong recommendation for DSA testing whenever criteria 1 and 2 are met

C4d Staining without Evidence of Rejection; All 4 Features Must be Present for Diagnosis

1. Linear C4d staining in peritubular capillaries (C4d2 or C4d3 by IF on frozen sections, or C4d>0 by IHC on paraffin sections)
2. Criterion 1 for active or chronic, active ABMR not met
3. No molecular evidence for ABMR as in criterion 2 for active and chronic, active ABMR
4. No acute or chronic active TCMR, or borderline changes.

Category 3: Borderline Changes

- Suspicious (Borderline) for acute TCMR
- Foci of tubulitis (t > 0) with minor interstitial inflammation (i0 or i1), or moderate- severe interstitial inflammation (i2 or i3) with mild (t1) tubulitis; retaining the i1 threshold for

borderline with t > 0 is permitted although this must be made transparent in reports and publications
- No intimal or transmural arteritis (v = 0).

Category 4: T Cell Mediated Rejection (TCMR)

Acute TCMR
- Grade IA: Interstitial inflammation involving >25% of nonsclerotic cortical parenchyma (i2 or i3) with moderate tubulitis (t2) involving 1 or more tubules, not including tubules that are severely atrophic
- Grade IB: Interstitial inflammation involving >25% of nonsclerotic cortical parenchyma (i2 or i3) with severe tubulitis (t3) involving 1 or more tubules, not including tubules that are severely atrophic
- Grade IIA: Mild to moderate intimal arteritis (v1), with or without interstitial inflammation and/or tubulitis
- Grade IIB: Severe intimal arteritis (v2), with or without interstitial inflammation and/or tubulitis
- Grade III: Transmural arteritis and/or arterial fibrinoid necrosis of medial smooth muscle with accompanying mononuclear cell intimal arteritis (v3), with or without interstitial inflammation and/or tubulitis.

Chronic Active TCMR
- Grade IA: Interstitial inflammation involving >25% of the total cortex (ti score 2 or 3) and >25% of the sclerotic cortical parenchyma (i-IFTA score 2 or 3) with moderate tubulitis (t2) involving 1 or more tubules, not including severely atrophic tubules ; other known causes of i-IFTA should be ruled out
- Grade IB: Interstitial inflammation involving >25% of the total cortex (ti score 2 or 3) and >25% of the sclerotic cortical parenchyma (i-IFTA score 2 or 3) with severe tubulitis (t3) involving 1 or more tubules, not including severely atrophic tubules; other known causes of i-IFTA should be ruled out
- Grade II: Chronic allograft arteriopathy (arterial intimal fibrosis with mononuclear cell inflammation in fibrosis and formation of neointima.

Reporting of Allograft Renal Biopsies

Specimen adequacy: 10 or more glomeruli in a biopsy with at least 2 arteries are sufficient for a diagnosis. 1 to 9 glomeruli with one artery are minimal requirements and an inadequate sample contains no glomeruli or arteries. Histopathological evaluation is performed on 3 micrometer, serial sections stained with H & E, PAS and JMS respectively and one extra section with Masson trichrome (for fibrosis) or Martius scarlet blue for fibrin when required.

Acute (Active) antibody-mediated rejection (AbMR): Occurs in 20-30% of biopsies with acute rejection and 20-48% of positive crossmatch patients. Diagnosis of AbMR includes diffuse peritubular capillary wall C4d staining, presence of donor specific antibodies in serum and histopathologic evidence of tissue injury. C4d, a terminal component of the classical complement cascade binds covalently to the capillary wall and persists in the graft as a surrogate marker of AbMR. Complement fixing alloantibodies are implicated in endothelial activation and lysis, coagulation, complement activation and influx of macrophages and neutrophils.[3-6]

Renal Transplant Diseases

Hyperacute rejection occurring within minutes or hours after transplantation, due to presensitization by preformed circulating donor antibodies, is a form of humoral rejection that now rarely occurs in about 0.5% of transplants, necessitating immediate graft nephrectomy. The microscopic features included neutrophil margination in glomerular and peritubular capillaries, fibrin thrombi, interstitial hemorrhage and cortical necrosis with positive C4d. This entity is replaced by the term Acute AbMR in the current Banff diagnostic categories. "Accelerated acute rejection" is a term that has also been deleted from the current Banff classification.[2-4]

Microscopic Features of Acute AbMR [3,4]

Type/grade I: Acute tubular necrosis with mild interstitial inflammation and C4d positive.

Type/grade II: Margination of neutrophils or mononuclear cells in peritubular capillaries and/or glomeruli, fibrin thrombi (C4d + and DSA present).

Type/grade III: Arterial transmural inflammation/fibrinoid change, C4d+.

Quantitative Criteria for Peritubular Capillaritis[1,6]

- ptc 0 No significant cortical ptc, or <10% of PTCs with inflammation
- ptc 1 ≥10% of cortical peritubular capillaries with capillaritis, with max 3 to 4 luminal inflammatory cells
- ptc 2 ≥10% of cortical peritubular capillaries with capillaritis, with max 5 to 10 luminal inflammatory cells
- ptc 3 ≥10% of cortical peritubular capillaries with capillaritis, with max >10 luminal inflammatory cells.

One comment on the composition (mononuclear cells vs. neutrophils) and extent (focal, ≤50% vs. diffuse, >50%) of peritubular capillaritis.

Quantitative criteria for early graft glomerulitis ("g" score): Transplant glomerulitis is defined as intracapillary endothelial enlargement with mononuclear cell infiltration occlusion/narrowing of one or more capillary lumina and is graded as follows:
- g(0): No glomerulitis
- g1: involving <25% of glomeruli
- g2: Segmental or global glomerulitis in 25–75% of glomeruli
- g3: Glomerulitis (global) in >75% of glomeruli.

C4d Scoring: (1)
The percentage of linear staining of peritubular capillary walls by IF or IHC is graded as follows:
- Scoring of C4d staining (% of biopsy or 5 high-powerfields)
- C4d0: Negative: 0%
- C4d1: Minimal C4d stain/detection: 1 to <10%
- C4d2: Focal C4d stain/positive: 10–50%
- C4d3: Diffuse C4d stain/positive: >50%.

Correlation of C4d staining by IF/IHC: Diffuse positive staining by IF and IHC correlates with circulating DSA with a sensitivity of 95% and specificity of 96% by the IF technique.

Diffuse positive C4d on the IF is possibly equal to focal positive on IHC as the former is more sensitive by one grade. Focal C4d positive on the IF is equal to minimal C4d positive on IHC but the clinical significance of the latter is unknown.

In daily reporting practice, focal staining for C4d on IHC in paraffin embedded tissue, combined with presence of donor specific antibodies and morphological features is considered positive for antibody-mediated rejection.[7]

C4d deposition without morphological evidence of active rejection can occur with presence of DSA or ABO incompatibility and has clinical implications.[1,8]

Cardinal Features of Acute (Active) AbMR[3,4]

1. **Morphological features** of acute tubular injury, peritubular capillaritis and glomerulitis and/or capillary thrombosis; intimal arteritis/arterial fibrinoid necrosis/intramural or transmural inflammation (Figs 15.1 to 15.6).
2. **Immunologic features** of antibody activity including C4d and/or rarely immunoglobulin in peritubular capillaries or immunoglobulin and complement in arterial fibrinoid necrosis (Figs 15.7 and 15.8).
3. **Serological evidence** of circulating antibodies to donor HLA or endothelial antigens.

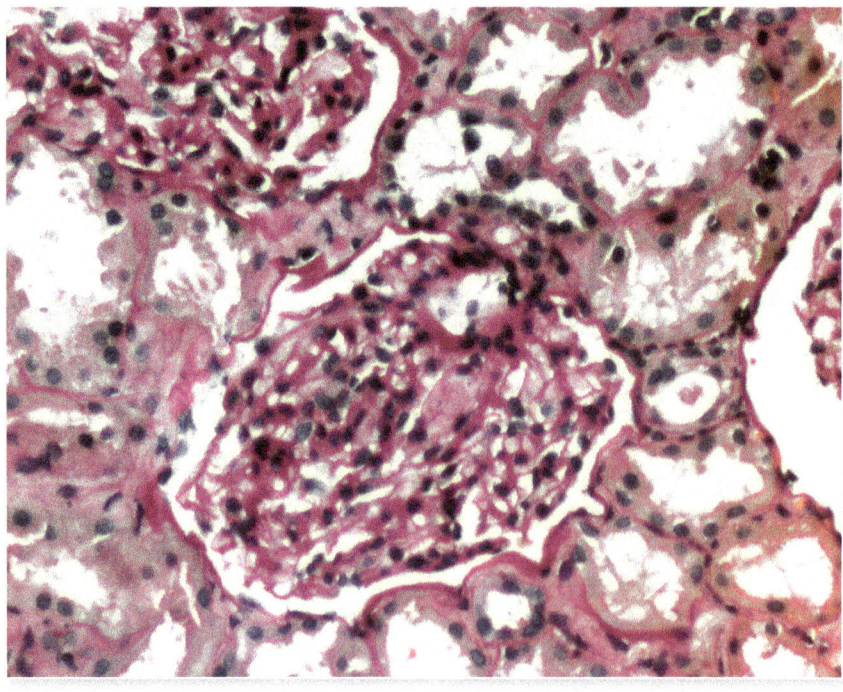

Figure 15.1: Transplant glomerulitis (PAS x 200)

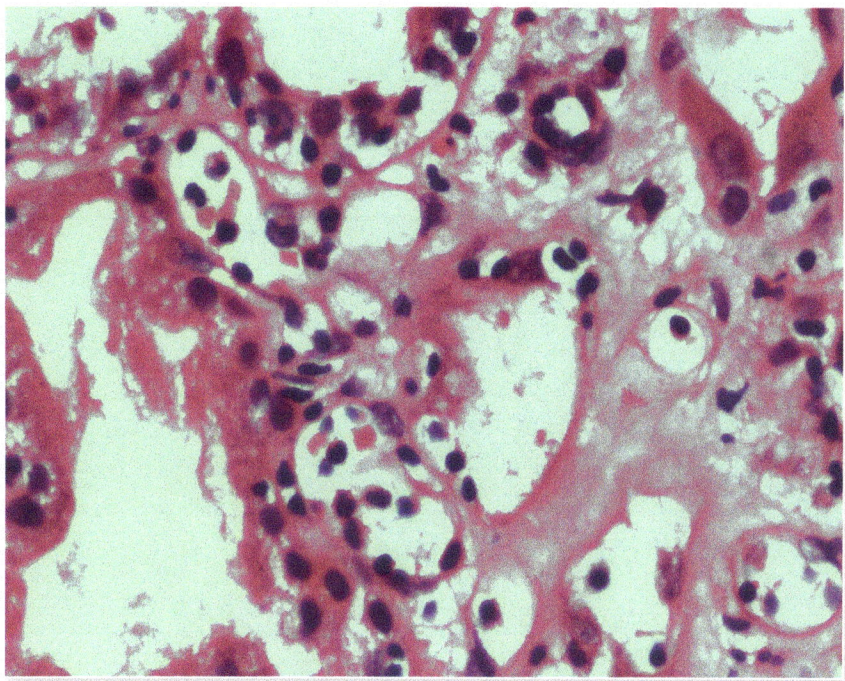

Figure 15.2: Moderate peritubular capillaritis (H & E x 400)

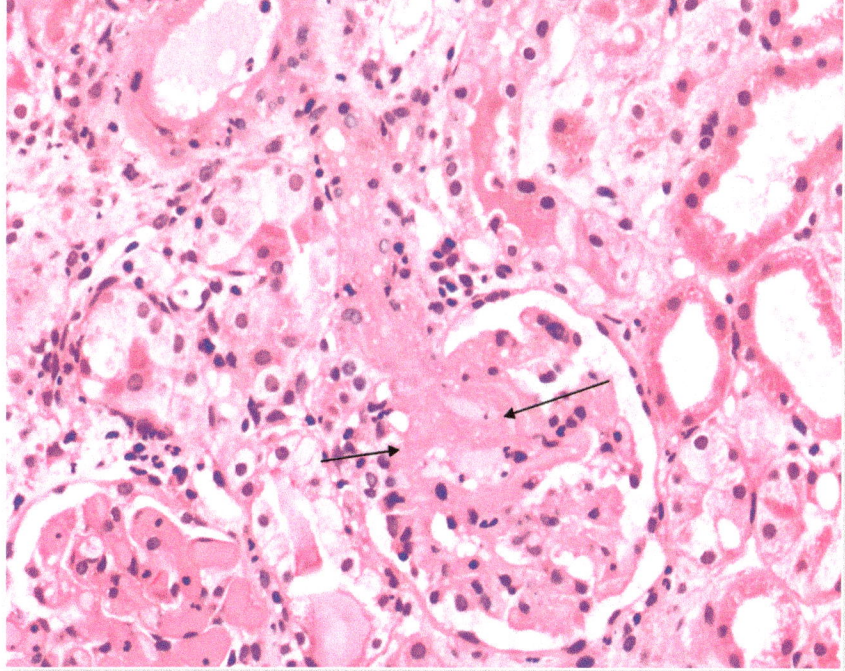

Figure 15.3: Acute antibody mediated rejection: Type III with afferent arteriolar and glomerular capillary (arrows) fibrinoid necrosis (H & E x 200)

Renal Biopsy Interpretation

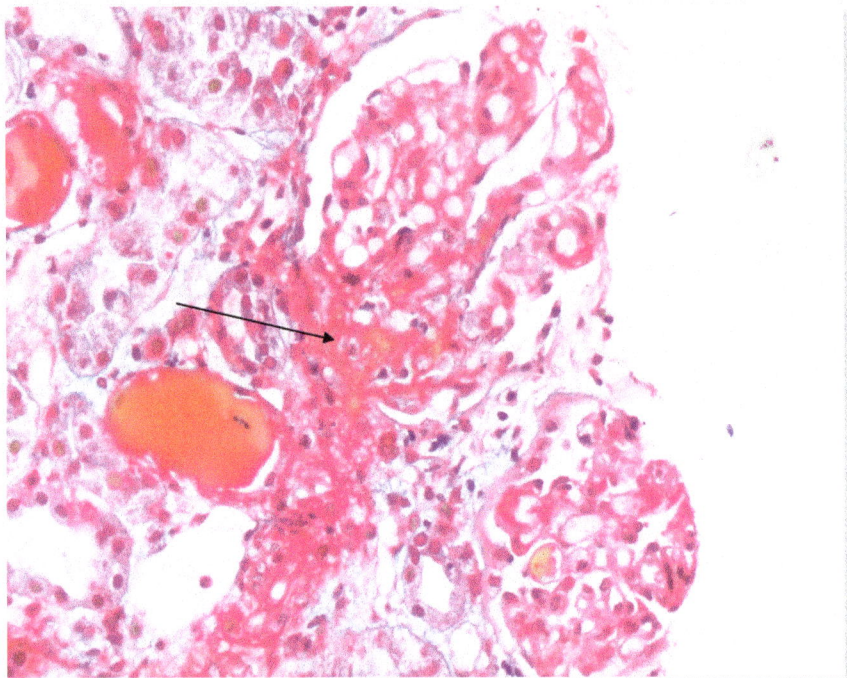

Figure 15.4: Focal segmental arteriolar and glomerular capillary fibrinoid necrosis (MSB stain x 200) (arrow)

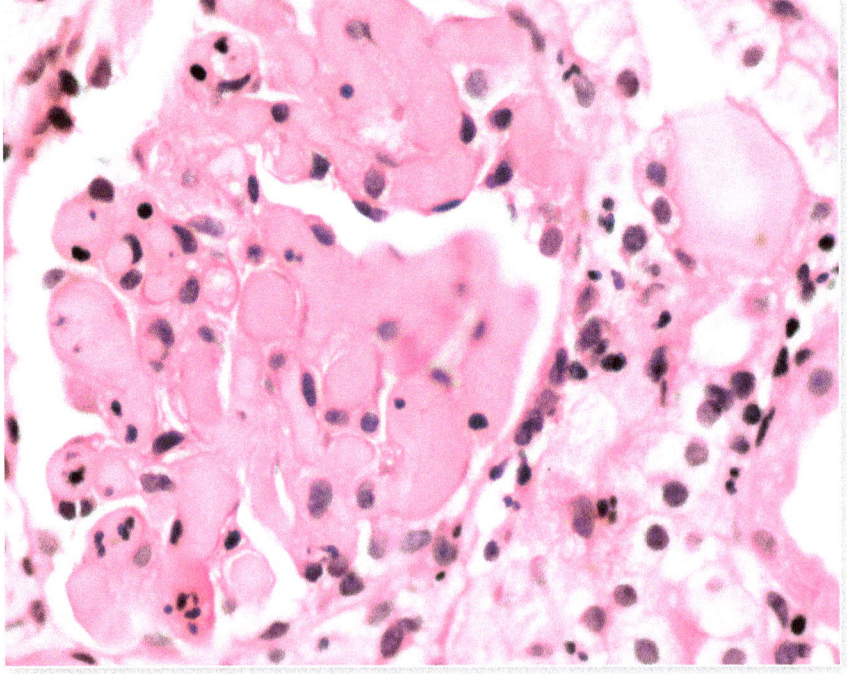

Figure 15.5: Glomerular capillary fibrin thrombi in acute antibody-mediated rejection (H & E x 400)

Renal Transplant Diseases

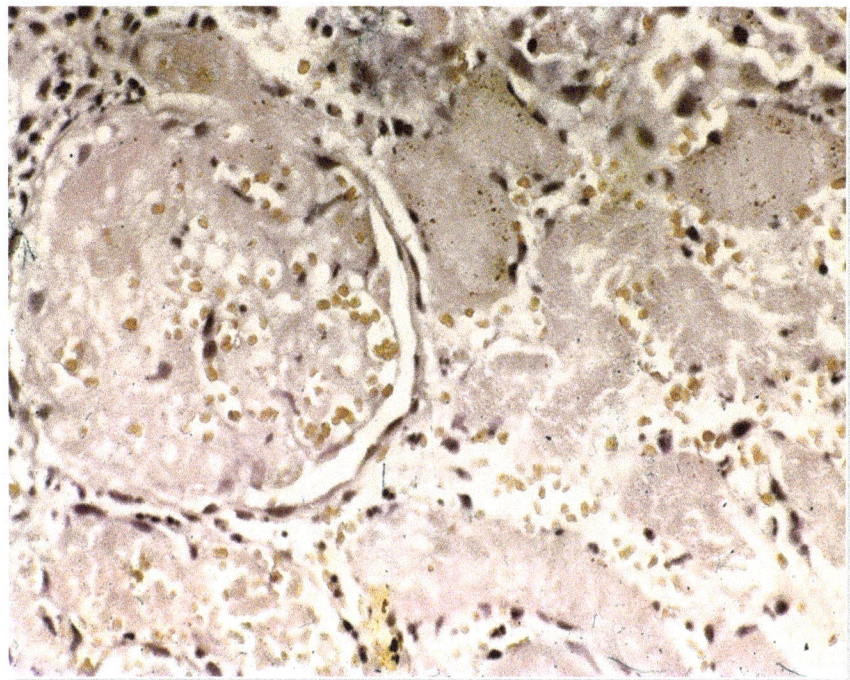

Figure 15.6: Cortical parenchymal necrosis in type III AbMR (H & E x 200)

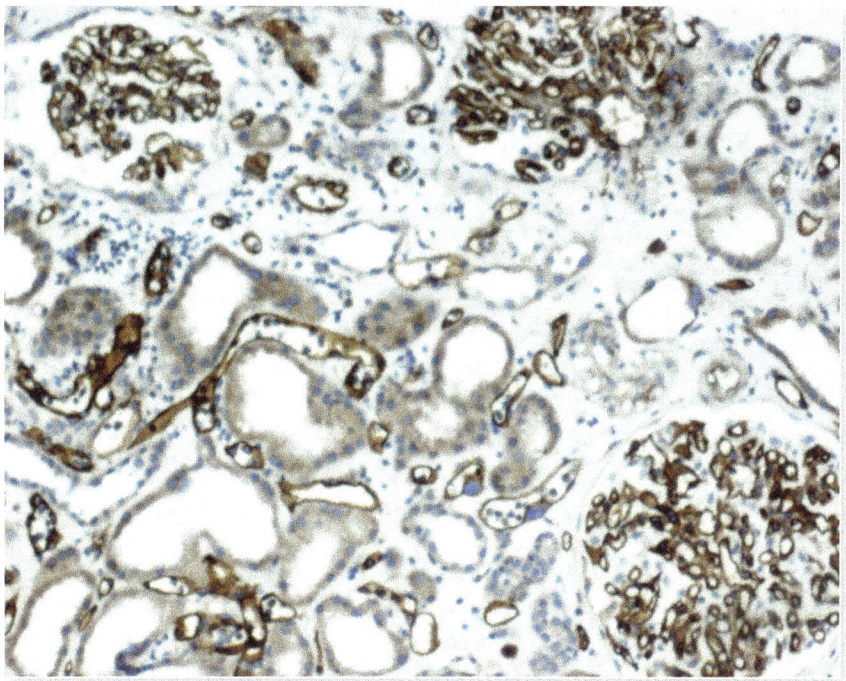

Figure 15.7: Glomerular and peritubular capillary wall C4d deposits (IHC x 200)

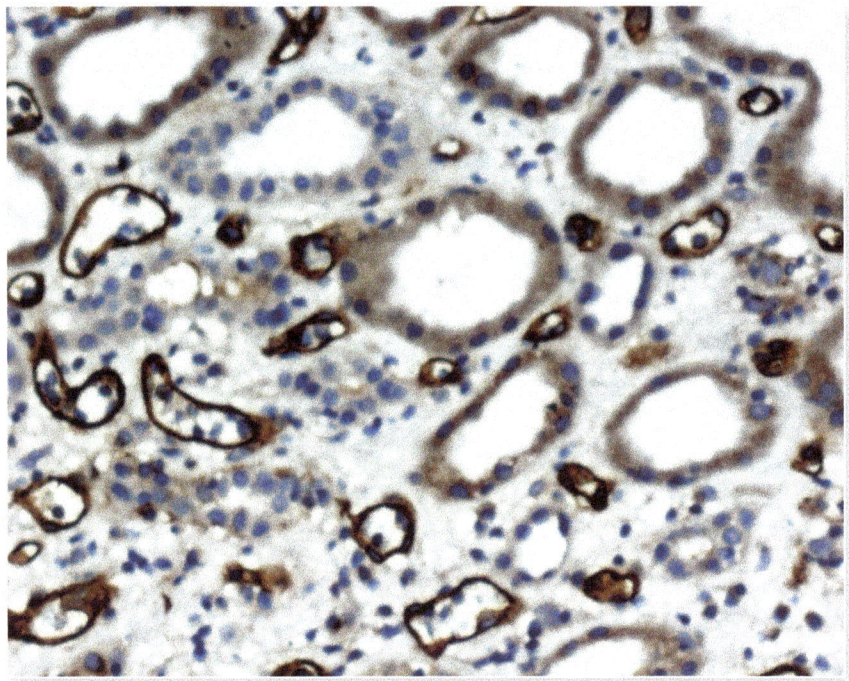

Figure 15.8: Peritubular capillary wall C4d deposits (IHC x 200)

Differential Diagnosis

Thrombotic microangiopathy due to calcineurin inhibitor microvascular toxicity, can show similar features with entrapped fragmented erythrocytes and involvement of glomerular vascular pole, but is C4d negative. Recurrent HUS in the allograft is also C4d negative.

Prognosis

Acute AbMR usually responds to plasmapheresis and intravenous immunoglobulin/anti CD20 (Rituximab) therapy and intensive immunosuppression with variable results.[7,9]

Chronic active Ab mediated rejection: Involves the glomeruli, peritubular capillary walls, arterial and tubulointerstitial compartment, presenting with late onset of graft dysfunction with proteinuria in the nephrotic range and hypertension. The diagnostic criteria of chronic AbMR[4,5] includes:
1. Morphological evidence of chronic injury with at least 2 of the following features:
    - Duplication of GBM
    - Arterial intimal fibrosis without duplication of internal elastica
    - PTC basement membrane, multilamination (PTCBMML)
    - Interstitial fibrosis and tubular atrophy (IF/TA)
2. Evidence of antibody action/deposition in tissue (C4d in tissue)
3. Serological evidence of anti-HLA or other anti-donor antibody.

Microscopic Features of the Four Major Components

Transplant Glomerulopathy

Transplant glomerulopathy (TG) is induced by chronic antibody-mediated endothelial injury with reactive lamellation of GBM.[10-12]

Light microscopy (Fig. 15.9)
- Glomerular mesangial matrix expansion
- Thickening of capillary walls with reduplication
- Graded "cg 1-3" (double contours in 1-25%, 26-50%, to > 50% of peripheral capillary loops in most affected of nonsclerotic glomeruli)
- Concomitant transplant glomerulitis with intracapillary mononuclear cells
- Secondary focal and segmental sclerosis with hyalinosis.

Early transplant glomerulopathy[12] is currently graded as follows:
- cg0: No GBM double contours by light microscopy or EM
- cg1a: No GBM double contours by light microscopy but GBM double contours (incomplete or circumferential) in at least three glomerular capillaries by EM with associated endothelial swelling and/or subendothelial electron-lucent widening
- cg1b: One or more glomerular capillaries with GBM double contours in ≥1 nonsclerotic glomerulus by light microscopy; EM confirmation is recommended if EM is available.

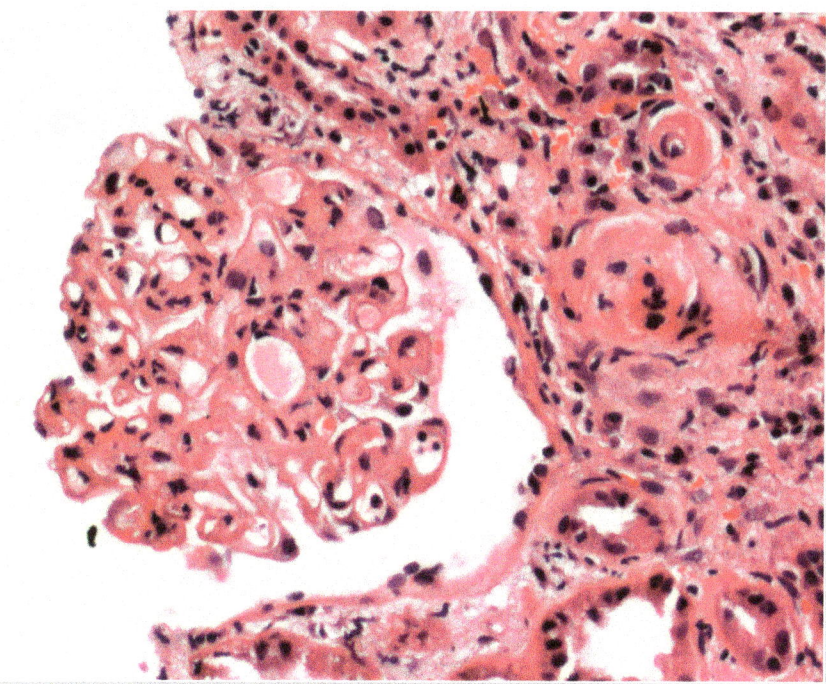

Figure 15.9: Transplant glomerulopathy (PAS x 200)

Electron microscopy
- Mesangial interposition
- Circumferential duplication or multilamination of GBM
- Endothelial hypertrophy with loss of fenestrations.

Transplant Capillaropathy

- Loss of peritubular capillaries with reduced capillary density
- Multilamination of capillary basement membrane (5 or more layers), on EM.

Transplant Arteriopathy

Intimal fibrosis with sparse mononuclear cell infiltration and no elastosis.

Extraglomerular Compartment

Interstitial fibrosis and tubular atrophy (IF/TA).

Immunohistochemical Interstitial Fibrosis (IHC/IF)

- C4d positive on glomerular capillary endothelium and peritubular capillaries, in varying proportion
- IgM and C3 deposits on glomerular capillary walls and mesangium.

Differential Diagnosis

Recurrent membranoproliferative glomerulonephritis, Type I: Marked glomerular enlargement with centrilobular mesangial matrix expansion and circumferential reduplication of capillary walls with perilobular capillary wall deposits of IgG and C3, mesangial interposition and subendothelial immune deposits on EM.

Course and Prognosis[2,4,6,12]

Review of protocol biopsies done immediately after transplantation has shown that C4d positivity correlated with a positive cross match and DSA leading to subclinical or overt AbMR in about 30% cases and transplant glomerulopathy after 1 year post-transplant. Anti-HLA class I and II antibodies had the highest risk of developing TG and 50% of TG was associated with acute AbMR. Glomerulitis correlated with onset of TG. IF/TA associated with transplant arteriopathy and TG in biopsies within 1 year had a worse prognosis. TG has a poor long-term prognosis with graft failure. C4d has been reported negative in >40% of cases of TG. Endothelial transcripts on molecular studies combined with DSA show a greater sensitivity for antibody mediated rejection including chronic AbMR and less specificity than C4d.[7,12]

Quantitative criteria for tubulitis: "t" score and interstitial mononuclear infiltrates: "I" score[1,2]
- t0: No mononuclear cells in tubules
- t1: Foci with 1–4 cells/tubular CS (or 10 tubular cells/LS)
- t2: Foci with 5–10 cells/tubular CS

- t3: Foci with >10 cells/tubular CS, or parenchyma with at least two areas of tubular BM destruction accompanied by i2/i3 (>25%) inflammation and t2 tubulitis elsewhere in biopsy
- i0: No or trivial inflammation (<10% of unscarred renal parenchyma)
- i1: 10–25% interstitial involvement
- i2: 25–50% interstitial involvement
- i3: >50 % interstitial involvement.

Scoring of the total parenchyma (scarred and unscarred) is the new lesion "ti" score[11] for mononuclear cell infiltrates infiltrating the renal cortex including subcapsular, perivascular regions and in areas of interstitial fibrosis/tubular atrophy: ti1 to ti3 (<25% to >50%). The "ti" score of the sum of persistent interstitial inflammation of any type is considered to have an adverse long-term outcome.

Borderline rejection: This category includes biopsies with mild tubulitis (t1) (Fig. 15.10) or any degree of tubulitis with minor interstitial inflammation (at least i1) and has to be interpreted in the clinical context, whether this is associated with stable renal function, subclinical rejection or seen in biopsies after initiation of treatment, with renal dysfunction.[1,2]

Acute/Active T Cell-mediated Rejection (TCMR)

Type IA
Microscopic features:
- Moderate tubulitis (t2) with lymphocytic infiltration between tubular epithelial cells (Fig. 15.11)

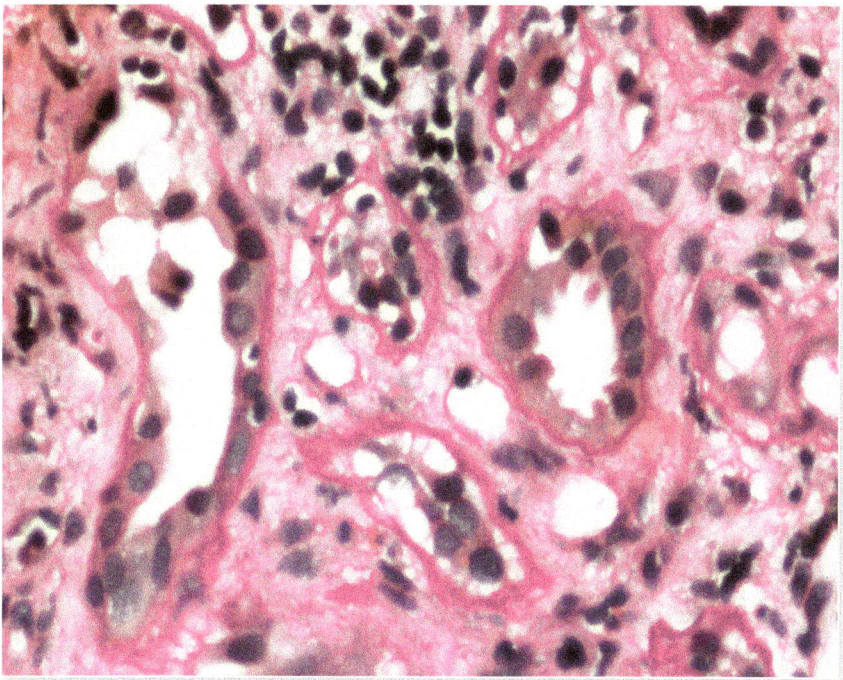

Figure 15.10: Acute cellular rejection with mild tubulitis (PAS x 400)

198 Renal Biopsy Interpretation

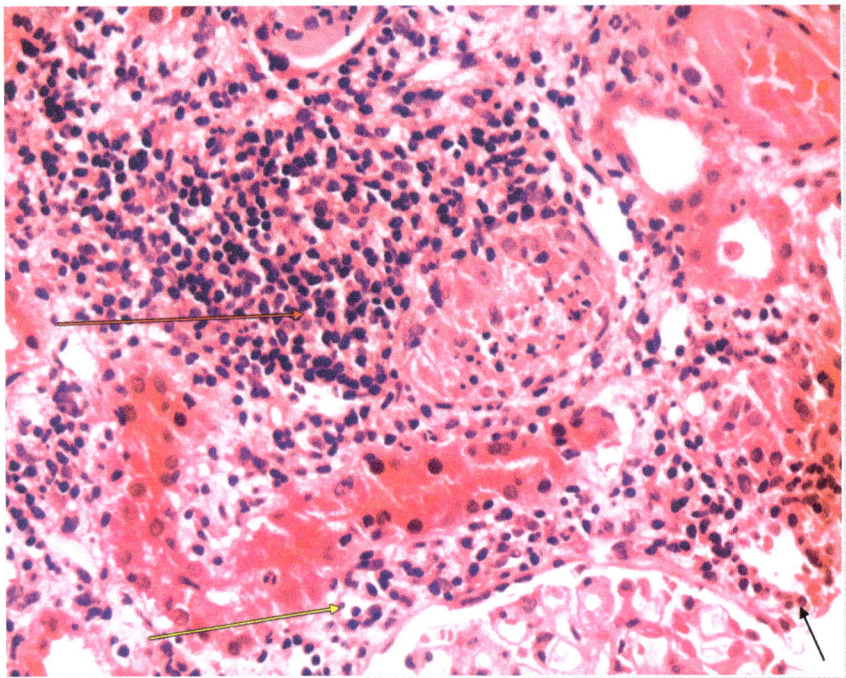

Figure 15.11: Acute cellular rejection with moderate (black arrow) to severe tubulitis (red arrow) and peritubular capillaritis (yellow arrow) (H & E x 200)

- Interstitial infiltrates of activated T lymphocytes with basophilic cytoplasm, enlarged nuclei, visible nucleolus
- Admixed, small lymphocytes with dense nuclear chromatin, plasma cells and scattered eosinophils
- CD8 +/> CD4 + T cells and fewer CD 20+ B cells
- Cytotoxic T cells expressing perforin and granzyme present
- Acute tubular necrosis with flattening and regeneration of lining epithelium
- Concomitant transplant glomerulitis ("g1-g3": <25% to >75% involvement)
- Enlarged glomerular endothelial cells and lymphocytic infiltrates.

Type IB

Microscopic features:
- Severe tubulitis (t3) with tubular BM loss in at least 2 tubules (Fig. 15.11)
- Dense interstitial lymphocytic infiltrates (t2–t3) replacing tubules (on PAS/JMS)
- Tubular necrosis and moderate tubulitis in other foci are usually seen.

Type IIA

Microscopic features (Figs 15.12 and 15.13):
- Mild to moderate lymphocytic endothelialitis with intimal infiltration (v1)
- Early lesion shows sparse lymphocytes subjacent to or lifting the endothelium
- Involvement of medium size to large arteries and few arterioles
- Any degree of concomitant tubulitis is usually present.

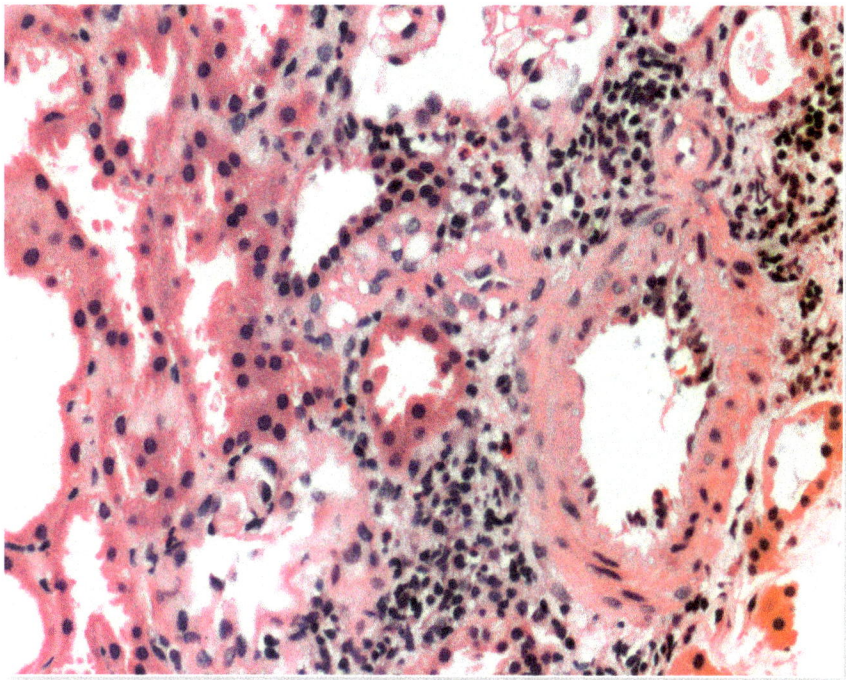
Figure 15.12: Acute lymphocytic endothelialitis (H & E x 200)

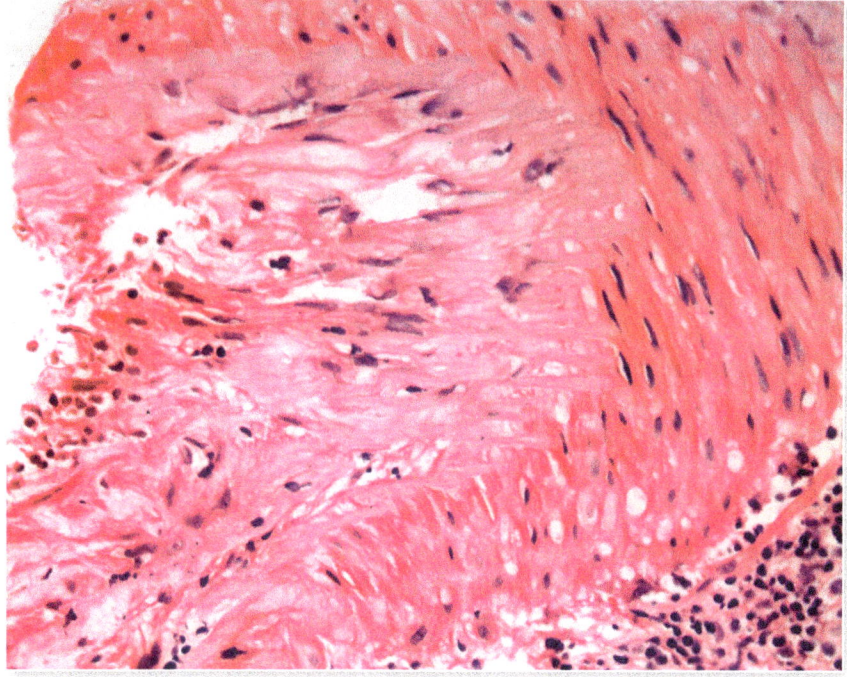
Figure 15.13: Acute vascular rejection with lymphocytic endothelialitis (H & E x 400)

Type IIB
Severe intimal arteritis involving >25% of luminal area ("v2").

Type III
- Transmural lymphocytic infiltrates/fibrinoid necrosis/Medial smooth muscle necrosis ("v3")
- Interstitial hemorrhage and infarction when extensive.

Course and Prognosis

Acute T cell-mediated type I rejection responds to steroids, whereas Type II vascular lesions are steroid resistant, associated with decreased graft survival.[1,2]

Isolated intimal arteritis/isolated "v" lesion in the absence of tubulointerstitial inflammation is currently under evaluation[2] and preliminary studies suggest that this factor has a poor prognosis.

CHRONIC ACTIVE T CELL-MEDIATED REJECTION (GRADE II)

Predominantly involves arterial compartment and is known as chronic allograft arteriopathy.[1,2]

Microscopic Features

- Intimal fibroplasia of medium—sized to large arteries
- Luminal narrowing or occlusion and formation of neointima
- Foam cells and mononuclear cells in fibrotic intima (Fig. 15.14)
- Concentric reduplication with disruption of internal elastic lamina (Fig. 15.15)
- Lesions graded from cv1 to cv3 (<25%, 26-50% to >50% involvement)
- Superimposed acute lymphocytic endothelialitis can occur
- Concomitant tubulitis can persist and is graded in mildly atrophic or non-atrophic tubules
- Associated with interstitial fibrosis and tubular atrophy (ci0–ci3; ct0–ct3 grades)
- Secondary focal segmental and diffuse global glomerular sclerosis can occur.

Differential diagnosis of chronic allograft injury associated with interstitial fibrosis and tubular atrophy: The term "Chronic allograft nephropathy" is obsolete[2,6] and has been replaced by specific diagnostic lesions that have to be excluded in the graft, as follows:
- Chronic active antibody and T cell-mediated rejection
- Chronic hypertensive nephrosclerosis
- Chronic calcineurin inhibitor vascular and interstitial toxicity
- BK polyomavirus nephropathy
- Chronic graft bacterial pyelonephritis/ureteric obstruction
- Recurrent chronic glomerulonephritis.

Banff 2013 Update[12]

The Banff 2013 meeting report of the 12th Banff Conference in Brazil sought to establish:
- Consensus criteria for diagnosing antibody mediated rejection (ABMR) with the presence and absence of detectable C4d deposition with definite criteria for C4d- negative ABMR.
- The significance of isolated intimal arteritis ("v" lesion) and association with antibody mediated acute rejection
- Standard definitions of glomerulitis and transplant glomerulopathy with double contours

Renal Transplant Diseases

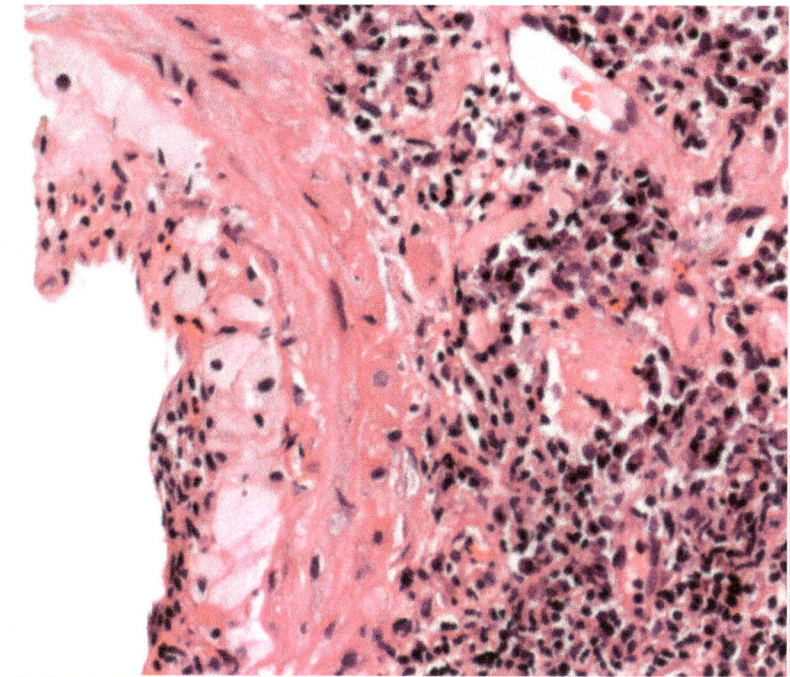

Figure 15.14: Acute on chronic vascular rejection (H & E x 200)

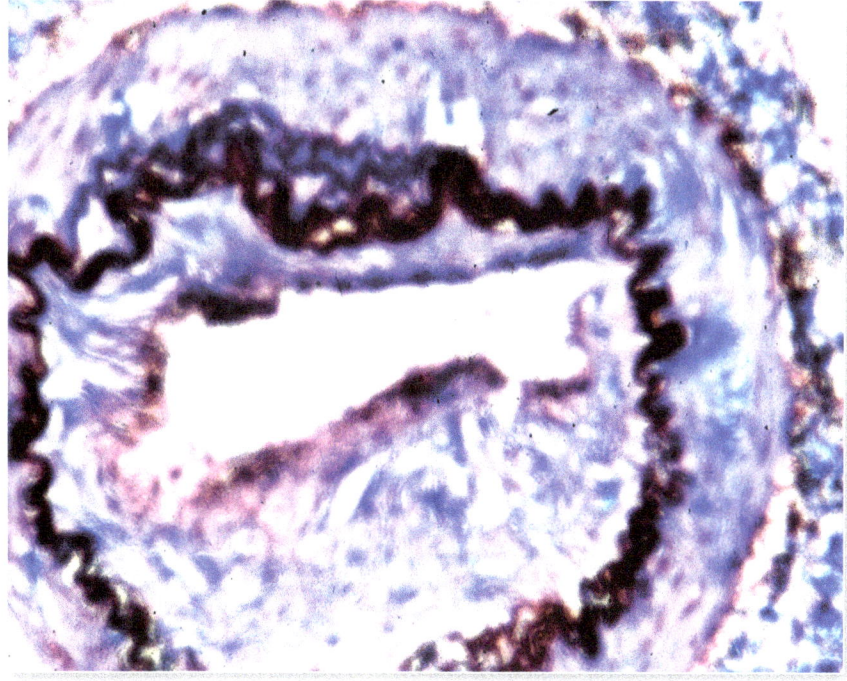

Figure 15.15: Chronic allograft arteriopathy (Elastic trichrome x 400)

- Methodologies to evaluate interstitial fibrosis and implantation protocol biopsies in order to facilitate reproducibility and prediction of graft function
- To define and prognosticate the morphological sub-classification of polyomavirus nephropathy.

Molecular studies of gene transcriptomes and gene expression profiles[13,14] with high density DNA microarray or real time PCR of renal biopsy material has shown T cell activation in TCMR and endothelial activation in ABMR, with the identification of C4d negative forms of ABMR.[15] Microvascular injury with glomerulitis and peritubular capillaritis in the presence of donor specific antibodies is strongly associated with interstitial fibrosis/tubular atrophy, transplant glomerulopathy and graft loss even in the absence of C4d deposits.[16-18] In the assessment of long term graft survival with de novo DSA, microvascular inflammation score (sum of glomerulitis and peritubular capillaritis scores) of ≥2 was associated with the highest risk of graft failure.[12] Recent evidence suggests that intimal arteritis and arterial intimal fibrosis may also be DSA-induced manifestations.[17] Integration of molecular genomics into the current Banff classification will overcome the limitations of the existing histopathological parameters in the prospective evaluation of renal allograft biopsies and to monitor treatment of active ABMR, chronic active and chronic ABMR.[15]

CALCINEURIN INHIBITOR TOXICITY

Cyclosporine and tacrolimus are potent immunosuppressants that have greatly improved graft survival. They inhibit calcineurin, a phosphatase that is required for the transcription of interleukin-2 and upregulation of cytokines during T cell activation by antigen presenting cells.

Calcineurin inhibitor (CNI) toxicity can occur in the therapeutic range of serum concentration of either of the two drugs and their structural effects are similar, diagnosed only by a renal biopsy. There are acute and chronic morphological features of CNI toxic injury involving the tubular, vascular and glomerular compartments.[19,20]

Functional Toxicity

Toxicity occurs early in the post-transplantation phase induced by vasoconstriction, with rise in serum creatinine and reduction in the GFR, with no definite structural lesion and is reversible on decreasing the dose.

Acute CNI Toxicity

Tubulopathy

Light microscopic features:
- Isometric vacuolization with uniform small, clear cytoplasmic vacuoles (Fig. 15.16)
- Involvement of straight segment of proximal tubules
- Concomitant individual cell necrosis due to prolonged warm and cold ischemia.

Electron microscopy:
- Markedly dilated empty smooth endoplasmic reticulum
- Giant mitochondria with sparse cristae are rarely seen
- Focal microcalcification of necrotic cells.

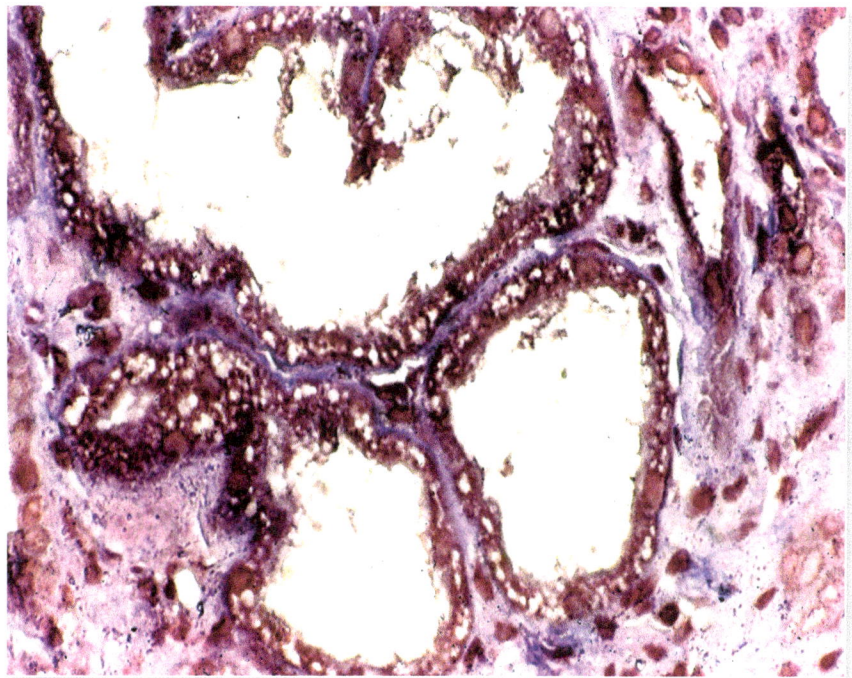

Figure 15.16: Isometric vacuolar change: CNI tubulopathy (Masson trichrome × 200)

Acute arteriolopathy:
- Endothelial swelling
- Ballooning of media with eosinophilic globules and focal necrosis.

Thrombotic microangiopathy:
- Fibrin thrombi in glomerular capillaries and afferent arterioles
- Mesangiolysis with segmental fibrinoid necrosis of glomerular tufts.

Differential Diagnosis

Osmotic nephrosis due to hyperosmolar solutions (mannitol and dextran) can show similar features of cytoplasmic isometric vacuolization as seen in CNI tubulopathy, by light microscopy. On EM prominent phagolysosomes are noted in the former. TMA due to acute AbMR and recurrent HUS in the allograft are identical to CNI-induced microvascular toxicity by LM but C4d is negative on IHC in the latter.

Chronic CNI Toxicity

- Arteriolar hyalinosis (Aah): PAS positive beaded or nodular hyaline deposits replacing necrotic cells in media and along the adventitia
- Grading of "aah1 to aah2": Focal replacement of necrotic/degenerate media of 1 to more than 1 arteriole
- Circumferential involvement of any number of arterioles with hyaline deposits (aah3).

Glomerulopathy

- Segmental duplication of capillary walls
- Secondary focal segmental glomerulosclerosis.

Interstitial Toxicity

- Striped fibrosis involving medullary rays containing atrophic tubules is nonspecific
- Associated hyalinization of arterioles and arteries.

Differential Diagnosis

Hypertensive arteriolosclerosis is associated with arteriolar hyalinosis with subendothelial hyaline deposits with atrophy of the media, in contrast to medial nodules and adventitial deposits in CNI-induced arteriolopathy. These lesions are often seen to coexist in the allograft.

Diabetic arteriolar hyalinosis is very similar and cannot be differentiated with certainty and can be associated with insudative lesions of glomerular capsular drops and fibrin caps.

Transplant glomerulopathy can be differentiated from CNI-induced glomerulopathy by the circumferential duplication and lamination of the GBM, mesangial interposition and C4d positivity on glomerular endothelium. Concomitant chronic allograft arteriopathy is often present.

Course and Prognosis

The arteriolar lesions regress on withdrawal of the CNI and repeat biopsies after 6 to 18 months. Renal limited TMA, devoid of systemic symptoms, such as hemolytic anemia, schistocytes and thrombocytopenia responds to dose reduction or change in immunosuppression and plasmapheresis with graft salvage of 80-90% and 60-90% in systemic variants. Tacrolimus or sirolimus in the present regimen has an overall lower incidence of TMA than cyclosporine.[21]

INFECTIONS IN RENAL ALLOGRAFT

Polyomavirus nephropathy (PVN) is the most common viral infection caused by the double-stranded DNA Polyoma BK-virus, occurring 8-13 months after transplantation and a prevalence of 1-9%, with intensive immunosuppression.[22] A high incidence of 9.3% has been reported among Indian transplant recipients, in a case series from North India.[23] Viral reactivation from a latent phase involves the urothelium and renal tubular epithelial cells, associated with free viral particles and/or intranuclear viral inclusions of shed urothelial "decoy" cells in the urine. A resurgence of BK virus transplant nephropathy has been reported with high dose tacrolimus and *mycophenolate-mofetil* immunosuppressive regimen in USA and Europe.[24,25]

Microscopic Features

The defining features include intranuclear viral inclusions and viral cytopathic tubular epithelial cell injury and cell lysis.[21] A minimum of 2 cores of renal cortex and medulla is required for a diagnosis, to avoid sampling errors, as the lesions are often focally localized.[22]

There are four types of intranuclear viral inclusions as follows:
1. Classical basophilic or ground glass inclusion with margination of chromatin and nuclear enlargement, clustered in focal tubules, often involving renal medullary collecting ducts (Figs 15.17 and 15.18).
2. Eosinophilic granular inclusion with incomplete halo is less common.
3. Finely granular eosinophilic inclusion devoid of halo is infrequent and nonspecific.
4. Vesicular variant with clumped chromatin and occasional nucleoli, cannot be distinguished from regenerated nuclei.

Cytopathic Features[21,22]

- Individual cell necrosis with lysis and denuded, intact basement membranes
- Regeneration of nuclei
- Glomerular parietal epithelial cells rarely show viral replication and crescents.

Electron Microscopy

Intranuclear parallel arrays of electron dense, rounded virions, 40–45 nm in diameter.

Morphological Stages of Polyomavirus Nephropathy

There are three stages ranging from early mild or limited involvement to florid viral activation with cell necrosis/lysis and a late sclerosing phase[22,26-28] as follows:

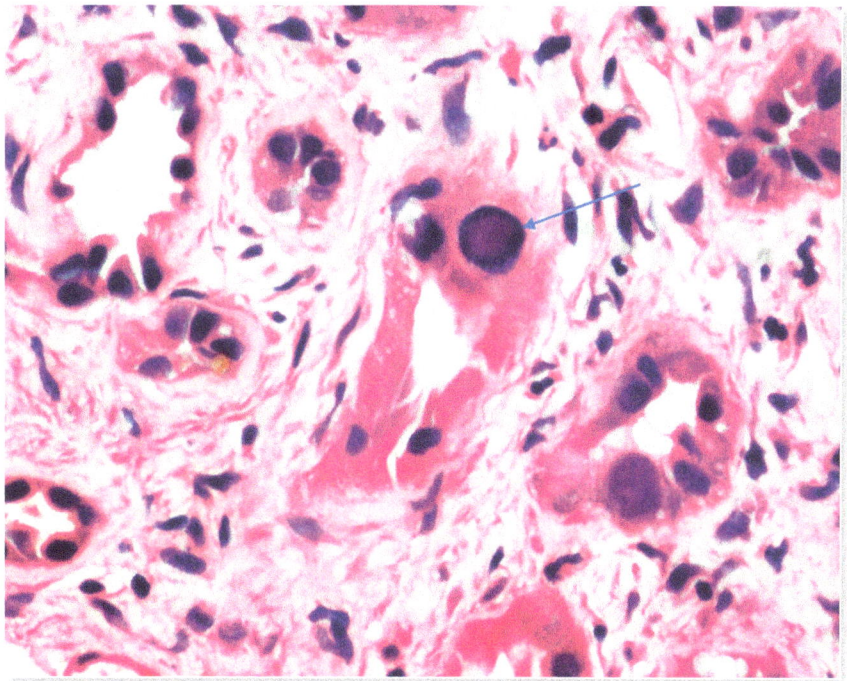

Figure 15.17: Polyomavirus tubulopathy with intranuclear inclusion (arrow) (H & E x 200)

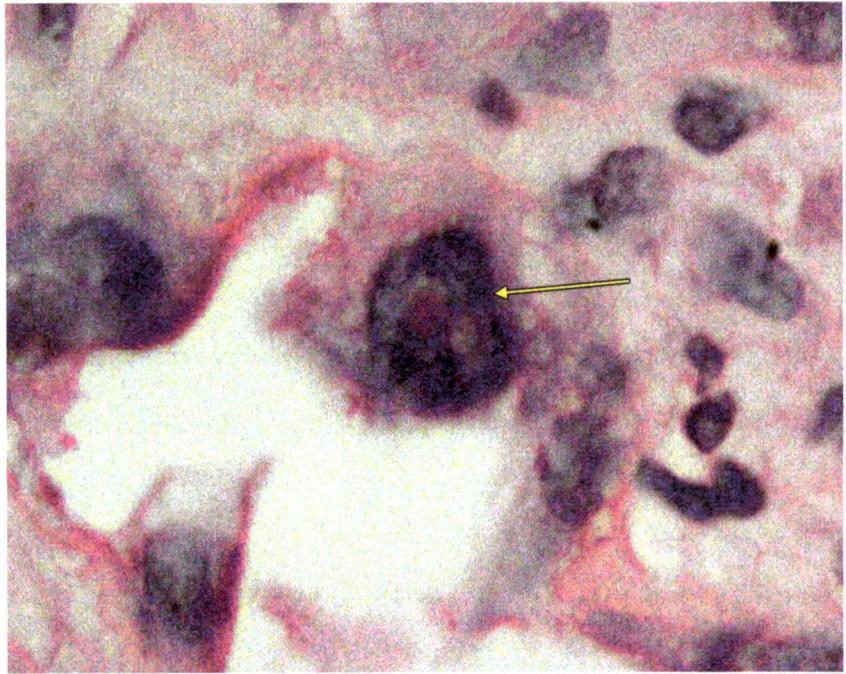

Figure 15.18: Polyomavirus intranuclear inclusion with margination of chromatin (H & E x 1000)

Stage A: Represents the **early phase** with viral activation in cortex and/or medulla with intranuclear inclusion bodies AND/OR positive immunohistochemistry or in situ hybridization signals.

There is no evidence of or minimal cell necrosis/lysis, no or minimal denudation of BM and no or minimal interstitial inflammation with edema and no or minimal (≤10%) interstitial fibrosis and tubular atrophy.

Stage B: The **florid phase** shows marked viral activation and replication in cortex and/or medulla with marked cell necrosis/lysis with denudation of tubular BM. There is mild to marked interstitial inflammation with lymphocytes and many plasma cells associated with tubulitis and minimal to moderate interstitial fibrosis and tubular atrophy (≤50%).

Stage B1, B2 and B3: Involvement of ≤25%; 26-49% and 50% or greater, of biopsy cores respectively (Interstitial fibrosis with tubular atrophy in particular, should not exceed 50%, in this stage).

Stage C: Viral activation in cortex and/or medulla with secondary diffuse interstitial fibrosis and tubular atrophy, in more than 50% of biopsy cores. Cell necrosis or lysis and inflammation are minimal to marked in severity.

Confirmation of Diagnosis

- *Decoy positive cells in urine* >10 cells/Thin Prep, liquid base cytology or a single decoy cell in Papanicolaou stained conventional cytology, are sufficient for evaluation in low risk cases, for a possible diagnosis of Polyomavirus nephropathy.[29,30] Repeat cytology and additional tests or monitoring are also required.

- *Quantitative PCR of plasma or urine samples* of significant viral loads (>10,000 copies/mL of plasma) for a presumptive diagnosis of high risk category PVN have a greater positive predictive value,[26] but has to be followed by renal allograft biopsy for a definitive diagnosis and close surveillance.
- Immunohistochemistry of formalin fixed paraffin embedded sections of renal allograft biopsy with antibody to SV40 large T antigen shows nuclear positivity, confirming the histopathologic diagnosis (Fig. 15.19).
- In situ hybridization of viral SV40 antigens in tubular epithelial cell nuclei is less often performed for diagnosis of early viral replication.
- PCR of viral DNA or RNA in renal biopsy tissue requires a strong amplification signal of >10 BK viral copies/cell for diagnosis of PVN.
- *Electron microscopy of urine sample*: Negative staining on EM of free virions in low risk and large three-dimensional viral aggregates ("haufen" clusters) in high risk cases is significant in decoy positive renal allografts, requiring further monitoring by plasma PCR quantification to predict progression.[22]

Differential Diagnosis

Cytomegalovirus and adenovirus nephropathy have different cytomorphologic features and are less frequent in the renal allograft.

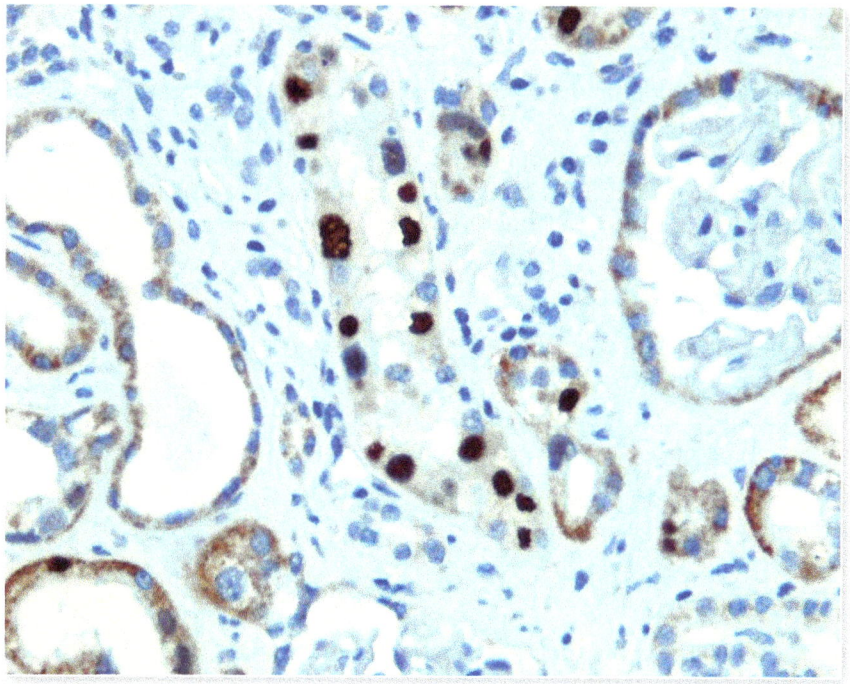

Figure 15.19: Polyomavirus nephropathy: IHC for SV40 large T antigen

Concomitant acute rejection: Supportive diagnostic features include transplant glomerulitis, intimal arteritis (v1 to v3 lesions), peritubular capillaritis and C4d positivity, along with tubulitis, particularly in areas without viral activation.[31]

Course and Prognosis[22,31-33]

Polyomavirus nephropathy occurs 6 days to 6 years after transplantation and presents with variable renal dysfunction and mild to marked rise in serum creatinine. Stage A PVN is diagnosed early, responds favorably to treatment with long term graft survival, stable graft function and resolution in >70% cases. Progression of viral replication can occur in about one third of these cases to Stages B and C. Regression from Stage B, mainly B1 to Stage A can occur and Stage C is irreversible, leading to graft loss. Early diagnosis and lowered immunosuppression and change to conventional drugs (cyclosporine and azathioprine) is recommended for PVN, with antiviral therapy (leflunomide) and careful monitoring by quantitative plasma PCR and urine cytology for decoy cells at 4 weeks intervals. Reduced immunosuppression for over 12 weeks is required for viral clearance from the renal allograft. Concomitant acute rejection requires transient anti-rejection therapy prior to specific antiviral medication.

CYTOMEGALOVIRUS NEPHROPATHY

Cytomegalovirus nephropathy in the allograft is uncommon with currently available modalities of screening and treatment in modern corporate Indian hospitals and has a reported prevalence of 1.9%.[21]

Microscopic Features

- Marked enlargement of tubular epithelial cells with intranuclear eosinophilic inclusions and distinct halo (Fig. 15.20)
- Multiple intracytoplasmic amphophilic inclusions (Fig. 15.20)
- Involvement of occasional glomerular endothelial cells with crescents
- Mononuclear inflammatory cell infiltrates with rare granulomas.

Electron Microscopy

Intranuclear and cytoplasmic virions, 150 nm in diameter with central electron dense core surrounded by an envelope.

Confirmation of Diagnosis

By immunohistochemistry, in situ hybridization and electron microscopy of renal biopsy material or CMV PCR of a blood sample.

Course and Prognosis

Cytomegalovirus nephropathy is complicated by concurrent acute rejection with tubulitis and acute allograft glomerulopathy that is treated with antiviral medication and immunosuppression.

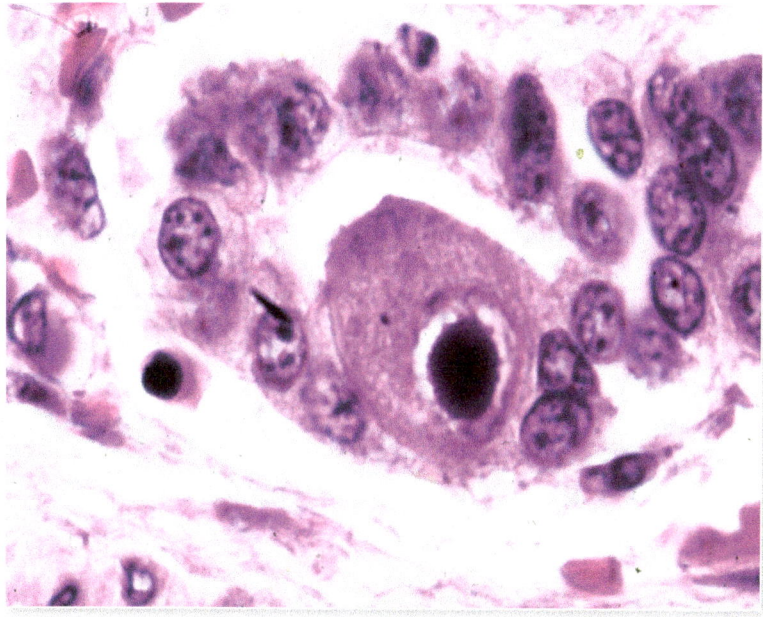

Figure 15.20: Cytomegalovirus tubulopathy (H & E × 1000)

ADENOVIRUS NEPHROPATHY

Adenovirus nephropathy is extremely rare in the allograft, with the following features:

Microscopic Features

- Acute necrotizing tubulointerstitial nephritis
- Smudged ground glass intranuclear inclusions in tubular epithelial cells
- Tubular necrosis with tubular rupture and granulomatous infiltrate
- Interstitial hemorrhage.

Electron Microscopy

Intranuclear virions, 75–80 nm, in tubular epithelial cells.

Confirmation of Diagnosis

Immunochemistry to adenovirus antigens in tubular epithelial cell nuclei.

Differential Diagnosis

Includes polyomavirus nephropathy and CMV nephropathy as described.

Bacterial infections in the allograft are identical to that of native kidneys associated with acute tubulointerstitial nephritis, leukocytic casts and microabscesses.

Fungal infections: In core renal allograft biopsies, these are rare and occurs with heavy immunosuppression or fungal sepsis with mycotic infiltration of arterial walls or granulomatous infiltrates.

RECURRENT GLOMERULONEPHRITIS

Recurrent glomerulonephritis occurs in 1-8% of renal allografts and include the following in order of frequency:
- Focal and segmental glomerulosclerosis (FSGS)
- Membranoproliferative glomerulonephritis (MPGN)
- IgA nephropathy (IgAN)
- Diabetic nephropathy
- Membranous nephropathy
- Hemolytic uremic syndrome
- Anti-GBM disease
- Antineutrophil cytoplasmic antibodies (ANCA) mediated vasculitis
- Monoclonal immunoglobulin deposition disease
- Fibrillary/immunotactoid glomerulopathy.

1. **Focal and segmental glomerulosclerosis:** It has a recurrence rate of 20-30% in the allograft and usually occurs after six months post-transplantation (average—7.5 months) in adults[21,34] and as early as 2 weeks after transplant in children,[35] leading to proteinuria and graft failure with graft loss in 30-40% cases.[36] The recurrence rate increases to 80% in the second renal transplant.[21,36] Recurrent FSGS in the allograft has been associated with a putative circulatory permeability factor[35] and podocin mutations.[37]

   Microscopic features are similar to that of primary FSGS, NOS of the native kidneys (Fig. 15.21). Collapsing variant of FSGS has a higher rate of recurrence.[21]

2. **Membranoproliferative glomerulonephritis: Type I, MPGN** recurs in 20-50% of allografts within the first four years and presents with proteinuria graft failure occurs in 10-50% cases.[34,36]

   Microscopic features include variable endocapillary proliferation with mesangial expansion and interposition with duplication of GBM, accentuated lobulation (Fig. 15.22) and crescents. Perilobular glomerular capillary C3 deposits on IF and subendothelial immune deposits on the EM are present, as in the native kidneys.

   Differential diagnosis: Transplant glomerulopathy can have similar membranoproliferative features but shows C4d glomerular endothelial positivity and multilamination of GBM on EM.[21]

   Type II, MPGN (Dense deposit disease): It recurs in >80% of allografts within two weeks of transplantation with rapid progression of renal failure and graft loss in 10-20% of cases.[34,36]

   Microscopic features are identical to that of native kidneys by LM, IF and EM.[38,39] Graft loss is due to recurrence of MPGN and related to severity of glomerular injury rather than type of original NKD[39] or isolated dense deposits in GBM. Presence of crescents has an adverse outcome.[38]

Renal Transplant Diseases

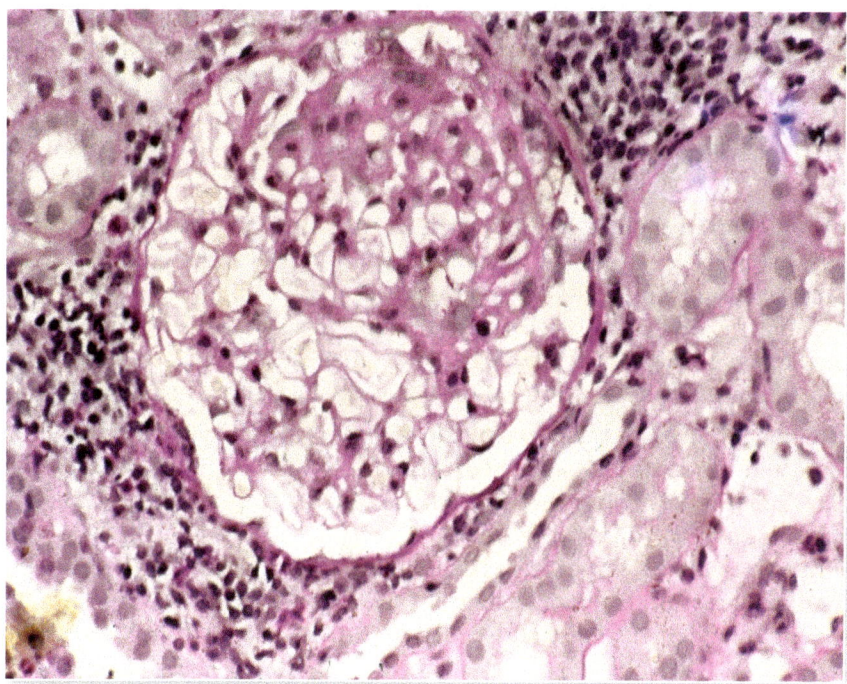

Figure 15.21: Recurrent focal and segmental sclerosis in renal allograft (PAS x 200)

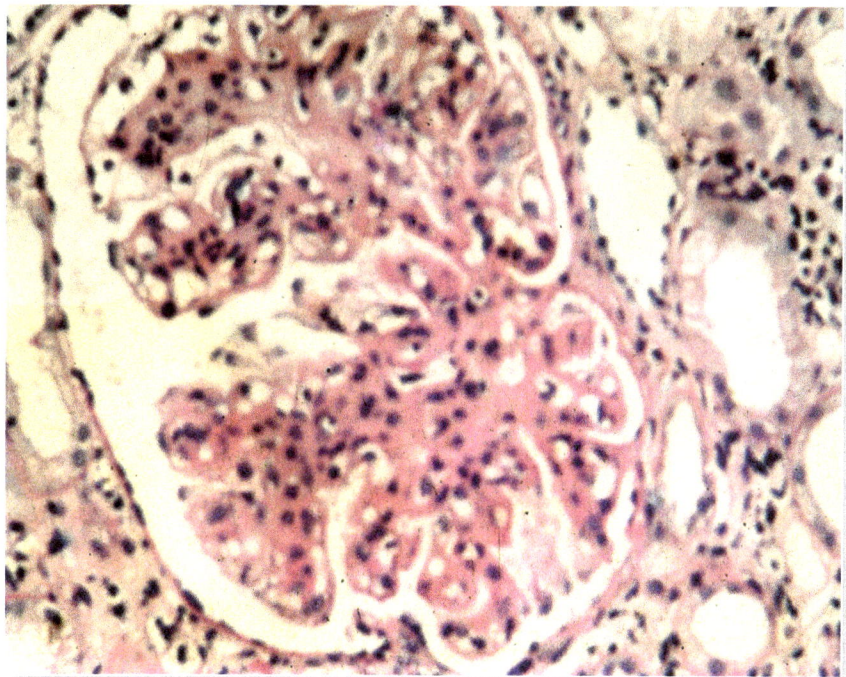

Figure 15.22: Recurrent membranoproliferative glomerulonephritis in renal allograft (H & E x 400)

3. **IgA nephropathy:** It has a recurrence rate of 25–60% after 2–4 years of transplantation with microscopic hematuria, proteinuria and graft dysfunction in about 10% of cases.[34,36,40] A higher rate of recurrence is noted among live related transplants, with an indolent course when compared to the native kidney IgA disease, in Indian patients, that has a malignant and rapid progression.[40] Latent IgA deposits in donor kidneys leads to an increased risk of recurrence.[41]

   Microscopic features show minimal or mild mesangial to endocapillary proliferation with segmental sclerosis and IgA mesangial deposits on IF and immune deposits on EM. Crescents are rare and graft loss due to recurrence of IgAN within 5 years of transplantation is uncommon,[34,36] when compared to graft survival in controls. After 10 years post-transplant graft loss occurs due to recurrence of IgAN and other causes.[34,36]

4. **Diabetic nephropathy:** It recurs in 30–40% of allografts within to 2–7 years of transplant.[21]

   Microscopic features are seen to develop after an average of 8 years with afferent and efferent arteriolar hyalinosis and intercapillary sclerosis with GBM thickening on EM. Nodular glomerulosclerosis is rarely seen in the allograft biopsy. Early lesions are known to be reversible on follow-up biopsies.

5. **Membranous nephropathy:** It recurs in about 30–40% of allografts within a few weeks to four months after transplantation, mainly in live related donors with severe proteinuria.[34,36] Graft loss occurs with concomitant rejection in 60–65% cases in 4 years after the diagnosis.

   Microscopic features are similar to that of the original kidney disease and IF is required to detect granular IgG deposits on glomerular capillary walls in early mild lesions.[42,43] PLA2R antibody has been reported positive in a renal allograft biopsy[43] that colocalized with IgG4 deposits and autoantibodies to PLA2R have also been detected in the serum[43,44] in association with very early recurrences, similar to primary membranous nephropathy in the native kidney.

6. **Hemolytic uremic syndrome:** It has a recurrence rate of about 15–40% in the allograft during the first year after transplantation due to the familial forms or scleroderma and rarely induced by *E. coli* infections.[21] The microscopic features of thrombotic microangiopathy are similar but can be more diffuse than that of calcineurin inhibitor toxicity and acute antibody mediated rejection and is C4d negative.

7. **Anti-GBM disease:** Recurrence can occur in the immediate post-transplantation time interval with the persistence of circulating anti-GBM antibodies in <5% cases, with no graft loss.[21] Current immunosuppressive therapy in transplant recipients is associated with prolonged graft survival and risk of later recurrence.[45]

Other recurrent glomerular diseases that are infrequently documented are ANCA-associated vasculitis,[36,46] lupus nephritis,[36,47] monoclonal immunoglobulin deposition disease, fibrillary glomerulonephritis, amyloidosis, primary oxalosis and Fabry's disease.[21]

DE NOVO GLOMERULAR DISEASES

De novo glomerular diseases are associated with the development of alloantibodies to donor specific antigens and include the following:
- De novo membranous nephropathy
- Anti-GBM disease in Alport syndrome recipients

- Focal and segmental glomerulosclerosis (FSGS)
- Congenital nephrotic syndrome.

De novo Membranous Nephropathy

De novo membranous nephropathy occurs in 1.8–9% of renal allografts in adult and pediatric cases respectively, within 2 years of transplantation, presenting with mild or nephrotic proteinuria. There is an association with antibody mediated rejection and transplant glomerulopathy with peritubular capillaritis and C4d positivity.[48,49] It differs from recurrent membranous nephropathy in that anti-human leukocyte antigen (HLA) donor specific antibodies can be present and PLA2 R antibody testing is negative.

Microscopic features show mild to moderate mesangial cell proliferation, segmental subepithelial deposits and heterogeneous stages by EM. On the IF a predominance of IgG1 or codominance with IgG4 immune deposits is noted. It has an indolent or rapid progression that can lead to graft loss. Concomitant hepatitis B or C viral infection, malignancy or other non-immune mediated diseases can present with exposure of cryptic autologous podocyte antigens with circulating autoantibodies and in situ subepithelial immune complex formation.[49]

Anti-GBM Disease in Alport Syndrome Recipients

In association with a X-linked genetic defect and lacking in alpha 5 chain of type IV collagen (COL4A5) can develop antibodies to this donor antigen, in a minority of renal allografts, in a few days to months after the transplant. A focal necrotizing crescentic glomerulonephritis is seen with typical linear IgG staining of glomerular capillaries on the IF. Graft failure occurs and the disease can recur rapidly in a second retransplant.[21]

Focal and Segmental Glomerulosclerosis

As a de novo disease is extremely rare. Secondary FSGS occurs due to glomerular hyperfiltration and loss of nephrons in association with chronic antibody or T cell-mediated rejection, calcineurin inhibitor toxicity and vascular stenosis. De novo collapsing variant of FSGS also can occur due to vascular hypoperfusion.

Congenital Nephrotic Syndrome

Congenital nephrotic syndrome of the rare, autosomal recessive Finnish type with NPSH1 gene mutation can recur in the transplant due to the formation of antibodies to nephrin in the graft.[21]

POST-TRANSPLANT LYMPHOPROLIFERATIVE DISORDER

Post-transplant lymphoproliferative disorder (PTLD) arises as a consequence of immunosuppression in a solid organ or bone marrow transplant recipient, in about 1% of all transplants PTLD, presents with renal graft dysfunction, 5 months to 1 year after transplantation involving the kidneys in >30% of cases and can be disseminated or localized to the renal parenchyma. PTLDs are usually Epstein-Barr virus (EBV) induced B cell polyclonal to monoclonal lymphoid proliferations and rarely of T cell/natural killer cell lineage.[50-54]

Children and EBV naïve patients who cannot initiate a cytotoxic T cell response are more prone to develop a PTLD. Early lesions with plasmacytic hyperplasia and infectious mononucleosis like infiltrates usually involve tonsils and lymph nodes than extranodal sites.[50,51]

Microscopic features vary from focal to expansile polymorphic to monomorphic lesions as follows:
1. Early focal lymphoplasmacytic infiltrate with many plasma cells and occasional immunoblasts.
2. Nodular or expansile polymorphous mixed infiltrates are seen as the most common form (Fig. 15.23).
    - Medium-sized atypical activated lymphoid cell with prominent nucleoli
    - Immunoblasts, plasma cells, large and small noncleaved cells, small lymphocytes
    - Variable necrosis is seen
    - Tubulitis is often present, with venular infiltration.
3. Monomorphic sheets of large lymphoid cells comprising one of the following types of B cell or T cell lymphomas:[51]
    - Immunoblastic, centroblastic or anaplastic B cell type with serpiginous necrosis
    - Plasma cell myeloma/plasmablastic type
    - Burkitt's lymphoma
    - T cell lymphomas: Peripheral T cell lymphoma, NOS type
    - Other types* (Hepatosplenic T cell lymphoma*) in extrarenal sites.
4. Hodgkin's like PTLD/Classical Hodgkin's lymphoma type PTLD, with rare renal involvement.

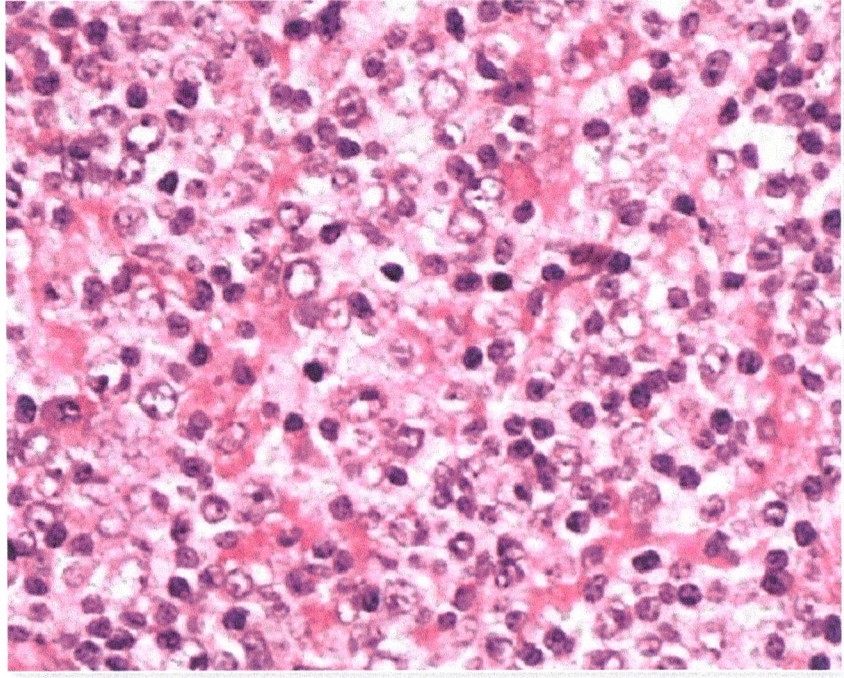

Figure 15.23: Polymorphous PTLD[50] (H & E × 200)

Confirmation of Diagnosis[55]

- In situ hybridization by EB encoded RNA (EBER) probes on formalin fixed paraffin embedded tissue can be done.
- **Immunohistochemistry** is less reliable with nuclei of neoplastic cells staining variably positive for EBV LMP1 and EBNA2.

Immunoglobulin, heavy chain gene rearrangement (IgH) to confirm clonality of B cell PTLD.

Differential Diagnosis

Severe cellular rejection is usually T cell predominant on IHC, including cytotoxic T lymphocytes, admixed with fewer B lymphocytes, granulocytes and macrophages and associated with transplant glomerulitis and intimal arteritis. IHC for EBV LMP/EBNA and in situ hybridization for EBER are negative. This can be difficult to distinguish from EBV negative cases of PTLD with non-neoplastic monoclonal T cell expansion of CD8 positive T cells, that can be admixed with a predominant B cell polymorphous PTLD.[50] Predominant clonal T cell infiltrates are found in the less common monomorphic T cell type of PTLD.[50,51]

Course and Prognosis

Early lesions usually regress with reduction of immunosuppression or spontaneously. Polymorphic PTLD shows a variable response to reduction to immunosuppression and antiviral agents and some progress requiring chemotherapy including rituximab. The monomorphic variant does not regress and usually progresses rapidly. The EBV negative PTLDs and those with BCL6 gene mutations are more aggressive and respond poorly to chemotherapy.[50]

REFERENCES

1. Solez K, Colvin RB, Racusen LC, Haas M, Sis B, Mengel M, et al. Banff '07 classification of renal allograft pathology: Updates and future directions. Am J Transplant. 2008;8:753-60.
2. Haas M, Loupy A, Lefaucher C, Roufosse C, Glotz D, Seron D, et al. The Banff 2017 Kidney Meeting Report: Revised diagnostic criteria for chronic active T- cell rejection, antibody-mediated rejection and prospects for integrated endpoints for next generation clinical trials. Am J Transplant.2018;18:293-307.
3. Racusen LC, Colvin RB, Solez K, Mihatsch MJ, Halloran PF, Campbell PM, et al. Antibody-mediated rejection criteria-an addition to the Banff '97 classification of renal allograft rejection. Am J Transplant. 2003;3:706-14.
4. Colvin RB. Antibody-mediated renal allograft rejection: diagnosis and pathogenesis. J Am Soc Nephrol. 2007;18: 1046-56, doi: 10.1681.
5. Colvin RB, Smith RN. Antibody-mediated organ-allograft rejection. Nat Rev Immunol. 2005;5:807-17.
6. Gibson IW, Gwinner W, Br"ocker V, Sis B, Riopeld J, Robertsl SD, et al. Peritubular capillaritis in renal allografts: prevalence, scoring system reproducibility and clinicopathological correlates. Am J Transplant. 2008;8:819-25.
7. Cohen D, Colvin RB, et al. Pros and cons for C4d as a biomarker. Kid Int. 2012;8(17):628-39.
8. Haas M, Segev DL, Racusen LC, Bagnasco SM, Locke JE, Warren DS, et al. C4d Deposition without. Rejection correlates with reduced early scarring in ABO-Incompatible renal allografts. J Am Soc Nephrol. 2009;20:197-204.
9. Bhowmik DM, Dinda AK, Mahanta P, Agarwal S. The evolution of the Banff classification schema for diagnosing renal allograft rejection and its implications for clinicians. Indian J Nephrol. 2010;20(1):2-8. doi: 10.4103/0971-4065.62086.
10. Sis B, Mueller T, Campbell P, Hunter C, Cockfield S, Solez K, et al. Transplant glomerulopathy, late antibody mediated rejection, and the ABCD tetrad. Am J Transplant. 2006;[Suppl]:469-70.

11. Solez K, Colvin RB, Racusen LC, Sis B, Halloran PF, Birk PE, et al. Banff '05 meeting report: Differential diagnosis of chronic allograft injury and elimination of chronic allograft nephropathy ('CAN'). Am J Transplant. 2007;7:518-26.
12. Haas M, Sis B, Racusen LC, Solez K, Glotz D, Colvin RB, et al. Banff 2013 meeting report: inclusion of c4d-negative antibody-mediated rejection and antibody-associated arterial lesions. Am J Transplant. 2014;14(2):272-83. doi:10.1111/ajt.12590.
13. Solez K, Racusen LC. The Banff classification revisited. Kidney Int. 2013;83:201-6.
14. Sis B, Jhangri G, Bunnag S, Allanach K, Kapland B, Halloran PF. Endothelial gene expression in kidney transplants with alloantibody indicates antibody-mediated damage despite lack of C4d staining. Am J Transplant. 2009;9: 2312-23.
15. Haas M. Molecular diagnostics in renal allograft biopsy interpretation:potential and pitfalls. Kidney Int. 2014:86,461-4. doi:10.1038/ki. 2014.12.
16. Haas M. Pathology of C4d–negative antibody-mediated rejection in renal allografts. Curr Opin Organ Transplant. 2013;18(3):319-26.
17. Haas M. Pathologic features of antibody-mediated rejection in renal allografts: an expanding spectrum. Curr Opin Nephrol Hypertens. 2012;21(3):264-71. doi: 10.1097/MNH. 0b013e3283520efa.
18. Haas M. An updated Banff Schema for diagnosis of antibody-mediated rejection in renal allografts. Curr Opin Organ Transplant. 2014;19(3):315-22. doi:10.1097/MOT. 0000000000000072.
19. Davies, David R, et al. Histopathology of calcineurin inhibitor induced nephropathy. Transplantation. 2000;69(12):8811-3.
20. Naesens M, Dirk RJ, Kuypers, Minnie Sarwal. Calcineurin inhibitor nephrotoxicity. Clin J Am Soc Nephrol. 2009;4:481-508 doi: 10.2215/CJN. 04800908.
21. Colvin RB, Nickeleit V. Renal transplant pathology. In: Jennette JC, Olson JL, Schwartz MM, Silva FG, (Eds) Heptinstall's Pathology of the Kidney, 6th Edition. Philadelphia: Lippincott-Raven. 2006;1347-1490.
22. Nickeleit V, Mihatsch MJ. Polyomavirus nephropathy in native kidneys and renal allografts: an update on an escalating threat. Transplantation. 2006;19:960-73.
23. Sachdeva MS, Nada R, Jha V, Sakhuja V, Joshi K. The high incidence of BK polyoma virus infection among renal transplant recipients in India. Transplantation. 2004;77: 429.
24. Randhawa PS, Finkelstein S, Scantlebury V, et al. Humanpolyoma virus-associated interstitial nephritis in the allograft kidney. Transplantation. 1999;67:103.
25. Mengel M, Marwedel M, Radermacher J, et al. Incidence of polyomavirus-nephropathy in renal allografts: Influence of modern immunosuppressive drugs. Nephrol Dial Transplant. 2003;18:1190.
26. Hirsch HH, Brennan DC, Drachenberg CB, et al. Polyomavirus-associated nephropathy in renal transplantation: interdisciplinary analyses and recommendations. Transplantation. 2005;79:1277.
27. Drachenberg CB, Papadimitriou JC, Hirsch HH, et al. Histological patterns of polyomavirus nephropathy: Correlation with graft outcome and viral load. Am J Transplant. 2004;4:2082.
28. Drachenberg CB, Hirsch HH, Ramos E, Papadimitriou JC. Polyomavirus disease in renal transplantation: review of pathological findings and diagnostic methods. Hum Pathol. 2005;36:1245.
29. Nickeleit V, Hirsch HH, Binet IF, et al. Polyomavirus infection of renal allograft recipients: from latent infection to manifest disease. J Am Soc Nephrol. 1999;10:1080.
30. Drachenberg CB, Beskow CO, Cangro CB, et al. Humanpolyoma virus in renal allograft biopsies: morphological findings and correlation with urine cytology. Hum Pathol. 1999;30:970.
31. Nickeleit V, Mihatsch MJ. Polyomavirus allograft nephropathy and concurrent acute rejection: a diagnostic and therapeutic challenge. Am J Transplant. 2004;4(5):838-9.
32. Vasudev B, Hariharan S, Hussain SA, Zhu YR, Breshnan BA, Cohen EP. BK virus nephritis: Risk factors, timing, and outcome in renal transplant recipients. Kidney Int. 2005;68:1834-9.
33. Bohl DL, Brennan DC. BK Virus nephropathy and kidney transplantation. Clin J Am Soc Nephrol. 2007;2: S36 –S46.doi: 10.2215/CJN. 00920207.
34. Ponticelli C, Glassock RJ. Posttransplant recurrence of primary glomerulonephritis. Clin Am Soc Nephrol. 2010;5: 2363-72 doi: 10. 2215/CJN. 06720810.
35. Schachter AD, Harmon WE. Single-center analysis of early recurrence of nephrotic syndrome following renal transplantation in children. Pediatr Transplant. 2001;5:406-9.
36. Choy BY, Chan TM, Lai KN. Recurrent glomerulonephritis after kidney transplantation. American Journal of Transplantation. 2006;6(11):2535-42.

37. Bertelli R, Ginevri F, Caridi G, et al. Recurrence of focal segmental glomerulosclerosis after renal transplantation in patients with mutations of podocin. Am J Kidney Dis. 2003;41:1314-21.
38. Little MA, Dupont P, Campbell E, Dorman A, Walshe JJ. Severity of primary MPGN, rather than MPGN type, determines renal survival and post-transplantation recurrence risk. Kidney Int. 2006;69:504-11.
39. Braun MC, Stablein DM, Hamiwka LA, Bell L, Bartosh SM, Strife CF. Recurrence of membranoproliferative glomerulonephritis type II in renal allografts: The North American Pediatric Renal Transplant Cooperative Study experience. J Am Soc Nephrol. 2005;16:2225-33.
40. Chacko B, George JT, Neelakantan N, Korula A, Chakko JK. Outcomes of renal transplantation in patients with immunoglobulin A nephropathy in India. Journal of Postgraduate Medicine. 2007;53(2):92-5.
41. Moriyama T, Nitta K, Suzuki K, et al. Latent IgA deposition from donor kidney is the major risk factor for recurrent IgA nephropathy in renal transplantation. Clin Transplant. 2005;19(Suppl 14):41-8.
42. Blosser CD, Ayalon R, Nair R, Thomas C, Beck JRLH. Very early recurrence of anti-phospholipase A2 receptor-positive membranous nephropathy after transplantation. Am J Transplant. 2012;12(6):1637-42.
43. El-Zoghbya ZM, Grandeb JP, Frailec MG, Norbya SM, Fervenza FC, Cosioa FG. Recurrent idiopathic membranous nephropathy: early diagnosis by protocol biopsies and treatment with anti-CD20 monoclonal antibodies. Am J Transplant. 2009;9:2800-7.
44. Stahl R, Hoxha E, Fechner K. PLA2R autoantibodies and recurrent membranous nephropathy after transplantation. N Engl J Med. 2010;363:496-8.
45. Khandelwal M, McCormick BB, Lajoie G, Sweet J, Cole E, Cattran DC. Recurrence of anti-GBM disease 8 years after renal transplantation. Nephrol Dial Transplant. 2004;19:491-4.
46. Geetha D, Eirin A, True K, Irazabal MV, Specks U, Seo P, et al. Renal transplantation in antineutrophil cytoplasmic antibody-associated vasculitis: A multicenter experience. Transplantation. 2011;91(12):1370-5.
47. Goral S, Ynares C, Shappell SB, et al. Recurrent lupus nephritis in renal transplant recipients revisited: it is not rare. Transplantation. 2003;75:651-6.
48. Kossi ML, Harmer A, Goodwin J, Wagner B, Shortland J, Angel C, et al. De novo membranous nephropathy associated with donor specific antibody. Clinical Transplantation. 2008;22(1):124-7.
49. Ponticelli C, Glassock R.J. De novo membranous nephropathy (MN) in kidney allografts. A peculiar form of alloimmune disease? Transplant International. 2012:1205-10.
50. Ibrahim HAH, Naresh KN. Post transplant lymphoproliferative disorders. Advances in Hematology Volume 2012, Article ID 230173, 1-11 doi:10. 1155/2012/230173.
51. Swerdlow SH, Webber SA, Chadburn A, Ferry JA. Post transplant lymphoproliferative disorders, In: Swerdlow SH, Campo E, Harris NL et al. (Eds) WHO Classification of Tumours of Haematopoietic and Lymphoid Tissues, 4th edition, IARC, Lyon, France. 2007:343-9.
52. Yin CC, Medeiros LJ, Abruzzo LV, Jones D, Farhood AI, Thomazy VA. "EBV-associated B- and T cell post-transplant lymphoproliferative disorders following primary EBV infection in a kidney transplant recipient. Am J Clin Pathol. 2005;123(2):222-8.
53. Kumar S, Kumar D, Kingma DW, Jaffe ES. Epstein-Barr virus-associated T-cell lymphoma in a renal transplant patient. Am J Surg Pathol. 1993;17(10):1046-53.
54. Kwong YL, Lam CCK, Chan TM. Post-transplantation lymphoproliferative disease of natural Killer cell lineage: a clinicopathological and molecular analysis. British Journal of Haematology. 2000;110(1):197-202.
55. Ibrahim HAH, Menasce LP, Pomplun S, Burke M, Bower M, Naresh KN. Presence of monoclonal T cell populations in B-cell post-transplant lymphoproliferative disorders. Mod Pathol. 2011;24:232-40.

Index

Page numbers followed by *f* refer to figure

A

Abscesses 48
Acid fast stains 160
Acyclovir 157
Adenovirus nephropathy 207, 209
Albuminuria 83
Allograft arteriopathy, chronic 201*f*
Allograft injury, chronic 200
Allograft renal biopsies 188
Alport's syndrome 2, 4, 129, 130*f*, 131*f*, 151, 213
    autosomal
        dominant 131
        recessive 131
    types of 129
American College of Rheumatology Criteria 63
Amyloidogenic precursor protein 103
Amyloidosis 4, 82, 103, 116, 136
    nodular 87
    primary 103, 105, 106, 106*f*
    secondary 82
        reactive 107
Angiokeratoma corporis diffusum 142
Antibody-mediated rejection, acute 188, 191*f*, 192*f*
Antigenemia, viral 30, 48
Antiglomerular basement membrane disease 4, 60, 100
Anti-human leukocyte antigen 213
Antineutrophilic cytoplasmic autoantibodies 89
Antiphospholipid antibody syndrome 76, 176, 182
    primary 79, 182
    secondary 182
Anti-retroviral therapy 127
Anti-rheumatic drugs 30
Anti-thyroid microsomal and thyroglobulin 80
Antitubular basement membrane
    antibodies 165
    disease 159
Antiviral medication 208
Apolipoprotein 104, 146

Arterial concentric intimal fibrosis 175*f*
Arterial fibrinoid necrosis 175*f*
Arteries
    arcuate 9
    interlobular 171
Arteriolar hyalinosis 9, 203
Arteriolar lesions 204
Arteriole 171
Arteriolonephrosclerosis, benign 173*f*
Arteriolopathy, acute 203
Arteriolosclerosis 85*f*
    hypertensive 204
Arterionephrosclerosis 172
Arteriopathy, transplant 196
Arteritis
    isolated intimal 200
    necrotizing 77*f*
Arthritis
    rheumatoid 4, 30, 48, 61, 77, 80, 81
    severe 78
Autoimmune chronic inflammatory multisystem disease 61
Autoimmune diseases 30, 48
Autoimmune thyroid disease 30
Autoimmune tubulointerstitial diseases 161
Autosomal dominant syndrome 135
Azathioprine 208

B

B cell lymphoma 117, 119
Bacterial infections 182, 210
Balkan nephropathy 159
Banded collagen fibrils 134, 136*f*, 137
Basement membranes, thickening of 8
Basket weave 131
Beta-hemolytic streptococcal infection 32
Biliary cirrhosis, primary 80
Blood pressure
    diastolic 176
    optimal 176
Blood vessels, extraglomerular 174

Bone marrow 176
  transplantation 48
Borderline rejection 197
Bowman's capsule 5, 6, 16, 22, 44, 105
Bowman's space 5, 44, 78

C

Calcineurin inhibitor toxicity 202
Calcium salts, tubular luminal concretions of 167
Capillary endothelial cells 8
Capillary lumina 22
  occlusion of 12
Capillary microaneurysm 84f
Capillary wall
  normal thickness of 6f
  rupture of 65
Capsular fibrosis 78, 80
Capsular synechiae 8, 17f, 42
Cells
  interstitial 154
  mediated rejection 186
Cellular rejection
  acute 197f, 198f
  severe 215
Central nervous system 90
Ceramide trihexoside 142
Cerebral hemorrhage 78
Cholesterol clefts 9
Chromatin, margination of 206f
Churg-Strauss disease 4, 89, 95
Churg-Strauss syndrome 45
Cock's combs 105
Collagen
  nephropathies 128, 128, 134
  vascular diseases 61
Colon 30
Congophilia 105
Corticomedullary junction 171
Crohn's disease 80, 114
Cryoglobulinemia 48
Cyclooxygenase inhibitors 157
Cyclosporine 176, 202, 208
Cystine crystals 166f
Cystinosis 159, 165
Cytomegalovirus 207
  nephropathy 208
  tubulopathy 209f
Cytopathic tubular epithelial cell injury 204
Cytotoxic therapy 102

D

Dense deposit disease 46, 49, 50f, 51f, 54, 210
De novo glomerular diseases 212
De novo glomerulonephritis 186
De novo membranous nephropathy 213
Dengue 182
Denys-Drash syndrome 150
Dermatomyositis 77
Diabetes mellitus 176
Diabetic glomerulosclerosis, advanced 86
Diabetic nephropathy
  development of 83
  glomerular classification of 85
Dialysis 102
Diarrhea, prodromal 176
Disease modifying anti-rheumatic drugs 82
Disseminated intravascular coagulation 182, 184
Distal interphalangeal joints 136
Dose steroids 102
D-penicillamine 30
Drug toxicity 186
Dysproteinemias 48, 165

E

Edema 9
Elastic lamina 171
Electron dense granules, focal 131f
Electron microscopy 8, 22, 23, 26, 29, 34, 36, 42,
  44, 48, 50, 51, 56, 59, 66, 71-73, 79, 95, 207
Endocapillary cell 20
  proliferation 36
Endocapillary hypercellularity 37, 39f, 73
  segmental 19, 36
Endocapillary proliferative glomerulonephritis,
  diffuse predominantly 32
Endocarditis, infective 48, 60
Endothelial cell nucleus 6f
Endothelial necrosis 74
Endothelial nuclei 5
Endothelialitis, lymphocytic 199f
Endothelium 6
End-stage renal
  disease 149
  failure 126, 136, 140
Enterococcus faecalis 161
Eosinophils 9
Epithelial cells 172
Epstein-Barr virus 213

Erythrocytes 132
Escherichia coli 161, 176
Esophageal dysfunction 78
Extracapillary cells, hyperplasia of 8
Extraglomerular compartment 36, 66, 196
Extraglomerular mesangial lacis cells 172

F

Fabry's disease 4, 142, 151
    diagnosis of 144
    end-stage renal 144
Familial lecithin cholesterol acyltransferase
    deficiency 145
Fanconi's syndrome 81, 165
Farber's disease 147
Fibrillary glomerulonephritis 45
Fibrillary glomerulopathies 106, 114, 115f, 136, 210
Fibrils, extracellular deposition of 103
Fibrin thrombi 189
Fibrinogen 104
Fibrinoid
    glomerular tuft necrosis 92f
    necrosis 73, 191f
Fibrosis 9
Finger print 71
Finnish type congenital nephrotic syndrome 148
Foam cells 9
Focal segmental
    glomerulonephritis 36
    glomerulosclerosis 16, 20f, 150
    necrotizing glomerulonephritis 91f
    proliferative lupus nephritis 65f, 66f
    sclerosis 17f, 19f
Foot deformities 136
Frasier syndrome 151
Fucosidosis 147
Fungal infections 48, 210

G

Ganglia, autonomic 142
Gangliosidosis 147
Garland pattern 34
Gaucher syndrome 144
Genetic
    autosomal mutations 23
    defects 152
    polymorphisms 176
Giant cell
    arteritis 90, 96
    reaction 164

Global mesangial sclerosis 130f
Globotriaosylceramide 142
Glomerular amyloidosis 105f
Glomerular basement membrane 5, 7f, 22, 44, 128
Glomerular capillary
    endothelial cells 142
    fibrin thrombi 192f
    fibrinoid necrosis 192
    lobule, ultrastructure of 6
    lumen 180f, 183
    staining of 84
    wall 33f
        deposits 70f
Glomerular compartments 202
Glomerular diseases 10, 158
Glomerular filtration rate 89
Glomerular immune complex disease, post-
    infectious forms of 32
Glomerular infarct 178f
Glomerular lesion 80, 81, 172
    concurrent 126
Glomerular mesangial deposits 104
Glomerular mesangiolysis 74
Glomerular retraction, ischemic 78
Glomerular tufts
    enlargement of 56
    ischemic atrophy of 23
Glomeruli 8, 36
Glomerulitis 189
    transplant 190f
Glomerulonephritis 4, 57, 114, 127
    chronic 4
    crescentic 3, 32, 44, 81
    cryoglobulinemic 4, 72, 114, 118
    diffuse endocapillary proliferative 3
    endocapillary proliferative 32
    familial membranoproliferative 54
    focal necrotizing 81
    IgA dominant postinfectious 40
    immune complex 127
    membranoproliferative 3, 32, 34, 45, 46, 48f, 49, 51, 72, 135, 140, 210
    membranous 45
    necrotizing 92f
    post-infectious 34, 45, 57, 60
    primary 10, 44
    proliferative 32, 60
    rapidly progressive 3
    recurrent 210
        membranoproliferative 196, 211f
    sclerosing 94f

segmental proliferative 60
subtype of 32
Glomerulopathy 204
   collagenofibrotic 116, 134, 134*f*, 136*f*, 137
   collapsing 20, 125*f*, 151
   fibronectin 139, 139*f*
   membranous 82
   non-immune derived fibrillary 116
   transplant 48, 195, 195*f*, 202
Glomerulosclerosis 20, 79, 165
   diabetic 85*f*, 106
   focal 3, 82, 151, 210, 213
   ischemic 173*f*
   nodular 84*f*
   secondary focal segmental 22
   segmental 3, 82, 151, 210, 213
Glomerulus, normal structure of 5
Glycogen storage disease 166
Glycolicaciduria 163
Glycoproteinoses 147
Glycosphingolipid, neutral 142
Glyoxylate 163
Gold salts 30
Gonadoblastoma 151
Goodpasture's syndrome 4, 44
Gout 159
Graft dysfunction, causes of 186
Granular
   immune deposits, focal 73
   perilobular capillary wall deposits 47*f*
   podocyte inclusions 142
   subendothelial deposits 140*f*
Granulomas 9
   interstitial 94*f*
Granulomatosis, eosinophilic 95
Graves' disease 114

H

Heavy chain
   deposition disease 4
   gene rearrangement 215
Hematoxylin bodies 69*f*
Hematuria 4, 60
   benign familial 129, 132
   degrees of 139
Hemolytic uremic syndrome 3, 176, 183, 184, 210, 212
Hemopoietic stem cell transplantation 106
Hemorrhage
   interstitial 189
   pulmonary 100

Hemorrhagic fever, viral 182
Henoch-Schonlein purpura 4, 45, 98, 98*f*
Hepatic enzyme, deficiency of 163
Hepatitis 80
   B 30, 48, 127
      viral infection 30, 213
   C 48, 80, 127
      viral infection 213
Hereditary osteo-onychodysplasia 136
Heredofamilial glomerulopathies 128
Human immunodeficiency virus 30
Hurler syndrome 144
Hyaline
   droplet 8
   thrombi 68*f*
Hyalinosis, diabetic arteriolar 204
Hyperacute rejection 189
Hypercalcemia 159
Hypercellularity, moderate mesangial 14
Hypergammaglobulinemia 80
Hyperosmolar solutions 203
Hyperoxaluria 159, 163
Hyperplasia 9, 23, 79
Hypertension 133
   malignant 175*f*
   primary pulmonary 78
   pulmonary 78
   renovascular 78
Hypertrophy
   glomerular 12, 23
   medial 78
   microvillous 13*f*
Hyperuricemia 166
Hypocomplementemia 50
Hypokalemia 159
Hypoxanthinine-guanine phosphoribosyl transferase 166

I

I cell disease 144, 147
Idiopathic membranous nephropathy 30
Immnofluorescence 72
Immune complex 45, 97
Immunofluorescence 26, 29, 32, 36, 42, 47, 50, 51, 56, 59, 60, 62-64, 66, 70, 73, 74, 77, 78, 84, 105, 172
Immunoglobulin 215
Immunotactoid glomerulopathy 114, 116, 117, 118*f*
In situ subepithelial immune complex formation 213

Indinavir 157
Inflammatory cell 157
  infiltrates 9
Interlobular artery, fibrinoid necrosis of 93f
Internal elastic lamina 171
  reduplication of 9
International Society of Nephrology/Renal Pathology Society Classification, modified 61
International Study of Kidney Disease in Childhood Criteria 12
Interstitial fibrosis 37, 74, 165, 200, 202
  diffuse 40f
  immunohistochemical 196
Interstitial foam cells 130f
Interstitial nephritis
  acute 3, 82, 87
  chronic 4, 82, 87
  cryptococcal granulomatous 160f
  granulomatous 4, 160
Intimal fibrosis 9
Intratubular oxalate crystals 164f
Intrinsic podocyte genetic mutational injury, sites of 152f
Ischemic nephropathy, chronic 174
Ischemic tubular injury, acute 156

J

Joint contractures 136
Jones methenamine stains 22, 35, 117
Juxtaglomerular apparatus 79, 172

K

Karyorrhexis 20, 74
Kawasaki disease 90
Keratoconjunctivitis sicca 80
Kidneys 104
  after transplantation 144
Kimmelstiel-Wilson's lesions 83
Klebsiella infection 161

L

Lambda conjugated antisera 8
Lamellated myelin 142, 144f
Lamina densa, lamellation of 131f
Leukemias 166
Leukocyte 20
  infiltration 8, 73
Light chain deposition disease 4, 87, 106
Lipid storage diseases 2, 4, 142

Lipoprotein glomerulopathy 4, 146, 146f
Liquid chromatography 55
Loops of Henle 155f
Luminal thrombosis 9
Lung 30
  disease, interstitial 78
Lupus nephritis 30, 45, 61-63, 65, 67, 69, 71f, 72, 73, 75f, 118
  minimal mesangial 63f
  necrotizing 66
  diffuse 69
Lupus vasculopathy 74, 75f
Lymphatic leukemia, chronic 117
Lymphocytes 9, 20
Lymphocytic
  endothelialitis, acute 199f
  leukemia, chronic 30
Lymphomas 166
Lymphoplasmacytic infiltrate 162f
Lymphoproliferative disorder 117
  post-transplant 186, 213
Lysosomal storage diseases 142, 147

M

Macrophages, foamy 20
Macula densa 172
Malaria 30
Mass spectroscopy 55
Masson trichrome stain 8, 9
Matrix, condensation of 17f
Membrane cofactor protein 55
Mesangial cell 6, 142
  interposition 180f
  nuclei 6f
  proliferation 42
Mesangial cellularity 38f
Mesangial collagen fibrils 135f
Mesangial expansion 86
Mesangial hypercellularity 13f
  grades of 14
  score 37
Mesangial interposition 80
Mesangial lambda deposits 106f
Mesangial matrix 6f
  expansion 12, 42, 56
Mesangium, normal cellularity of 36
Metabolic disorders 160, 163
Metabolic enzymes 151
Metal toxicity 165
Methicillin resistant *Staphylococcus aureus* 40
Microalbuminuria 83

Microangiopathy
  acute thrombotic 3
  chronic thrombotic 48, 174
  thrombotic 4, 74, 75*f*, 174, 176, 194, 203
Minimal change
  disease 3, 10, 11*f*, 12, 15, 82
  nephropathy 11, 82, 151
Mitochondria 151
Mitochondriopathies 166
Mitomycin drug toxicity 176
Mixed connective tissue disease 4, 48, 61, 78
Monoclonal gammopathy 48, 163
Monoclonal immunoglobulin deposition disease 4, 103, 140, 210
Monocytes 20
  intraluminal 125
Mucolipidosis 144, 147
Mucopolysaccharidosis 144, 147
Multiorgan failure, severity of 182
Multiple myeloma 163, 165
Multisystem autoimmune disease 78
Mural fibrinoid necrosis 9
Myeloproliferative disorders 166
Myocarditis 78

N

Nail-patella syndrome 135, 136, 151
Natural killer cell 213
Necrosis, cortical parenchymal 193*f*
Nephrin gene 148
Nephritic syndrome 3
Nephritis 45, 48, 98, 98*f*
  interstitial 158
Nephropathy
  analgesic 82
  diabetic 4, 83, 210, 212
  HIV-associated 2, 4, 124
  hypercalcemic 167, 168*f*
  hypertensive 87
  membranous 3, 10, 25, 28*f*, 29*f*, 82, 210, 212
  primary membranous 25, 25*f*, 28*f*, 30, 73
  radiation-induced 48
  secondary membranous 30
Nephrosclerosis
  benign 4, 172
  malignant 4
    hypertensive 79, 174
Nephrosialidosis 147
Nephrotic syndrome 3, 42, 60, 148
  complications of 148
  congenital 2, 4, 148, 149*f*, 213
  minimal change 150
  primary 10

Nephrotoxic acute tubular necrosis 157
Nephrotoxicity, drug-induced 82
Neutrophilic infiltrates 56, 65
Neutrophils 9, 20, 89
Niemann-Pick disease 147
Non-diabetic glomerular lesions 87
Non-infectious vasculitis, categories of 90
Non-inflammatory necrotizing vasculopathy 74
Non-muscle myosin heavy chain protein 150
Non-proliferative glomerulonephritis 10
Non-steroidal anti-inflammatory
  agents 30
  drugs 30, 82, 157
Normal glomerulus
  electron micrograph of 7*f*
  light micrograph of 6*f*
Nuclear ribonuclear protein 77

O

Obesity 176
Onion-skin thickening 174
Osmotic nephrosis 203
Oxalosis
  acquired 164
  primary 2
  secondary 164
  systemic 163
Oxford classification 37

P

Pain, abdominal 98
Pancreas 181
Papillary necrosis 82
Paraproteinemia 4, 103, 117
Parasitic infections 48
Parenchyma, cortical 171
Parenchymal infarction 171
Parietal epithelial cells 8
Penicillamine 82
Pericarditis 78
Periglomerular granuloma 92*f*
Periodic acid-Schiff 84
  reagent 6
Peritubular capillaries 189, 198*f*, 208
Perivascular granuloma 93*f*
Phospholipase C epsilon 150
Pierson syndrome 149, 150
Plasma cell 9
Plasma membrane 151
Plasmapheresis 102
Podocytes 18*f*, 144*f*, 153
  foamy vacuolization of 143*f*
  granular inclusions in 143*f*

hypertrophy 23
injury
    causes of 152
    distinct pathways of 152*f*
proliferated 125
Podocytopathies 2, 4, 11, 148, 151
    classification of 151
    diagnosis of 152
Polyangiitis 95
    granulomatous 4, 45, 89, 90
    microscopic 4, 45, 95
Polyarteritis nodosa 90
Polyarthralgia 98
Polydipsia 165
Polymyositis 77, 80
Polyomavirus nephropathy 204, 207*f*, 208
    morphological stages of 205
Polyomavirus tubulopathy 205*f*
Polyuria 165
Pre-eclampsia 183
Preglomerular arterioles, fibrinoid necrosis of 178*f*
Pregnancy-induced complications 182
Proliferative glomerulonephritis
    atypical 57
    diffuse 32, 33*f*, 36, 45*f*, 71
        mesangial 14
    focal 3, 60, 79, 81
    mesangial 3, 32, 36, 77, 81, 98*f*
    non-IgA mesangial 42, 42*f*
Proliferative lupus nephritis
    diffuse 35, 68*f*, 160*f*
        global 69
        segmental 69
    mesangial 62, 64, 64*f*
Prostate 30
Proteinuria 4, 60, 133
Proteinuric diseases 151
Proteus mirabilis 161
Pseudomonas 161

R

Raynaud phenomenon 78
Renal amyloidosis 104*f*, 107*f*
Renal arteries
    large 82
    segmental 171
    stenosis 174
Renal biopsies 1, 3, 6, 8, 34
Renal cortex 154
Renal disease 3, 98
    dysproteinemias-associated 103
    systemic 4

Renal dysfunction 4
Renal failure 129, 133, 139
    acute 3
        postpartum 176
    chronic 4
    mild 181
    severity of 102
Renal function
    deterioration 83
    mild impairment of 96
Renal medulla 155*f*
Renal papillary necrosis 87
Renal syndromes, pulmonary 101
Renal transplantation 140, 144, 164
Renal tubular acidosis, proximal 81, 165
Renal vasculature, normal structure of 171
Renal vasculitis 81, 96
Rituximab 194

S

Sarcoidosis 30
Schistocytes 175*f*
Schistosomiasis 30, 48
Scleroderma 4, 78
    renal crisis 79
Sclerosis 8, 9
    diffuse mesangial 150*f*, 151
    focal 10
    glomerular 74
    hypertensive segmental 23
    mesangial 42, 46
    nodular 86
    renal crisis, systemic 176
    secondary mesangial 80
    segmental 10, 37, 39*f*, 211*f*
    systemic 61, 77, 78
Scoliosis 136
Shigella dysenteriae, shiga toxin of 176
Sjogren's syndrome 4, 30, 48, 61, 77, 80, 159, 161
Smooth muscle 142
Solid tumors 30
South West Pediatric Nephrology Study 14
Sphingolipidoses 147
Staphylococcal infections 40
Staphylococcus aureus 40
    infection 32
Starry sky pattern 34
Stem cell transplantation 176
Steroid resistant genetic forms 152
Stomach 30
Subendothelial deposits, diffuse massive 69
Subendothelial floccular fibrin tactoids 74

Subendothelial region, electrolucent expansion of 179*f*
Sulfadiazine 157
Swollen endothelial cells 125
Syphilis 30
Systemic glomerular diseases 60, 61
Systemic lupus erythematosus 4, 30, 60, 61, 73, 77, 80
Systemic renal diseases, secondary 45
Systemic sclerosis, diffuse cutaneous 78

T

T cell 213
Tacrolimus 202
Takayasu arteritis 90
Thin basement membrane disease 4, 129, 132
Thrombocytopenia 114, 182
Thrombotic thrombocytopenic purpura 176, 181, 184
Thyroid 181
Toxemia, pre-eclamptic 183
Toxic injury 165
Toxicity, interstitial 204
Transplant rejection, chronic 79
Transplant renal diseases 4
Transthyretin 104
Triglyceridemia 176
True inflammatory vasculitis 76
Tubular atrophy 37, 40*f*, 74, 80, 165, 200, 202
    proximal 165
Tubular dilatation, microcystic 126*f*
Tubular injury
    acute 156, 186
    ischemic acute 157
Tubular necrosis, acute 3, 156, 156*f*, 179*f*
Tubules 8
Tubulitis 197*f*, 198*f*
Tubulointerstitial diseases 154
Tubulointerstitial lesions 80, 81, 86
Tubulointerstitial nephritis 157
    acute 157, 158, 158*f*
    chronic 158, 159, 159*f*, 174
    sclerosing 2
Tubulointerstitial nephropathy 161
    sclerosing 161*f*
Tubulopathy 202
Tumor lysis syndrome 166

U

Urate nephropathy 166, 167, 167*f*

V

Vascular diseases 4, 158
Vascular endothelium 142
Vascular lesions 73, 86, 87, 172
Vascular rejection
    acute 199*f*, 201*f*
    chronic 201*f*
Vascular renal diseases 171
Vasculitis 4, 60, 89, 90, 160
    acute necrotizing 76*f*
    large vessel 90
    rheumatoid 81
    small vessel 90, 102
Vessel vasculitis, medium-sized 90
Vitamin D resistant rickets 165
von Willebrand factor, dysfunction of 181

W

Waldenstrom's macroglobulinemia 103
Wegener's granulomatosis 4, 45, 89, 90, 160
Wilson's disease 159
Wire loops 67, 68*f*

X

Xerostomia 80

Z

Zebra bodies 142
ZMPSTE24 gene 151

Other Best-selling Books

CYTOPATHOLOGY REVIEW

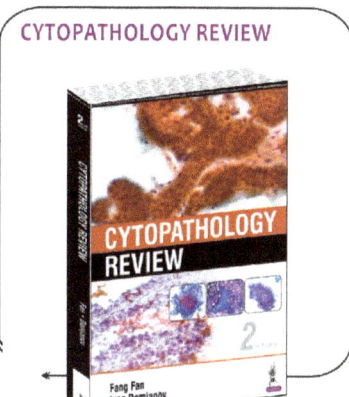

Fang Fan, et al.

Full Colour | Hard Cover | 2/e, 2017 | 8.5" x 11" | 210 Pages | 9789352700462

- A cytopathology review book based on multiple choice questions covering comprehensively the most important modern cytopathology
- Includes 416 multiple choice questions, more than half of them pertaining to images
- Answers with detailed explanatory notes emphasizing the key learning points of each question.
- Review and update book for practicing pathologists preparing from the specialty board recertification.

HANDBOOK OF CERVICAL CYTOLOGY

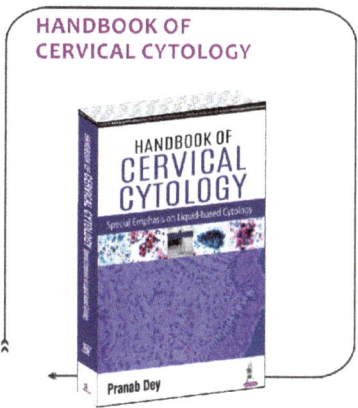

Pranab Dey

Full Colour | Soft Cover | 1/e, 2018 | 6.25" x 9.5" | 188 Pages | 9789352702657

- A concise practical handbook on cervical cytology.
- Presents salient diagnostic features of differential cervical lesions on cytology smears.
- Provides detailed discussion on differential diagnosis and management of the lesions.
- Emphasizes on cytomorphology in liquid-based cytology.
- Includes a large number of microphotographs to facilitate the recognition of the lesions.
- Useful for practising cytologists, students and cytoscreeners

CASE-BASED APPROACH IN FINE NEEDLE ASPIRATION CYTOLOGY

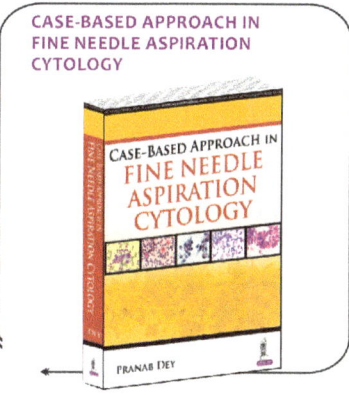

Pranab Dey

Full Colour | Soft Cover | 1/e, 2016 | 6.75" x 9.5" | 390 Pages | 9789352501809

- A unique collection of classical and interesting 250 real cases of last two decades of fine needle aspiration cytology that cover all the systems.
- Essential clinical history and multiple microphotographs have been provided with every case.
- Diagnosis and differential diagnosis for each case are discussed at the end of each chapter.
- Further reading list is also provided after each case.

ATLAS OF HISTOPATHOLOGY

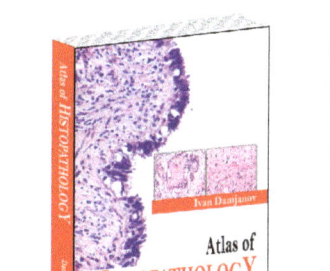

Ivan Damjanov

Full Colour | Hard Cover | 1/e, 2012 | 8.5" x 11" | 418 Pages | 9789350251881

- Illustrates the salient aspects of systemic pathology.
- It has 500 full colour microphotographs printed in large format.
- Useful in preparation for examinations.
- It acts as a desktop manual to be used next to the microscope in standard laboratory sessions.
- This book is immensely helpful for medical students, veterinary medicine students, and dental medicine students, students in laboratory medicine, junior pathology residents and teachers of pathology.

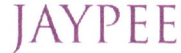

JAYPEE
The Health Sciences Publisher

Please visit our website
www.jaypeebrothers.com or Scan the QR Code

EU GSPR Authorised Reprsentative
Logos Europe, 9 rue Nicolas Poussin
1700, La Rochelle, France
Phone: +33 (0) 6 67 93 73 78
E-mail: contact@logoseurope.eu

www.ingramcontent.com/pod-product-compliance
Ingram Content Group UK Ltd.
Pitfield, Milton Keynes, MK11 3LW, UK
UKHW050243150426

5217IPUK00005B/117